Praise for Phoebe Lapine and her books

"Phoebe Lapine is an amazing self-taught cook who creates healthy takes on comfort food in her tiny Manhattan apartment."

—*Food & Wine*

"Making good food and lifestyle choices is the best medicine for curing what ails us. For those suffering from autoimmune or other chronic health problems, *The Wellness Project* is an invaluable look at how one woman learned to apply best health practices and still enjoy all that makes life sweet."

—Terry Wahls, MD, author of *The Wahls Protocol Cooking for Life*

"*The Wellness Project* is a smart, funny, and incredibly helpful guide to the complexities of not just what makes us sick, but what makes us well."

—Robynne Chutkan, MD, FASGE, integrative gastroenterologist & best-selling author of *The Microbiome Solution*

"I couldn't agree more with Phoebe Lapine when she says 'healthy choices can't happen in a vacuum.' This incredibly informative, delightfully human (and fun!) chronicle of her path to sustainable wellness is an inspiring read that makes living well feel approachable. Whether you're looking for support as you take an honest inventory of your health or are seeking inspiration for long-lasting changes, Phoebe has been there and done that and shares it all."

—Julia Turshen, author of *Small Victories*, on *The Wellness Project*

"If you're struggling to figure out why you're not feeling like you should, and are overwhelmed by all the wellness information online, then start your journey with *The Wellness Project*. You'll not only learn so much valuable information in this book, but you'll learn a lot about yourself and your potential for feeling good again!"

—Alisa Vitti, functional nutritionist, hormone expert, author of *WomanCode*, and founder of FLOliving.com

"A great, funny, and down-to-earth read. I loved every minute of it. There's something in there everyone can relate to (adjusting to moving in with a boyfriend, starting an exercise regimen, regulating your 'cycle'). The recipes are easy and approachable, just like Phoebe's writing!"

—Ali Maffucci, creator and best-selling author of *Inspiralized* and *Inspiralize Everything*, on *The Wellness Project*

─────────────

"An engaging memoir about creating your own path to wellness."

—*New York Post*, on *The Wellness Project*

─────────────

"Lapine's yearlong journey of self-care [is] funny, relatable, and ultimately hopeful."

—*Bustle*, on *The Wellness Project*

─────────────

"With a witty tone that'll have you laughing out loud, this book is a must for anyone wondering if drinking lemon water or giving up alcohol ACTUALLY makes a difference."

—*Mind Body Green*, on *The Wellness Project*

─────────────

"This inspiring story about one 20-something's journey from illness to wellness is perfect for natural-living newbies, those on the fringe of going all in, and anyone looking for simple ways to improve their health without sacrificing life's pleasures. Part memoir, part game-plan, all good."

—The Chalkboard, on *The Wellness Project*

─────────────

"Packed with brilliant advice and delicious recipes for anyone who wants to cook and entertain—no matter what size your kitchen."

—Ina Garten, on *In the Small Kitchen*

SIBO
Made Simple

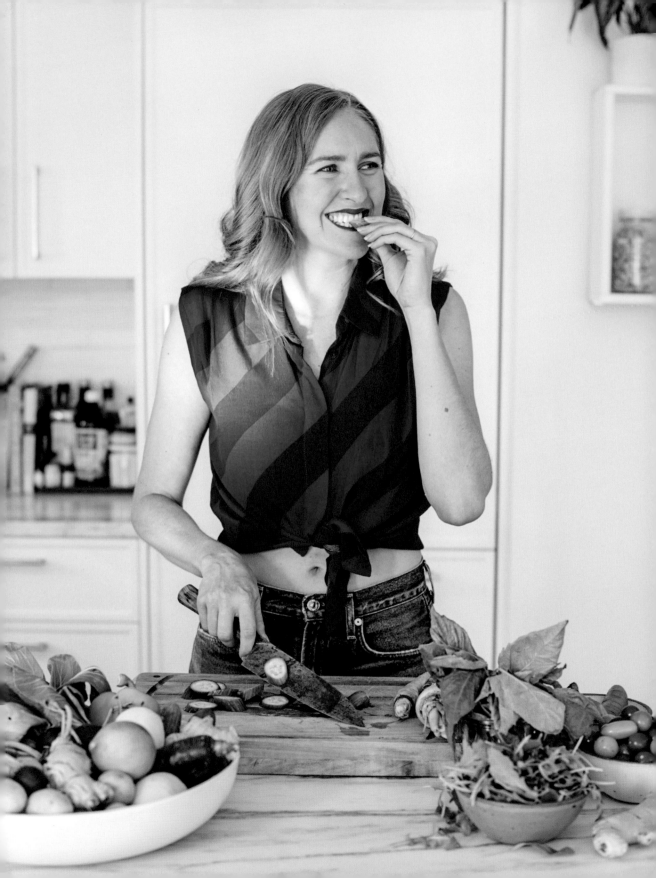

SIBO
Made Simple

90 Healing Recipes
& Practical Strategies
to Rebalance
Your Gut for Good

PHOEBE LAPINE

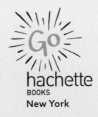

hachette
BOOKS
New York

Copyright © 2021
by Phoebe Lapine

Photography by Haley Hunt Davis

Cover design by Amanda Kain

Cover photographs by
Haley Hunt Davis

Cover copyright © 2021 by
Hachette Book Group, Inc.

Hachette Book Group supports
the right to free expression
and the value of copyright.
The purpose of copyright is to
encourage writers and artists to
produce the creative works that
enrich our culture.

The scanning, uploading, and
distribution of this book without
permission is a theft of the
author's intellectual property. If
you would like permission to use
material from the book (other
than for review purposes), please
contact permissions@hbgusa
.com. Thank you for your support
of the author's rights.

Hachette Go, an imprint of
Hachette Books

Hachette Book Group
1290 Avenue of the Americas
New York, NY 10104

HachetteGo.com
Facebook.com/HachetteGo
Instagram.com/HachetteGo

First Edition: January 2021

Hachette Books is a division of
Hachette Book Group, Inc.

The Hachette Go and Hachette
Books name and logos are
trademarks of Hachette Book
Group, Inc.

The publisher is not responsible
for websites (or their content) that
are not owned by the publisher.

Library of Congress Control
Number: 2020942861

ISBNs: 978-0-306-84616-8
(paperback); 978-0-306-84615-1
(e-book)

Printed in China

1010

10 9 8 7 6 5 4 3 2 1

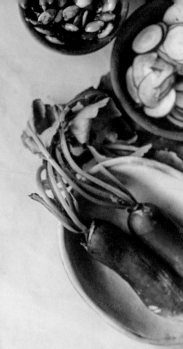

For all my SIBO Amigos and
members of the chronically ill crew—

I love your guts

• • •

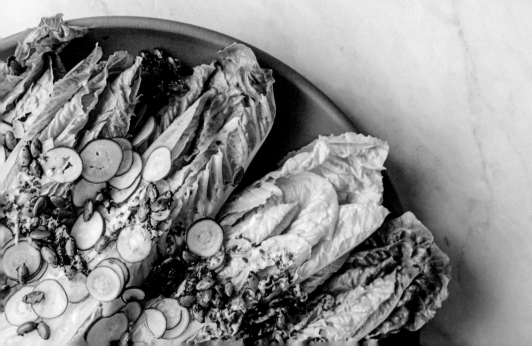

CONTENTS

Part Two
PUTTING YOUR SIBO DIET INTO PRACTICE

④ GET COOKING
*Stocking Your Kitchen
Medicine Cabinet*

⑤ THE RECIPES
*Really Delicious Dishes for Every Stage
of Your SIBO Journey*

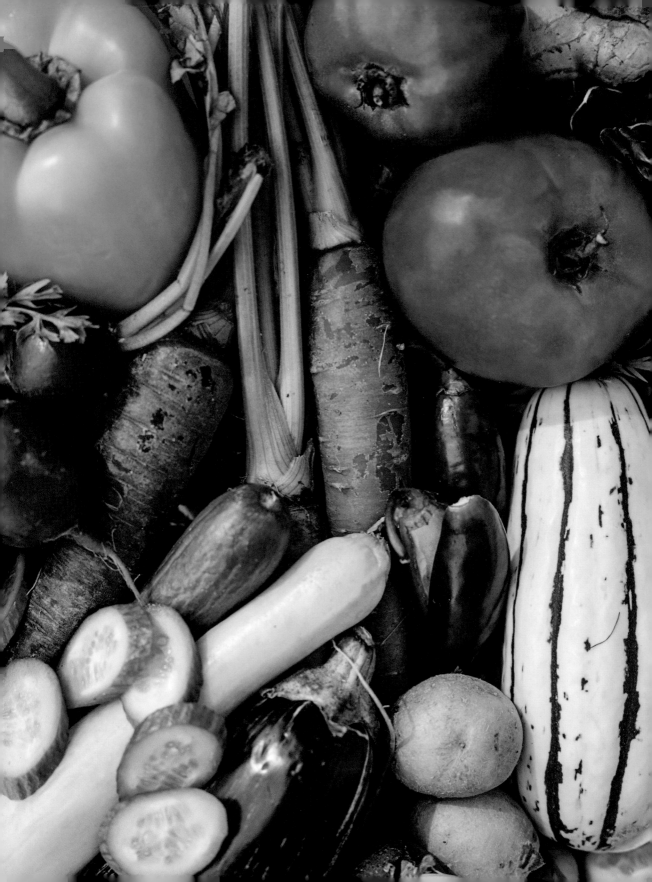

FOREWORD
by Dr. Will Cole

As a functional medicine practitioner who consults with people around the world, my heart and passion is immersing myself in complex health cases, uncovering their root facets. Being a part of someone's wellness journey is a sacred responsibility, one that I don't take lightly.

No matter who I am working with, I talk a lot about the gut and digestive system, because they are a core focus of health and the place where just about every chronic health problem has its roots. I'm often reminded that discussing bowel movements is not normal, when I ask my patients about them and get giggles, blushes, and embarrassment as a response. But in truth, the gut microbiome, the trillions of bacteria and yeast living in our digestive system, is one of the most fascinating health topics.

This bustling kingdom of bacteria living inside each one of us is vast and hugely critical to our overall well-being; this intelligent microbial ecosystem in your gut actually contains around 100 trillion bacteria, compared to your 10 trillion human cells. In other words, you are 10 times more bacteria than human—a sort of sophisticated (and beautiful) host for the microbiome. In addition, the genes of your microbiome bacteria outnumber your own by 100 to 1.

The bacterial diversity and balance of your microbiome is an important part of your health; the more balanced your microbiome, the better your health potential tends to be, and that balance comes from exposure to the down-and-dirty world, including not just the foods we eat but the dirt we work in outside, the animals that we play with, and the very air we breathe; even how and where we were born affects our microbiome. All these things determine the richness, diversity, and balance of our individual gut garden.

What sounds like science fiction is actually fact. These trillions of microbes and their colonies are the manufacturers and managers of how you look, how you feel, and how you think. Hippocrates, the father of modern medicine said, "all disease begins in the gut"; now research is catching up with antiquity. Scientists are quickly learning how much your microbiome regulates just about every system of your body.

For example, we now know that about 75 percent of your immune system is produced in your gut. It's no wonder that many immune issues, including autoimmune diseases, can be linked to underlying gastrointestinal problems.

An amazing 95 percent of your happy neurotransmitter serotonin is made and stored in your gut, not your brain. Your gut and brain were actually formed from the same fetal tissue when you were growing in your mom's womb and are inextricably linked for the rest of your life through what's referred to as the gut-brain axis, the vagus nerve, and the enteric nervous system. It's no wonder that the medical literature actually refers to the gut as the "second brain." It is for this reason that imbalances of the microbiome are linked to brain problems like anxiety, depression, fatigue, ADD, ADHD, and autism.

Even more seemingly unrelated health problems, such as diabetes and heart disease, are now being linked to underlying gut problems. We have seen the implications of gut health problems reach far beyond digestion, but digestion itself is paramount for our total health. A sort of "check-engine light," digestive problems are often a sign that something else in the body needs to be addressed, as well as needing to be dealt with directly. Small intestinal bacterial overgrowth—SIBO—is no exception to this principle.

SIBO is something that I see clinically on an almost hourly basis. Manifesting differently in different people, SIBO exists on a larger inflammation spectrum, from mild to extreme symptoms. My patients with SIBO report everything from mild digestive discomfort to painful bloating that they describe as making them look "eight months pregnant"; they also report everything from looser or sluggish bowel movements to the throes of an irritable bowel syndrome (IBS) flare, indigestion to extreme acid reflux, or GERD. SIBO can not only do a number on your digestion, but when your GI tract is weakened or damaged, it can trigger a number of potential autoimmune problems throughout the body. This is the SIBO spectrum.

Over the years, I have seen firsthand how living with SIBO can be an isolating existence. To everyone else, you look "normal," but others don't see the silent suffering behind closed doors or the struggle it takes just to get through the day. SIBO can mess with your emotions as much as your stomach.

Additionally, there can be great overwhelm with the endless vortex of conflicting information online. Dr. Google is one fickle, confused physician. Low-FODMAP, low-histamine, low-oxalate, SCD, GAPS, carnivore, plant-based, paleo, low-carb, high-carb, keto, pharmaceutical antibiotics, herbal antibiotics, no antibiotics . . . it's difficult to be both your own health advocate and the one suffering at the same time.

Phoebe Lapine is an angel in the time of health distress; she is a source of calm direction in a storm of disillusionment and frustration. In this book, she offers clear explanations for SIBO, as well as offering information on related conditions, how you can get an accurate diagnosis, how you can develop a plan to ease your symptoms, and how you can nourish your distressed gut with health-supportive, delicious food. She's been on the front lines with SIBO, and I believe her words certainly will be a light in a dark time in your wellness journey.

My friends, the book you are now holding is a priceless, practical road map for all your SIBO questions. Finally, *SIBO Made Simple*.

INTRODUCTION

How I Became Your SIBO Amigo

When I was diagnosed with SIBO in late 2017, I had already received an unofficial bachelor's degree in gut health studies from Life University.

Or so I thought.

A few years prior, after struggling for years with autoimmune disease, I decided to try a new approach to my health. Instead of resolutions, which had always left me feeling guilty and overwhelmed, I came up with a list of short-term monthly experiments that would help me tackle each of my wellness problem areas, one change at a time. The goal was to explore my limits in order to find a more sustainable middle ground going forward, something I call *healthy hedonism*.

My year of health became a series on my award-winning blog, and after the outpouring of support from fellow Hashimoto's sufferers and other members of the chronically ill crew trying to find that elusive "balance," it became a popular book called *The Wellness Project*.

As I learned the hard way, though, **being healed is very different from getting cured**. Although I managed to mitigate my worst thyroid symptoms—the skin havoc, the digestive woes, the mental monkeying—I made it known that even though my project might have been over, there never really was a finish line.

Perhaps it was the deep knowing that being someone with an autoimmune disease means that I may always be a little more sensitive to change or need a beat to recalibrate. Perhaps it was simply a premonition of the new path up Health Mountain that lay ahead.

It seemed like only a matter of months after my book hit stands that I started noticing some mysterious symptoms creeping back into my life. Having experienced a decade of digestive issues, I didn't pay much attention to the bloating and constipation. Didn't consider how my usual diet—full of fiber and fermented foods that, in theory, supported good gut health—was starting to make me feel off after every meal. I didn't even worry that my habitual burping, and more than occasional tooting, was becoming a regular companion soundtrack to my partner's and my nighttime Netflix binges.

There was so much easy rationalizing. Thanks to the learnings I gleaned during my wellness project, I was drinking more homemade kombucha, which was fizzy. Despite those learnings, I was going semihorizontal after meals (definitely not part of a "good gut diet," but eventually could be corrected). And I was getting more and more comfortable in my relation-ship, which meant that maybe it didn't matter if I just let 'er rip.

But after a few months of this, and having turned a more discerning eye on my daily habits, I could see myself more clearly. And what I saw was a spare tire in my abdomen. Once I started to put the physical pieces together—the outward, second trimester–level bloating with the inward distress—I decided to see a doctor for a full workup.

The diagnosis I received was one that would change everything I thought I knew about gut health and kick off an unofficial master's degree in small intestinal studies.

What to Expect When You're Not Expecting, but Look Like You Are

Small intestinal bacterial overgrowth is exactly what it sounds like.

It's a type of dysbiosis, which simply means an imbalance of the trillions of bacteria that take up residence in your gut. In the case of SIBO, however, the issue is not necessarily the ratio between good, beneficial bacteria and bad, pathogenic bacteria (though that could be part of it too). Rather, **the main problem is location, not type**.

Although critters colonize all sections of our alimentary canal, the majority of bacteria is found in the large intestine (also known as the colon). There, it assists in the final step of the digestive labyrinth and prepares waste matter for evacuation. The small intestine, on the other hand, is where your food intermingles with digestive juices, nutrients are absorbed into the bloodstream, and your body reaps the rewards of what you've just put into it. It's not a place where bacteria have much of a function. In fact, as is the case with SIBO, their presence can cause a lot of harm.

Since these are living organisms with their own cravings, high numbers of bacteria in your small intestine means there are other mouths at the table competing for your dinner. When there's not enough nourishment to be had, they turn to the next best thing: your intestinal lining. The result is an increased permeability, also known as leaky gut syndrome, whereby larger food particles (instead of just essential nutrients) seep into the bloodstream. The downwind effect is often systemic inflammation, food sensitivities, and autoimmunity. **Although you can have leaky gut, food intolerances, and an autoimmune disease without SIBO, it is not unusual for these conditions to be a package deal.**

Unwanted bacteria can also disrupt your quality of life in a host of other ways. As they eat your dinner, these critters release gas. Your small intestine was not designed to withstand the buildup, and it tends to get trapped (like a bicycle inner tube underneath your diaphragm), or released through burping, or out the other end. You can also experience nausea from slowed stomach emptying due to the traffic jam, and classic hallmarks of irritable bowel syndrome (IBS), such as constipation or diarrhea.

Even more insidious and sneaky are the changes that can occur to your weight and your mood. Depending on what type of bacteria is overgrowing, you might experience chronic weight loss or resistant weight gain—no matter how much or little you eat, pounds seem to fall off or stick stubbornly like a puffer vest you can never take off. Since 90 percent of your serotonin is made in the gut, a damaged intestinal tract can also mean descending into an inexplicable fog of depression or feeling as if your life is being run by a humming undercurrent of anxiety.

So, what happens when all these inexplicable symptoms add up? Usually, someone will be given a blanket diagnosis of IBS.

Thanks to the last decade of new research, experts in the field now estimate that over 60 percent of all IBS cases are being caused by SIBO. If this is true, **twenty-five million people** are finally being given a diagnosis they can dig into. For those suffering from these mysterious digestive symptoms, SIBO can be a beacon of hope—an answer that has escaped them during years of bouncing between doctors, and one that actually has a path to treatment.

The only problem? That path is so damn complicated...

Up Sh*t's Creek Without a Road Map

There's no one approach to SIBO, which is what often makes patients so confused. I should know, since I was one of them.

Even the best doctors, who are brilliant at the *what*, often forget about or don't have time to explain the *why* or the *how*. This was the case when I first got my Hashimoto's thyroiditis diagnosis, and it was also what happened when I tested positive for SIBO. While I saw an extremely capable functional MD who knew to dig deeper, once I got the diagnosis of SIBO, I walked away with a single piece of paper advising a low-FODMAP diet, meal spacing, and a regimen of herbal antimicrobials. And I knew I was lucky to even get that much advice.

Since I just can't help but make my medical struggles ammunition for a whole new stream of resources for my audience, I immediately went home and hopped down the SIBO internet rabbit hole. What I discovered was a mountain of options, many of which contradicted one another. I began digging further, attending virtual seminars, and even going so far as to take an online course to become a SIBO certified practitioner. As I researched, I curated and I synthesized. And as always, I shared my findings with my readers on my website, *Feed Me Phoebe*.

The response was instantaneous and overwhelming.

I received hundreds of comments, messages, and emails from chronic SIBO sufferers and the newly diagnosed. Notes telling me that they, too, had once gone to the ends of the internet to find solutions, and that my series was one of the most comprehensive, thoughtful, and easy to navigate of any they'd found. There were also notes saying that my writing prompted them to get tested for SIBO—which they'd never heard of—and after years of uncertainty, they received a clear answer.

Around this time, I also got an email from my biggest fan.

"Phoebe, how amazing that you're already attracting an audience around SIBO—I'm so impressed," wrote my mother. To which I replied: "Mom! I'm not attracting them. It turns out my audience already has a raging case of SIBO!"

Like my HashiPosse—the millions of women struggling with Hashimoto's thyroiditis (which, as it so happens, is a risk factor for SIBO)—I realized how badly my newfound SIBO Amigos needed more than what they were getting from their doctors.

They needed a complete SIBO self-care tool kit. They craved an array of sustainable strategies and healing recipes. And they wanted a clear picture of how to choose their own SIBO adventure without it feeling like a complete, social-life-killing drag.

Taking SIBO from Complicated to Simple

With SIBO, the struggle is *real*. The road map up Health Mountain is far from linear and streamlined. Rather, it involves many forks, detours, and steep uphill climbs that often lead you to exactly where you started.

These are just a few of the nuances for getting to the bottom of your SIBO, the most confusing element being that even after sifting through much of today's research, there are still a lot of unknowns. Here are some of the issues and contradictions we'll unpack in this book:

- To treat an overgrowth properly, **you need a breath test to determine which of the three gas types you have**: methane, hydrogen, or hydrogen sulfide. The latter isn't yet directly captured on breath tests, so practitioners are left guessing.

- SIBO has similar symptoms to SIFO—small intestinal fungal overgrowth—and they often present together in the same patient. **Roughly half of SIBO sufferers also have SIFO.** But it's harder to test for the latter, so again, practitioners are left guessing.

- The conventional **antibiotics and herbal antimicrobials used to treat SIBO differ depending on the type of gas** you test positive for. For example, allicin, an extract of garlic, has been shown to be effective on methanogen overgrowths, which tends to be the harder of the types to eradicate.

- Whole garlic eaten in food, because it contains high concentrations of certain carbohydrates in the FODMAP acronym, is often one of the biggest contributors to SIBO symptoms. Meaning, **garlic itself can be part of both the suffering and the solution.**

4

- Although both conventional and herbal antibiotics have been shown to be 80+ percent effective at treating SIBO, **the condition often comes back within two weeks of treatment because the root cause has not been dealt with**.

- Many times, the root cause cannot be fully cured or eliminated, which makes **chronic SIBO** that much more likely.

- Diet can be a big alleviator of the worst symptoms of SIBO. But **food alone is not necessarily causing or curing SIBO**.

- While studies have shown that a low-FODMAP diet is extremely effective at mitigating symptoms of IBS, research also indicates that **being on this diet long-term can be damaging** to the balance of bacteria in the large intestine, which we need for good ongoing gut health and SIBO prevention.

- Unsurprisingly, the diet advice of top microbiome specialists directly contradicts popular SIBO diets. Everything on their "yes" list—prebiotic inulin-rich vegetables, fibrous legumes, fermented probiotic foods—are on the "no" list for SIBO.

- SIBO can cause leaky gut, which can lead to autoimmune disease. And yet, some **autoimmune diseases, such as Hashimoto's thyroiditis and celiac disease, are big risk factors for SIBO**. There's still a lot to learn about the chicken-or-the-egg relationship.

If this list makes your chest tighten with anxiety or causes you to feel disheartened about the journey before you've even begun—take a breath.

This isn't just another health book that overpromises and underdelivers, which is why it's important to start with a good dose of *realism*. That said, despite these considerations, **the road ahead is far from hopeless**. In fact, there is an incredible array of strategies that can put you in the driver's seat of your own healing.

Today, practitioners across the globe have made it their mission to treat complicated, stubborn cases of SIBO, and they are uncovering more tools for our arsenal every day. The goal of starting my podcast, *SIBO Made Simple*, was to collect as much of their advice as possible. Since research studies on the subject of SIBO and IBS are a constant work in progress, these clinical perspectives (meaning, what doctors see every day in their practices) are essential to understanding what we can do to treat our own SIBO. The nuggets of wisdom I gleaned from interviews with dozens of the top functional medicine minds and SIBO-specific practitioners have become the backbone of this book. Only, as your SIBO Amigo, I'll be distilling their medical advice in a way that most laypeople, like myself, can actually digest.

Since I am an obsessive researcher and curator of information, rather than a clinical practitioner with a singular approach, **this book synthesizes and explains the varied ways that doctors, dietitians, bodyworkers, psychiatrists, and nutritionists approach gut healing**.

In Part 1, I'll take you through the *what* and the *why* of SIBO so you can suss out what your underlying causes might be. As you may have noticed if you, too, fell down the internet rabbit hole, reading about SIBO can sometimes feel like a foreign language. To kick things off, you'll find a helpful digestive system cast of characters and explanation of key terms. Within each chapter, you'll also get tips and takeaways to make occasionally dense information super actionable in your own life. And, finally, at the end of each section I've given you the SIBO Amigo Digest with the most important rules of thumb.

In Chapter 2, we will get into treatment options, natural therapies, and lifestyle interventions that will help you clear your bacteria and dismantle some of the digestive obstacles that might have contributed to your SIBO in the first place.

I've also dedicated an entire section to the diet piece. In Chapter 3, I'll take you through an in-depth analysis on the pros and cons of each dietary approach and who they are best for. Dr. Allison Siebecker, dubbed "the Queen of SIBO," has said that the most important part of any SIBO diet approach is simply to pick one and stick with it. *SIBO Made Simple* will help you choose your lane, while offering alternate paths forward, should you have to try again.

In Part 2, we will get intimate with your kitchen together and discuss how to put your SIBO diet into practice. This section includes invaluable information on "hero ingredients" that aid in healing and how to remove others that might be adding insult to injury. **But what truly sets *SIBO Made Simple* apart is not just the comprehensive overview of information. It's the recipes.**

I've worked as a professional on all sides of the food space for over a decade. As a private chef, cookbook author, culinary instructor, and recipe developer for some of the largest brands in the health food aisle, I've prided myself on always getting comforting, nourishing meals on the table, no matter how restrictive the diet or tough the culinary puzzle.

In Chapter 5, you'll find **90+ delicious low-FODMAP recipes** that can be tailored to any of the leading SIBO practitioner diets, or the biggest concerns that dovetail with SIBO, including low-histamine and yeast-friendly dishes. All the recipes are **soy-optional** and **completely free of gluten, corn, refined sugar, and dairy** (with the exception of ghee and 24-Hour Yogurt, page 163). More importantly, the recipes are built around nutrient-dense, anti-inflammatory ingredients so that you can actually give your body ammunition to heal.

For SIBO sufferers, this book isn't about short-term fixes. It's about finding a new way of living with your gut health in mind. Because of this, each recipe has an ONWARD variation, which includes ingredients that may be on the way back in through the process of reintroduction. The long-term goal of any SIBO diet is to get you eating the most diverse array of plants possible, since ultimately, the diverse, robust ecosystem in your gut counts on it.

My hope is that this book becomes a trusty road map that allows you to become your own intestinal detective, gut problem solver, and critter-free kitchen crusader. The silver lining of SIBO (and, trust me, there is one), is that it will force you to learn more about your body and digestive system than you ever knew possible. When I was through with my "year of health" and had written *The Wellness Project*, I thought I had a handle on my gut health. SIBO was my wake-up call that I had just glimpsed the tip of the iceberg.

So, before we begin wading through the SIBO weeds, I want to share with you the most important lesson I learned during my unofficial master's degree in small intestinal studies: **Healing is not a straight line between point A and point B. Progress is often one step forward, two steps back.** And it doesn't matter when you reach your destination, as long as you've learned something about your mind, body, and spirit along the way.

This book may not be a silver bullet or seamless solution—if there was one to be had, I would have found it by now. But it's my hope that by reading along, you'll be better able to choose your own path up the SIBO Summit of Health Mountain, wherever it may lead.

So, let's roll up our sleeves and start our climb together.

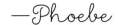

—Phoebe

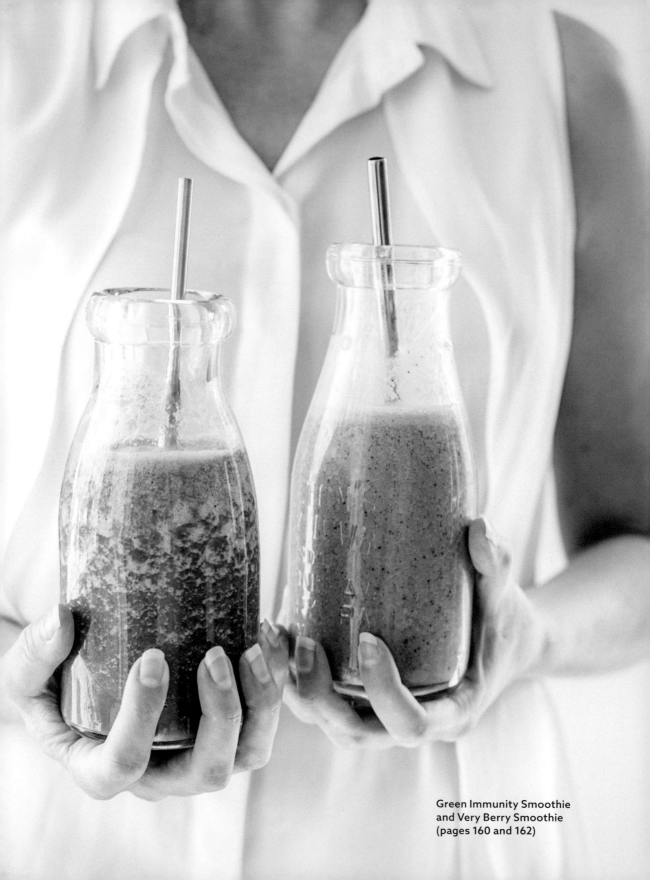

Green Immunity Smoothie
and Very Berry Smoothie
(pages 160 and 162)

Part One

SIBO 101

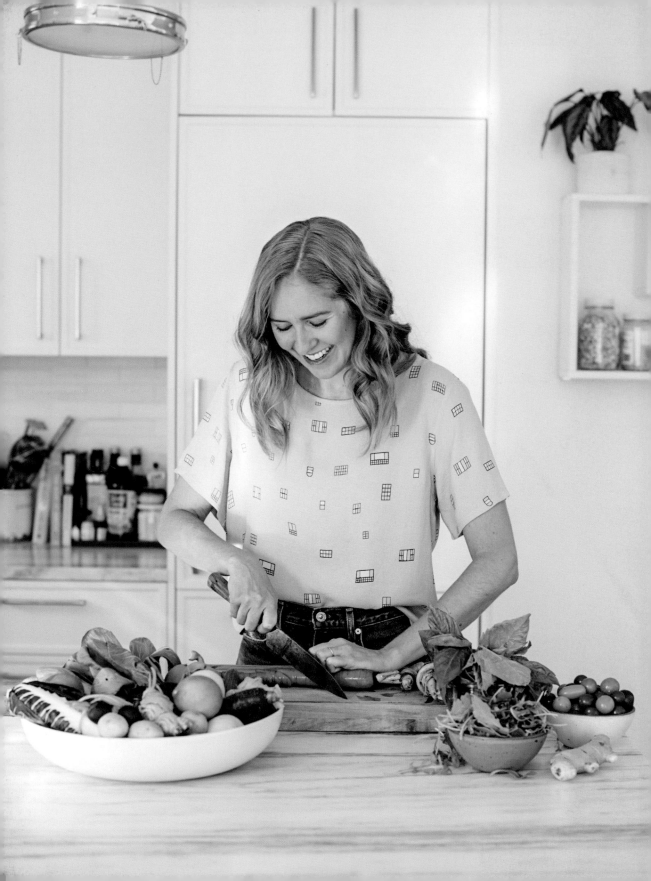

Chapter One

SIBO BASICS

Symptoms, Root Causes, and Testing

Your Digestive System Cast of Characters (in Order of Appearance)

The GI tract is a series of organs joined in a long, winding path from the port of entry (your mouth) to the exit ramp (your anus). There are hollow organs that transport and process food—such as the stomach, small intestine, and large intestine, and solid organs—such as the liver, pancreas, and gallbladder—that don't deal with food directly, but aid in breaking it down. Here's a brief description of the main players and how they come together in this ensemble cast to keep your body fueled and healthy.

MOUTH AND TEETH In the first leg of the digestive labyrinth, all that chomping is responsible for mashing food into more manageable pieces, while allowing powerful digestive enzymes in your saliva to begin breaking them down.

↓

VAGUS NERVE
This pair of nerves forms the superhighway between your brain and gut. It dictates when your body switches into rest-and-digest mode—or its opposite, fight or flight—and tells the muscles in your stomach to contract and push food into the small intestine, among many other functions.

→

STOMACH
Where hydrochloric acid and peptic enzymes further work on your meal, softening hard vegetable skins, breaking down proteins, and killing off any bacteria that have entered through the nose or mouth. It usually takes about one to five hours for a medium-size dinner to become a nicely digested slurry that gets fully emptied into the small intestine.

→

PANCREAS
One of the main workhorses responsible for producing digestive enzymes that break down carbohydrates, fats, and proteins—a cocktail that gets delivered directly to the small intestine.

LIVER
Your most scrappy, industrious organ, responsible for filtering your blood, removing toxins, metabolizing drugs, regulating hormones, micromanaging your energy reserves, storing nutrients, and synthesizing bile for safekeeping in your gallbladder.

→

GALLBLADDER
This small storage pouch sits just under the liver, ready to deliver bile to the small intestine to process parts of your meal, particularly fats.

→

SMALL INTESTINE/ SMALL BOWEL
The longest leg of the digestive maze, this twenty-foot length of tubing is where major food groups are broken down into their essential elements—amino acids, sugars, and fatty acids—that are then absorbed into the bloodstream. It can take between two and four hours for a meal to be processed in the small intestine.

↓

LARGE INTESTINE/COLON Finally, we've reached the five-foot-long exit ramp where water is absorbed from remaining food matter and all excess waste is ushered out of the body. It's also where the majority of your gut bacteria reside and feast off undigested fibers during your food's five- to seventy-hour residence before evacuation via the rectum.

"Sorry, I Don't Speak SIBO": A List of Essential Terms

Reading about SIBO can sometimes make you feel as if you need to learn a new language. This section contains bare-bones definitions of some of the most referenced conditions, bodily functions, and processes in this book. If you ever find yourself confused or want to work on your SIBO literacy, flip back here.

IRRITABLE BOWEL SYNDROME (IBS)
The most common gastrointestinal diagnosis in the world, affecting up to 15 percent of the global population. It is characterized by symptoms of bloating, abdominal pain or discomfort, constipation, diarrhea, or a combination.

SMALL INTESTINAL FUNGAL OVERGROWTH (SIFO) When fungi or yeast, most notably *Candida*, exceed their typically small numbers in the small bowel, often leading to IBS symptoms. Experts estimate that 50 percent of all SIBO sufferers also have SIFO.

POST-INFECTIOUS IBS (PI-IBS)
The onset of IBS symptoms weeks after a case of food poisoning or traveler's diarrhea due to a process of acute autoimmunity. Only 10 percent of people who get food poisoning will develop PI-IBS. It is diagnosed by a blood test that measures the presence of certain antibodies. Experts say that PI-IBS is the root cause of the majority of IBS-D or diarrhea-dominant SIBO cases.

MOTILITY
The process of moving food through your digestive tract. The small bowel and large intestine each have their own separate functions and speeds.

SMALL INTESTINAL BACTERIAL OVERGROWTH (SIBO) When normal populations of bacteria begin to colonize and multiply too far up the digestive canal, often leading to IBS symptoms. Experts estimate 60 percent of IBS sufferers have SIBO.

INFLAMMATORY BOWEL DISEASE (IBD) Autoimmune diseases, such as Crohn's and ulcerative colitis, are characterized by chronic inflammation of the gastrointestinal (GI) tract. Many IBD suffers have IBS symptoms, but only a small subset of IBS sufferers has an inflammatory bowel disease.

MIGRATING MOTOR COMPLEX (MMC)
The street sweeper mechanism responsible for clearing undigested food and cellular debris from the small intestine. It occurs during a fasting state, like washing the dishes after a meal.

PERISTALSIS
The constriction and relaxation of muscles that move food through the GI tract. It's a slow mixing, versus the quick, propulsive movement of the MMC. In the small intestine, the process of peristalsis churns our food so we can reap the rewards of our meal and the MMC cleans up afterward.

INFLAMMATION
Your body's normal reaction to infection or injury that signals to the immune system that it's time to repair damaged tissue or defend against foreign invaders, such as viruses or bacteria.

AUTOIMMUNE DISEASE
When an inflammatory response is triggered despite no real foreign threat present, often due to a case of mistaken identity (see molecular mimicry, below). This can cause the immune system to repeatedly attack and damage your body's own tissues.

HISTAMINE
An essential neurotransmitter involved in local inflammatory responses, as well as gut and brain function.

DIAMINE OXIDASE (DAO)
A digestive enzyme produced in your kidneys, your thymus, and the intestinal lining of your digestive tract, responsible for breaking down excess histamine.

MOLECULAR MIMICRY
When a foreign compound looks similar to your own tissue. This often leads to a form of autoimmunity, when your body accidentally attacks itself.

PARASYMPATHETIC NERVOUS SYSTEM
Your body's rest-and-digest mode, when the heart rate slows and your digestive organs kick into high gear.

SYMPATHETIC NERVOUS SYSTEM
Your fight-or-flight mode, when the heart rate increases, stress hormones start pumping, and you can respond to threat or injury.

HYDROCHLORIC ACID (HCL)
Gastric juices formed in the stomach; used in tandem with the term *stomach acid*.

HYPOCHLORHYDRIA
Low stomach acid.

ILEOCECAL VALVE (IV)
The back door connecting your small intestine to your large intestine. Material can only flow one way, unless you have a defective or nonexistent IV.

ADHESION
A band of internal scar tissue binding together two areas that would ordinarily have movement.

HERXHEIMER REACTION (DIE-OFF)
Your immune system's response to toxins that are released when pathogens are killed off, which can lead to another set of symptoms if the body does not eliminate them quickly enough.

PROKINETIC
A type of drug or natural agent that enhances motility. It can help move food through the small intestine, but is not the same as a laxative.

INTESTINAL PERMEABILITY (LEAKY GUT)
When the tight junctions of the intestinal wall become compromised and allow larger particles to pass through into the bloodstream, often leading to systemic inflammation.

VISCERAL HYPERSENSITIVITY
An altered response to the normal functions of our digestive organs—most notably, intestinal contractions or gas pressure in the colon—that gets read by the brain as intense pain.

VILLI
Hairlike threads on the intestinal wall that increase surface area and facilitate absorption of fluid or nutrients into the bloodstream.

BIOFILM
A colony of organisms (bacteria and fungi) living together under one slimy roof that allows these critters to share resources, evade your immune system, and resist antibiotics or antifungals.

GI, Interrupted: Getting to the Bottom of Your IBS Symptoms

Irritable bowel syndrome has long been thought of as a mystery, symptom-based disorder—what many physicians refer to as a "wastebasket diagnosis" that should only be reached after all other possibilities are ruled out and thrown in the trash.

Over forty conditions could cause the keystone symptoms of IBS: abdominal bloating, abdominal pain, constipation, diarrhea, or a combination. But more often than not, someone will walk into a doctor's office with two or more of these issues, and with no further investigation they are diagnosed with IBS and sent on their not-so-merry, gassy way.

If this scenario sounds familiar, you are not alone.

IBS is the most pervasive gastrointestinal condition in the world, affecting anywhere from 10 to 20 percent of the global population, whereas GI diseases, such as celiac, make up only around 1 percent. IBS sufferers are twice as likely to be female, and therefore, that much more likely to be told that the distress is all in their head and the best medicine is a chill pill.

For this camp, learning about SIBO can be a welcome light at the end of the IBS tunnel. Before the twenty-first century, this type of overgrowth was only discussed in medical literature in isolated instances—usually when a section of the small intestine was removed. It wasn't until the last decade that we've come to understand that SIBO is far more pervasive, and now estimated to be responsible for more than half of IBS cases.

Still, as awareness for SIBO grows, it risks becoming a similarly catch-all diagnosis, when in reality, it is really **a symptom of a larger problem in your digestive tract, not a disease in and of itself**. If you have SIBO, there's always *a reason* the bacteria are overgrowing, and often several. It could be that endometriosis or a tumor is pressing down on your intestines. It could be inflammatory bowel disease—Crohn's or colitis—which makes someone nine times more likely to develop SIBO. Similar to IBS, **with SIBO, it's not the *what* we should be after, but the *why***. Because a more serious problem can go ignored if we feel SIBO is the one answer we've been looking for after many years of suffering.

On the following cheat sheet, you'll see the many disparate symptoms that might be a result of SIBO. As we get into the nuances of the different organisms that can colonize the small intestine (page 26), you may better understand why certain seemingly opposite symptoms (e.g., constipation or diarrhea, chronic weight loss, or stubborn weight gain) are present in some people and not others.

Women with SIBO will often report that they wake up feeling normal, but after breakfast, their abdomen balloons to the point of looking visibly pregnant. The timing, frequency, and location of your symptoms is one of the biggest indicators of whether you have an issue in your small intestine or another type of gut imbalance. Distension, that feeling of wearing an internal inner tube below your ribs, is one of the hallmark symptoms of SIBO. It's a different sensation than what a woman might experience during her period. With SIBO, that bloating happens much higher, the pressure is harder, and it's chronic.

Most SIBO sufferers will feel the impact of their meal within the first hour of eating, whereas GI symptoms six hours after your bean burrito are likely due to gas in the colon. If you find you're experiencing pain or discomfort after *every* meal, that is more indicative of SIBO than are intermittent bouts of IBS, which may be due to an intolerance or exposure to a specific ingredient. The sample Symptom and Activity Tracker (page 300) should help you better identify where and when symptoms occur and whether food triggers could be at play.

In other words, just because you experience gas, bloating, diarrhea, or brain fog, it doesn't mean you have SIBO—or, that it's *only* SIBO.

The most important element of unpacking your symptoms is ruling out additional causes. SIBO is associated with many other disorders, and we are still in the process of understanding the chicken-or-the-egg relationship between them. Chapter 1 is all about helping you parse through your symptoms, test properly for SIBO, consider or rule out coinfections, uncover the malfunctions within your digestive system, and overall, discover a more complete picture so you can formulate the appropriate treatment plan in Chapter 2.

We'll discuss the role that something as common as food poisoning can play in your intestines' ongoing functionality (page 20) and why women may be more susceptible to foreign invaders than men are (page 33). Lastly, we'll talk about the beast that is yeast and how *Candida* overgrowth can be an equally formidable foe for your small intestine (page 30).

SIBO SYMPTOM CHEAT SHEET

Use the daily worksheet on page 300 to track the rate and severity of any of the following symptoms.

• Abdominal bloating and distension	• Gas: belching and flatulence	• Abdominal pain and cramps	• Constipation, diarrhea, or both
• Heartburn	• Acid reflux or GERD	• Nausea or feeling overly full after eating	• Intestinal permeability (leaky gut syndrome)
• Food sensitivities	• Headaches	• Brain fog	• Fatigue
• Joint pain	• Skin irritations: eczema, rosacea, rashes, itching, etc.	• Anxiety or depression	• Malabsorption (fat or fructose)
• Histamine intolerance	• Nutrient deficiencies	• Chronic weight loss or resistant weight gain	

Playing Gut Detective: Uncovering Your Root Causes and Risk Factors

To be able to wrap your head around how bacteria can overgrow in the small intestine, you first need to understand your digestive system's fundamental anatomy and functions.

We are constantly ingesting bacteria through our nose and mouth via the food we eat and our most basic interactions with the world around us. The labyrinth of our alimentary canal is designed to ward off the bad guys before they have a chance to join the bacterial ecosystem of our large intestine and potentially throw its delicate balance into disarray. To accomplish this, **our digestive organs work together to produce a cocktail of naturally antibacterial substances**. These include the industrious HCl in our stomach, bile from our gallbladder, and digestive enzymes from our pancreas. The latter two are secreted into the small intestine and act as safety nets, killing and arresting growth of whatever critters manage to get past the stomach.

The most robust safety measure, of course, is our own immune system. What doesn't get killed by acid, bile, or enzymes must then face our immune cells, 70 percent of which live in our intestinal lining. When a foreign invader seems to be gaining ground, this battalion unleashes its own patented brand of antimicrobial toxins to fight it.

If all else fails and bacteria manage to survive these measures, your body can rely on its own anatomy to at least get rid of them in a timely manner. The migrating motor complex (MMC) is our small intestine's local dishwasher, responsible for clearing the decks and street sweeping undigested food and unwanted critters through the canal after each meal. Because of this role, **the MMC only kicks in during a fasting state of ninety minutes or more**. If you have a noisy or gurgling gut in between meals, that's a good sign that your MMC is not falling down on the job.

Once your small intestine is sufficiently cleared for the next round of nourishment, your trusty ileocecal valve forms a barrier that prevents any backflow of bacteria from your large intestine. When functioning properly, the hinge on this back door allows traffic to pass through in only one direction.

At least one, but more often several, of these protections need to fail in order for SIBO to occur. **Although low stomach acid, deficient bile, or a compromised immune system may be significant risk factors, research points to a defective MMC or a structural blockage as being the two biggest underlying causes.**

STAGNATION: A Malfunctioning Migrating Motor Complex

There are plenty of examples in nature for what happens when free-flowing water becomes inert. Think of a rapid, flowing river. There's hardly any scum on the top, whereas a still pond or swamp quickly becomes murky as numerous species overgrow.

The breakdown of the migrating motor complex sets a similar scene, and it can stop doing its job for a myriad of reasons. The most basic lifestyle issues are stress (coupled with lack of sleep) and snacking. Stress has not only been shown to limit small intestinal motility, but it also hampers the production of stomach acid. We'll get into how to combat the unconscious stressors of the digital age on page 33. And it's not by reaching for a bag of chips every few hours.

The myth of needing to eat around the clock is another way our MMC is constantly halted in our modern world. Even if your snacks are "healthy" on paper, a handful of almonds between meals is enough to shut down that housekeeper wave. Drinking a beverage too quickly in a single chug can switch off that function as well, albeit for a shorter amount of time than an actual snack or meal. Even artificial sweeteners devoid of calories can bind to gut receptors and indicate that a meal is coming. Luckily, meal spacing is a fairly easy lifestyle change that we'll get into more on page 102.

Another way your MMC can go off the rails is via the gut-brain axis. The vagus nerve is the CEO of the parasympathetic nervous system, which dictates our ability to "rest and digest." Any sort of head or spinal injury, even a mild concussion, can shut down the vagus nerve, halting signals to our MMC that it's time to kick into gear. Habitual use of certain types of medications can also impair motility, most notably antibiotics, opiates, and smooth muscle relaxants—ironically, pills that may likely be prescribed after a serious accident or injury.

Many of the diseases on the risk factor list (page 19) create a halo of gut dysfunction that includes the MMC. Notable examples include hypothyroidism or Hashimoto's, celiac disease, diabetes, Ehlers-Danlos syndrome, Parkinson's, Lyme, and postural orthostatic tachycardia syndrome (POTS).

Finally, the biggest root cause of a malfunctioning MMC is a common ailment not often lumped into the disease category: food poisoning. We'll do a deep dive on this on page 20.

BLOCKAGES AND BACKFLOW: Structural Anatomy Issues

Even if your migrating motor complex is functioning properly and moving food and bacteria through your intestines, it's possible that there's a wall, loop, nook, or cranny causing bacteria to hide out and build up. This partial obstruction might not be significant enough to be life-threatening—you might not even notice it.

A recent study showed that even minor abdominal surgeries cause adhesions that could lead to SIBO. Whether that's a laparoscopy for endometriosis, cesarean, hysterectomy, or appendectomy—these surgeries can all form internal scar bands in your abdomen. You might be left with only a trace of the event on the outside, but on the inside, sinewy fascia has bound in a way that prevents your organs from moving unencumbered.

Many practitioners have likened adhesions to plastic wrap gone awry, thin bindings that force your organs together in unnatural ways. Even if they form outside the intestines, adhesions can bear down on your tubing, causing it to narrow. Like a clogged freeway when several lanes are out of commission, the slower food and bacteria move through, the more likely they are to pull off the road, check into a motel on your intestinal wall (called a biofilm), and stay for a while.

Other structural abnormalities include a volvulus, which is a twisting or kinking of the small intestine, or a narrowing due to a vein, artery, organ, or tumor squeezing your organs. Blind loop syndrome occurs when part of the small intestine forms a kink that food bypasses during digestion, but can still harbor stagnant pockets of bacteria. Any type of compression or stricture like this means more roadblocks and possible bacterial buildup.

Then there are the structural issues that cause back migration of bacteria from the large intestine. An abnormal connection called a fistula might develop between the small and large intestine, allowing bacteria to move through. And if you've had your ileocecal valve removed, that means the back door is gone entirely.

PIECING THE PUZZLE TOGETHER

People often have multiple root causes that have one foot in the structural bucket and the other in motility issues. For example, you may have fallen off a horse as a child and landed on your tailbone. Whiplash or spinal damage could stunt the vagus nerve and, by extension, the MMC. You might have been given pain medications that limited motility even further. Even more insidious, though, could be the way your body formed internal adhesions as it healed. Luckily, neurofeedback and bodywork techniques exist to help undo even the hardest-to-locate damage (more about this on page 62). Other root causes, such as the absence of an ileocecal valve, might be permanent.

As you discover the various pieces of your SIBO puzzle—and there may be three or four—you'll be better able to work your way through them, correcting what you can, and putting in place your own safety measures through lifestyle choices that compensate for what you cannot change. Use the following checklist to identify all your risk factors and root causes. For an abbreviated list of SIBO-concurrent diseases and conditions, see page 302.

SIBO ROOT CAUSE AND RISK FACTOR CHECKLIST ✓

STRUCTURAL ISSUES

- ☐ Abdominal or pelvic injury
- ☐ Abdominal cancer (ovarian, uterine, pancreatic, liver, gallbladder)
- ☐ Abdominal surgery (C-section, bariatric, blind loop, hysterectomy, gastrectomy, laparoscopy for endometriosis, ileocecal valve resection)
- ☐ Adhesions
- ☐ Blind loops
- ☐ Cystic fibrosis

- ☐ Diverticulosis
- ☐ Endometriosis
- ☐ Fistula
- ☐ Ileocecal valve dysfunction
- ☐ Internal hemorrhage
- ☐ Intestinal mechanical or pseudo-obstruction
- ☐ Pelvic inflammatory disease
- ☐ Short bowel syndrome
- ☐ Volvulus

MOTILITY ISSUES

Lifestyle

- ☐ Antibiotic use
- ☐ Food allergies
- ☐ NSAIDS (Advil, etc.) use

- ☐ Opiate or smooth muscle relaxant use
- ☐ Stress

Disease or Injury

- ☐ Celiac disease
- ☐ Crohn's disease
- ☐ Diabetes
- ☐ Ehlers-Danlos syndrome
- ☐ Food poisoning/traveler's diarrhea
- ☐ Hashimoto's/hypothyroidism
- ☐ Intestinal permeability (leaky gut syndrome)
- ☐ Lyme disease
- ☐ Muscular dystrophy

- ☐ Obesity
- ☐ Parasites
- ☐ Parkinson's disease
- ☐ Postural orthostatic tachycardia syndrome (POTS)
- ☐ Scleroderma/systemic sclerosis
- ☐ Traumatic brain or spinal cord injury
- ☐ Ulcerative colitis

FAILED PROTECTIVE MEASURES (BACTERIA NOT KILLED)

- ☐ Cholelithiasis (gallstones)
- ☐ Enzyme or bile deficiency
- ☐ Gastroparesis
- ☐ HIV
- ☐ *H. pylori*
- ☐ Hypochlorhydria/low stomach acid
- ☐ Immunosuppressant use
- ☐ Immuno-compromise or deficiency (from disease or coinfection)

- ☐ Lactose intolerance
- ☐ Liver disease
- ☐ Lyme disease
- ☐ Mast cell activation syndrome (MCAS)
- ☐ Mold illness/environmental toxin exposure
- ☐ Pancreatitis
- ☐ Proton pump inhibitor use

FOOD POISONING: The Root Cause of the Root Cause

SIBO is an issue of location, not type. Meaning, our main worry isn't whether our bacteria are "good" or "bad," per se. Just that they're in the wrong place.

That said, in the last five years, we've come to better understand how pathogenic bacteria are often the first players in a chain of events that eventually leads someone to develop SIBO. Many of these discoveries have been made by Dr. Mark Pimentel, whose research at Cedars-Sinai in Los Angeles has revealed that the most common way our motility becomes slowed is through an acute case of food poisoning, traveler's diarrhea, or stomach flu—**a new diagnosis category called post-infectious IBS**.

What happens in the scenario of post-infectious IBS is that an opportunist enters the small intestine—say, a salmonella exposure, parasite, or virus—and our immune system is kicked into action. It releases its patented response to the invader's toxins, a compound called CdtB. Producing anti-CdtB antibodies is a healthy response—one that our immune system has been training for its whole life. But for some people this catalyzes a case of mistaken identity: in the process of fighting off the bad guys, our immune system attacks our own cells. We call this **molecular mimicry**. Our migrating motor complex is powered by nerve cells that are made up of a protein called vinculin. Since vinculin is similar in makeup to part of the bacteria's toxins, the process of fighting it can damage our own tissue, leading to slowed MMC function, and an increased likelihood that other bacteria entering the body will become stagnant and overgrow.

The tricky part about post-infectious IBS is that often you feel better within a few days. The battle against the invader is won. But after a month or so of slowed motility, bacteria begin to build up, and IBS symptoms creep into your everyday life. Because of the time lag and slow onset, very few people put the pieces together that their symptoms might have been caused by that bout of food poisoning.

Luckily, there is now a blood test—called the IBS Smart Test—to determine whether food poisoning is one of your root causes. It works by checking for the presence of anti-vinculin and anti-CdtB antibodies. If anti-CdtB antibodies are present, that's an indication that you've had a case of food poisoning in the last year. If anti-vinculin antibodies are present, you have confirmed a diagnosis of post-infectious IBS. This means you have developed an autoimmune reaction as a result, the effects of which could last much longer than a year.

According to research by the Mayo Clinic, the vast majority—90 percent—of people with various genetic protections experience a bout of food poisoning and never develop long-term IBS symptoms. The other 10 percent, however, have anti-vinculin antibodies present in their bloodstream that make overcoming an overgrowth that much more difficult.

Luckily, our ICC nerve cells repair quickly. This means that once antibodies go down, your gut can easily return to normal. But this is often when other underlying causes and risk factors work their way into your overall SIBO picture. Sketchy street meat in a foreign country might have been the trigger, but low stomach acid or adhesions could have made you more susceptible to the aftermath. And those same factors could also make you more likely to develop SIBO as a result of food poisoning, long after those nerve cells have repaired themselves.

In other words, most people with a history of SIBO have root causes that will make them more susceptible to food poisoning. But **those diagnosed with the autoimmune component of post-infectious IBS will suffer the consequences more easily and for longer**. The antibiotics or antimicrobials used to clear SIBO don't affect the presence of these antibodies—they will linger long after your overgrowth has been temporarily relieved. **And as long as these anti-vinculin antibodies are elevated, the MMC is impaired.** This will make a patient that much more susceptible to chronic SIBO and future bouts of food poisoning that can start the autoimmune cycle all over again.

> Post-infectious IBS = You acquire a pathogen > Invader releases toxins > Your immune system releases anti-vinculin antibodies > Antibodies accidentally attack your nerve cells > Slowed MMC = Overgrowth

INFLAMMATION, LEAKY GUT,
AND THE AUTOIMMUNE CONNECTION

Post-infectious IBS is just one example of how a foreign player can trigger local inflammation in the gut. To understand why so many autoimmune diseases are risk factors for SIBO and why, conversely, SIBO is a risk factor for so many autoimmune diseases, **you need to wrap your head around how instances of local inflammation in the gut can spiral into a case of system-wide immune dysfunction**.

Let's break it down.

Our body is both a highly advanced and an utterly primal operating device. We are built to live in harmony with our surroundings, yet also to ensure that our environment doesn't kill us. The main workhorses tasked with differentiating between friend and foe, foreign invader and cherished guest, are our immune cells.

Now, let me explain why this is such a tricky job. In case treating SIBO made you biased and fearful toward all forms of bacteria, you should know that we are all one big walking cesspool of foreign matter. Our body is riddled with bacteria. In fact, **foreign organisms outnumber our own cells three to one**! For the most part, these species are friends who help our body function properly—even giving our immune cells a leg up so they can do their job better. But this relationship relies on a few built-in protections to ensure "tolerance."

Seventy percent of our immune cells live in the gut, and similarly, the majority of our bacteria live in the gut as well, primarily in the large intestine. To keep both parties working in harmony, the immune cells reside in your intestinal wall, which is separated from other matter by a protective layer of mucus. In the large intestine, where the majority of your bacteria are housed, this mucus layer is thick, making it unlikely that your bacteria will intermingle with your immune cells. In the small intestine, the bacterial population is meant to be much smaller, and therefore, the protective mucus layer is quite thin.

In a healthy gut, this all works in harmony. Incoming bacteria get killed by your stomach acid. Any stragglers get neutralized by digestive enzymes in the small intestine. Soluble fiber gets sent to the large intestine, where industrious bacteria happily munch on the remaining debris and break it down further. Your mucus layer keeps each team on their own side, and the immune cells are only sent in to break up a fight when necessary.

But what happens in the case of SIBO?

When there are too many bacteria in the small intestine, they eat food that is ordinarily meant for you. This creates many of the symptoms we discussed earlier in this chapter. But they can also eat through the thin mucus layer, which is made of polysaccharides (a word you might recognize from the FODMAP acronym). Once the bacteria breach that layer of protection, they are in direct contact with your immune cells.

"Bacteria are not ourself," says Dr. Susan Blum, the author of *The Immune System Recovery Plan*. "We have tolerance for our own tissues, but we don't have tolerance for the microbes that live in the gut. That's why nature gave us this barrier."

When the immune cells meet the bacteria, they register them as foreign. As a reaction, they release cytokines and inflammatory compounds—a firing squad to try to damage the bacteria. This local inflammatory response—the fireworks display—has the potential to harm your own tissue in the crossfire, similar to what I described in the case of post-infectious IBS.

To add insult to injury, the gas that the bacteria produce also damages the gates in your intestinal wall, known as tight junctions. What was once a fine-mesh sieve is now a colander that allows larger particles to pass through. When the immune cells are sending out their bullets, they end up breaking bacteria into pieces. If the tight junctions aren't so tight anymore, these pieces of bacteria can enter the bloodstream. **This is known as leaky gut. And it's the main mechanism that can lead someone with SIBO to develop an autoimmune disease.**

To recap: Once the mucus layer is damaged, the immune system gets exposure to bacteria that it wouldn't normally have. Once the gates are damaged, those bacteria can slip through into the bloodstream. **What was only a local inflammatory response then becomes a system-wide inflammatory response, causing pain and strange symptoms in distant sites.** For example, studies have found bacterial cell wall proteins in the joints of people with rheumatoid arthritis. "If you think about this happening day in, day out for months, the immune system can run the risk of becoming broken," says Blum. "As a result of this chronic, ongoing irritation, you can develop a loss of tolerance to your own tissues."

In other words: SIBO is more than just a little bloating and discomfort. Living with this gut imbalance for too long can create bigger problems that then make chronic SIBO that much more likely. Just look at the list on pages 19 and 20 for all the autoimmune diseases that are risk factors for SIBO. It's a vicious cycle.

> SIBO = Bacteria damage SI mucus lining > Exposure to immune cells > Local inflammation > Tight junctions damaged > Leaky gut > Bacteria pass to bloodstream > Systemic inflammation > Immune system dysfunction = Autoimmune disease

Finally, leaky gut is not just a phenomenon tied to SIBO—this damage to your intestinal wall can evolve from many lifestyle factors: long-term use of NSAIDS (e.g., Advil) and exposure to pesticides, antibiotics, and chronic stress. Certain foods, such as gluten, can also fuel leaky gut. At the same time, **food sensitivities (thanks to food particles that also pass through the damaged intestinal wall) are one of the biggest symptoms of both leaky gut and SIBO**. For more on this relationship and why I believe removing big allergens is so important for healing SIBO, see page 85. For a list of supplements to help heal the intestinal wall, see page 54.

As you can see, even for those not dealing with antibodies from post-infectious IBS, the halo effect of SIBO for your gut wall and immune function means healing involves so much more than just killing bacteria.

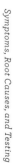

Testing Options & How to Interpret Your Results

The small intestine is not the easiest place to access or culture. Even via traditional scoping—endoscopy or colonoscopy—physicians are only able to reach a small section of one end or the other. Because it is expensive and invasive, and because it misses a large section of small bowel (around seventeen feet of the middle), endoscopy is not the primary method used to diagnose SIBO.

Although most people think of stool sampling as the leading way to test for microbiome imbalances, it reflects only what's going on in the large intestine. If you've been told you have SIBO as a result of a poop analysis, you should know that there's no stool test for SIBO and, therefore, that diagnosis is questionable at best.

In the last section, we chatted about the IBS Smart Test—a blood test that checks for anti-vinculin and anti-CdtB antibodies. This is useful for determining part of the "why"—whether your root cause was food poisoning and you need to factor that into treatment—but it doesn't necessarily tell you *what* is overgrowing. Although post-infectious IBS is common for diarrhea types, it's also much less likely for those who experience symptoms of constipation.

To get a thorough reading on what's going on throughout the entirety of your small intestine, the gold standard is a **hydrogen and methane breath test to diagnose SIBO**.

When I did my first SIBO breath test at home, I felt a little bit like a mad scientist. Included were several vials, a straw, and a colorful syrup. After a twenty-four-hour period of preparation—during which I ate nothing but rice and chicken, then fasted overnight—on test morning, I drank the sugar solution (bacterial fast food), then breathed through a straw into one of the vials every fifteen minutes.

Once back at the lab, technicians use these samples to measure the levels of hydrogen and methane in your breath as the sugar solution makes its way through your intestines. These gases can only be produced by bacteria as they eat, so their presence means critters are alive and feasting off the fast food you just swallowed. The timing is what indicates whether they are in your small or large intestine; that is, whether their presence is normal or an indication of SIBO.

SIBO breath tests differ by the sugar solution used. Glucose and lactulose are the two most prominent types, and there are pros and cons to each. Some doctors, if it's within the patient's means, will perform both separated by a day. All bacteria eat glucose, which means it will capture a greater variety of species present in your digestive tract. However, glucose will absorb into the body in the first two to three feet of the small intestine, leaving over twenty feet unaccounted for.

A 180-minute lactulose breath test is what many SIBO experts recommend. Since it's a nonabsorbable laboratory-created sugar, lactulose will make it all the way to the large intestine, letting you get a read on the whole digestive tract. It may not be consumed by some bacterial species, but it will cover about 80 percent of what's present and, more important, will report on the lower portion of the small intestine (known as the distal end), where overgrowths are most common. Although transit times vary according to each individual's motility, **it usually takes two hours to progress to the large intestine**.

You can get a negative result on a glucose breath test and still have SIBO. But if you prep properly (according to the advice on page 29) for a lactulose breath test and get a negative result, that's usually a true negative. Lastly, with lactulose you don't get the same glycemic push that you would with glucose, which is preferable for those with blood sugar issues.

WHAT DOES A POSITIVE TEST LOOK LIKE?

Interpreting SIBO breath tests is still a little bit of the Wild West. Each lab uses a different set of criteria as to what gas levels constitute a positive result and at which cutoff time. But in broad strokes, you're looking for a significant rise in one gas, or a combination of the two, before the sugar solution reaches the large intestine.

Aerodiagnostics, one of the leading labs for SIBO breath testing, uses the following diagnostic criteria:

- A rise in hydrogen of 20 parts per million (ppm) or greater within 120 minutes after ingesting lactulose

- A rise in methane of 12 ppm or greater within 120 minutes after ingesting lactulose

- A rise in the combined sum of hydrogen and methane of 15 ppm or greater within 120 minutes after ingesting lactulose

Historically, **a sharp rise in gases past the 120-minute mark is considered normal**, since the solution would have moved into the large intestine, where bacteria are typically rampant. The North American Consensus (a panel of expert gastroenterologists and researchers) and some other labs use a more conservative cutoff time at the 90-minute mark since one of the notable side effects of the lactulose solution is that it has laxative effects, meaning transit time can be speedier than usual.

In general, the variance in an individual's digestion is one reason that interpreting breath tests can be more of an art than a science. Patients who are severely constipated may see a rise past the 120-minute mark, followed by a second peak once the solution reaches the large intestine. Because of this variance in symptoms and transit times, SIBO experts recommend the 180-minute test to get a complete picture. The recent discoveries around a third gas, hydrogen sulfide, has also made insights during the third hour of the test more important. We'll get into the nuances of these three gases in the next sections.

METHANE & HYDROGEN

The gas that peaks more dramatically is what will diagnose you as either hydrogen or methane dominant. You can have excesses of both gases, but this indicates which is more significant than the other.

These two types of gases can tell you different things about what might be overgrowing. For example, hydrogen-producing bacteria commonly found in SIBO include *E. coli*, *Klebsiella*, and *P. mirabilis*. On the other hand, compounds that create methane in the body are called methanogens and include archaea, a group of ancient single-cell organisms, as well as some types of bacteria. And what do these methanogens like to eat? Hydrogen!

Yes, I know. Another way that SIBO can create more brain fog than it already has.

When archaea consume hydrogen, they produce methane as a by-product. Cows are a great example of having an archaea-dominant digestive system. They produce a huge amount of methane because of all the bacteria in their stomach that ferment grass. The archaea love the hydrogen from this fermentation process, so they proliferate and produce methane. If you have methanogens present, it can mean a reduction in hydrogen peaks on your breath test, even if there are in fact hydrogen-producing bacteria present as well. It also explains why you can have a false negative hydrogen test result and yet still have hydrogen SIBO.

Methane SIBO is a misnomer since it is not really bacteria, and the overgrowth is not always limited to the small intestine. For this reason, a new set of guidelines published in January 2020 rebranded the condition as intestinal methanogen overgrowth (IMO). But for the purpose of this book and to limit confusion, I am going to continue to refer to methane overgrowth as a type of SIBO.

Carbohydrates feed bacteria > Bacteria produce hydrogen > Hydrogen feeds archaea > Archaea produce methane

Hydrogen dominance is more commonly associated with diarrhea, whereas methane gas is known to cause constipation, or a mixed pattern where constipation is more predominant. You will often hear the terms SIBO-C (for constipation) and SIBO-D (for diarrhea), with the former usually associated with methane dominance. When the methane gas hits, your intestines cramp and can't function normally. This slower transit time is why the bloating, abdominal pain, and lack of bowel movements can be so frustrating with this type. Because methanogens cause a higher production and absorption of short-chain fatty acids, they are also linked to obesity and weight gain.

In other words, methanogens are more effective at breaking down food and extracting calories from them, so those with an overgrowth of methane SIBO might be prone to packing on pounds that someone eating the exact same meal without methane SIBO wouldn't. On the other hand, hydrogen SIBO can include types of bacteria that prevent you from absorbing necessary nutrients and therefore make putting on weight hard.

To add insult to injury for methane sufferers, the archaea that produce methane are resistant to many antibiotics. Because of this, methane SIBO is the more difficult type to treat. You'll need a slightly different approach, with an extra agent to fight the methanogens, as explained on page 42.

HYDROGEN SULFIDE

The reason that extending your breath test into the third hour is important is because of the gas hydrogen sulfide (H_2S).

Hydrogen sulfide–producing bacteria compete with methanogens in consuming hydrogen. "Think of hydrogen as the rabbits," says Dr. Mark Pimentel, who is currently developing a hydrogen sulfide test at his lab. "They're the food source for the wolves or the coyotes. The wolves are the methane and the coyotes are the hydrogen sulfide. If the wolves are winning, the coyotes move onto new territory. One of them has to win and the one that wins, that's your dominant symptom."

If your lactulose breath test looks like a flat line, what Dr. Allison Siebecker classifies as no more than a 6 ppm rise in hydrogen or 3 ppm rise in methane by the 120-minute mark, this could be an indication that hydrogen sulfide is overgrowing in your intestines. By the two-hour mark, the sugar solution should have reached the large intestine, where there is normally a lot of bacteria that cause gas numbers to peak. Without that hydrogen peak, something else is at play.

A flat line is not always a confirmation of HS SIBO. In fact, studies show that it is only the case 25 percent of the time. Another common explanation? You forgot to drink the sugar solution before taking the breath test, something that Gary Stapleton, founder of Aerodiagnostics, sees often in his lab. Although the specific test for hydrogen sulfide is in the works, the interpretation of a flat line result coupled with symptoms is the only current path to diagnosis.

So, what are those symptoms?

In small amounts, hydrogen sulfide is a vital molecule that is needed for living organisms to survive. **Sulfate plays an important role in a number of daily processes that occur within our body**, such as maintaining the viscosity of our blood and lining our connective tissues. We need a constant supply to function properly, but if our sulfur metabolism is not working correctly, and our body recognizes that we are low in sulfate, it can adapt and grow more H_2S-producing bacteria to compensate.

When that delicate balance has been exceeded, people might experience the hydrogen sulfide gas's toxic effects: brain fog, memory issues, fatigue, numbness or tingling in the hands and feet, sensitivity to noise, muscle pain, bladder irritation, and digestive issues, such as diarrhea and constipation. Many of these symptoms are similar to other types of SIBO, but those with hydrogen sulfide might experience them more intensely or notice that gas passed will have the not-so-pleasant odor of rotten eggs.

Besides the usual treatment tactics for hydrogen-dominant SIBO discussed in Chapter 2, those dealing with a hydrogen sulfide overgrowth will benefit from a low-sulfur diet free of garlic, eggs, and brassica vegetables. Reducing your intake of sulfur-containing foods, for even a small amount of time, can help your body detox from a clogged sulfur pathway. Epsom salts baths, while ordinarily therapeutic, might cause hydrogen sulfide SIBO sufferers to feel worse because of the magnesium sulfate. For a full list of high-sulfur foods, see page 297. You'll also want to note the HS label of recipes in this book that are low in sulfur.

THE GREAT BREATH TESTING DEBATE: Is it worth it?

Breath testing is an imperfect science, but it remains the only way to get a positive SIBO diagnosis. If you've just picked up this book, looked at the symptom cheat sheet, and are convinced you have SIBO, you might be wondering, what's the point of even getting a test?

Let's look at both sides of the debate.

Some doctors have disagreed with the central hypothesis of breath testing: that rising levels of gas must mean SIBO. Some argue that the presence of these gases might be coming from bacteria in the mouth. Others say that a positive breath test is more likely an indicator of fast transit time, meaning the sugar solution has reached the large intestine faster in positive tests than controls. But given what we know about intestinal motility and its connection to SIBO, the latter seems unlikely.

If we look at all the data, we see that a meta-analysis of eleven SIBO breath-testing studies shows a correlation between patients with abnormal breath tests and IBS symptoms. They also show that both gas levels and symptoms improved after treatment. Whether or not we can call this SIBO, what is clear is that breath tests tell us we have some sort of imbalance in our intestines and give us a path to right it.

More important, it's easier to choose the right treatment plan when you know what type of bugs you're trying to kill. Those who self-diagnose and go through a round of antimicrobials without moving the needle might not have SIBO at all. Or they could have methane-dominant SIBO without having used the necessary antimicrobials to deal specifically with archaea. Another scenario is that their SIBO was caused by post-infectious IBS. Although not all practitioners will recommend an IBS Smart Test on top of a SIBO breath test, the results can help design a more tailored treatment plan. If anti-vinculin antibodies are extremely elevated, that will tell you that your SIBO will be more stubborn, you should take extreme precautions while traveling abroad, and a prokinetic agent to stimulate the MMC might be necessary until those antibodies are cleared (more about this on page 53).

If you want to go the conventional antibiotic route, getting insurance to cover treatment makes testing a vital step. And even if you're proceeding with over-the-counter herbs, plant medicine is not innocuous. You want to make sure something in your intestines actually needs to be eradicated before going on a killing spree.

That said, breath testing is often not innocuous either. Sometimes people's symptoms get worse after consuming the lactulose solution. Since it's fast food for microbes, it can inflame an overgrowth or make you much more aware of the fact that you have one, for better or worse. **A big learning in this book, and on any type of health journey, is that anything that can help also has the potential to do harm.**

What both sides of the argument tell us is that **a positive breath test result is meaningless in isolation**. Some perfectly healthy people will test positive for SIBO. Some incredibly sick people may not. Your symptoms need to match the numbers. If your breath test is negative, it's possible that you have normal gas levels, but are highly sensitive to the pressure in your colon—a condition called visceral hypersensitivity. In this case, your treatment plan wouldn't need to include anything to kill your bacteria, but simply some diet modifications to reduce gas output, and potentially probiotics that can improve your sensitivity. If paying for a breath test, or a doctor to interpret it, isn't in the cards, anyone with IBS symptoms can start by seeing how a low-FODMAP diet (page 79) improves their quality of life. They can also do an allergen elimination diet to rule out food sensitivities (page 85), or try a few different types of probiotics and prebiotics (page 58) to see whether shifting the populations of bacterial species does the trick.

The bottom line: SIBO is the easiest thing to find. That doesn't mean that it's the only issue. If you treat your SIBO and still have symptoms but come up negative on a breath test, there's likely another diagnosis at play. Most of the time we have more than one digestive problem (see page 30 for how yeast can play a role), and with SIBO, often several underlying causes that need to be uncovered before we can truly heal.

BEST PRACTICES FOR BREATH TEST PREP

Breath tests are usually performed in the morning, since they need to be preceded by twelve hours of eating a very limited diet, then twelve hours of fasting (usually overnight).

The purpose of a prep diet is to make sure you don't have any fiber or fermentable foods lingering in your intestines. This is the only way to ensure a clear reaction to the sugar solution and not just normal digestive processes still happening in your gut. If you change the breath test prep, you potentially will change your results.

Instructions will vary from lab to lab, but a typical prep diet is limited to white rice, fish/poultry/meat, clear beef or chicken broth (not bone broth or bouillon), light oil, and minimal salt (my Pre–Breath Test Chicken Congee recipe, page 224, covers all the bases). I realize this is much harder for vegetarians, but one day of eating white rice is still better than a day of not eating anything at all!

If you're highly constipated or have a poky digestion, two days of the prep diet may be needed to get your gases down to their actual baseline. Antibiotics should not be used for at least two weeks prior to a test, although some sources recommend four weeks. If you're looking to retest after treatment, it's a best practice to wait a few weeks after you've finished your course.

☐ **Two weeks before**…Stop taking herbs, botanicals, nutraceuticals, antibiotics, or antimicrobial medications.

☐ **Four days before**…No vitamin C, magnesium, or any laxative that might increase transit time. This could lead to a false positive as the sugar solution might reach the large intestine faster.

☐ **24–48 hours before**…No fiber, lactose-containing foods, or spices. Consume only clear broth, lean meats, and white rice with minimal salt. Limit fats and oils. Our goal is to prep the small intestine so it doesn't have any food in it by the time we send in the glucose or lactulose. My Pre-Breath Test Chicken Congee (page 224) is all you need the day before.

☐ **12 hours before**…Full water fasting. This usually happens overnight. Also, no exercise. Vigorous exercise changes the whole biochemistry of the gut. People who exercise before the test may have their bacteria masked by the production of lactic acid, leading to a false negative.

☐ **Morning of**…No smoking prior or during. Don't forget to drink the sugar solution in your testing kit! Try to breathe normally and don't puff too hard during the test. When someone blows as if they're blowing up a balloon or inhales really deeply, they end up breathing in room air and depositing it back into the tube. This is most commonly an issue for children and men.

Yeast Is Also a Beast:
The SIBO-Candida Connection

Let me take you through a common SIBO Amigo scenario: You are diagnosed with SIBO and go through treatment. You're feeling 40 or so percent better, so you retest and discover the SIBO is gone. But your symptoms—the chronic bloating, belching, nausea, diarrhea, and gas—persist, even if they're to a lesser degree.

It would be nice if there was one problem causing all our IBS issues, and many put all their hopes and dreams on SIBO's being that ticket. But unfortunately, many times, a few coinfections are in play. And one of the most common overlaps is a yeast or fungal overgrowth, also known as candidiasis or, more colloquially, candida.

Much like bacteria, the presence of yeast in the body is fairly normal. For the most part, it colonizes our skin and mucous membranes. The problem arises—often from the same risk factors as SIBO, such as recurrent antibiotics—when our immune system or microbiome gets thrown out of balance. This can lead to either an overgrowth or a loss of tolerance for these organisms, or both.

There are three main scenarios that can cause problems. The first is an infection—the type of thing that might be taken care of with over-the-counter medications (think: a vaginal yeast infection or fungal infection in a toenail). Excess estrogen is one of the potential triggers for recurrent yeast infections, especially if they tend to get exacerbated around midcycle or before your period, due to fluctuating hormone levels (more about estrogen dominance on page 33).

The second scenario is the one we see most commonly with SIBO: an overgrowth in the gut. SIFO means there is an excessive number of fungal organisms in the small intestine as opposed to SIBO, which is an excessive number of bacterial organisms. The term was coined by Dr. Satish Rao, one of the leading researchers on the relationship between SIBO and SIFO. Through his studies, which involve taking samples of juices from the small bowel via endoscopy, Dr. Rao has seen that when patients exhibit IBS symptoms, **a quarter will have just SIBO, another quarter just SIFO, and roughly half will have both**.

The third yeast scenario, which might happen in conjunction with an overgrowth, is when your immune system turns on your fungal friends and becomes intolerant of them. We discuss the connection between leaky gut and systemic inflammation on page 23. This is another instance where your immune system can be having cross-reactivity issues between different proteins.

For example, people with this type of candida intolerance may also have a sensitivity to the gluten protein or full-blown celiac disease. There's also a high correlation between loss of yeast tolerance and mast cell activation syndrome, eczema and other skin issues, and inflammatory bowel disease (IBD). Several studies have found that patients with Crohn's disease have a higher percentage of colonization of yeast, as well as high levels of anti-yeast antibodies. The immune response to the yeast may actually trigger Crohn's and associated symptoms in some patients. Similarly, using antifungals in treatment of ulcerative colitis patients has been shown to improve symptoms and remission rates.

What makes differentiating between SIBO and SIFO tricky is that the symptoms are relatively the same, as are many of the risk factors. The testing options for determining yeast are much less reliable and accessible than the SIBO breath test, so your best bet is a process of elimination. If the SIBO test is negative and all signs in your health history point toward yeast, a round of antifungals or dietary modifications are an easy next step.

☞ Tips & Takeaways

▷ **Do a diet test.** When you have a fungal overgrowth, it can cause a sensitivity to mold or yeast in your diet. A yeast challenge involves removing yeast and mold-containing foods, plus yeast-feeding foods for five days. This includes sugar, baking yeasts, vinegar, dried fruit, fermented alcohol (wine, beer, cider), fermented vegetables, kombucha, teas, coffee, aged meats, bottled juices, bone broth, and really anything aged. For a full list, see page 296. On the sixth day, add one of these foods back and gauge your reaction. For example, start with fermented vegetables and see how you feel for the next one to three days. Use the Symptom and Activity Tracker (page 300) and the Elimination Diet Reintroduction Worksheets (page 299) to plan your test and keep notes on the results.

▷ **Tease out whether it's also a histamine issue.** If you react to fermented foods, it could also mean histamine dysregulation (more about that on page 95). You may have noticed that the yeast-containing foods listed here are quite similar to foods that contain a lot of histamine (page 295). Test again with distilled vinegar or fresh lemon juice, both of which are high in histamine but not in yeast or molds, to parse out which group is irritating you.

▷ **Watch cross-reactivity with other food groups.** If you develop an immune resistance or allergy to candida, those antibodies can cross-react with the gluten protein. Other things to avoid if you're trying to reduce your yeast symptoms: all sweeteners (table sugar, honey, maple syrup, agave, juice concentrates, etc.), eggs, soy, and corn. Or better yet, do a full elimination diet to find your triggers (more about this on page 85). Keep whole grains in your diet if you tolerate them. Many candida diets on the internet will say to eliminate all starches and starchy vegetables, but this may not be necessary for SIFO. "White rice is going to have less mold than if you're eating a flour product that's been ground up and has been sitting on the shelf for a while," says Dr. Ami Kapadia, who specializes in SIFO in her practice. "There have been studies that show, if you remove all starches, fungi can start to feed on other food groups." For a full list of foods to watch out for with a yeast sensitivity, see page 296. To cook from this book during your testing period, note the YC for yeast- and candida-friendly at the bottom of each recipe that fits the bill.

▷ **Look at nutrient deficiencies.** Low magnesium, B vitamins (including biotin and folate), vitamin A, zinc, essential fatty acids, and iron have all been associated with yeast-related problems.

▷ **Check for coinfections.** Tick-borne illnesses (such as Lyme) and environmental toxins (such as mold, heavy metals, fragrance, and endocrine disruptors in household products) can affect your immune system's tolerance and overall gut health. Parasites (such as *Giardia intestinalis*, *Entamoeba histolytica*, *Cyclospora cayetanensis*, and *Cryptosporidium* spp.) are another biggie.

▷ **Pay attention to die-off.** If you have a strong reaction to antifungal agents, such as those found in many compound herbal protocols for SIBO (see page 44), that might be a tip-off that your immune system is no longer tolerating those organisms. It may also be helpful to add a biofilm buster to your treatment plan, since bacteria and fungi use biofilms as a joint form of protection from antibiotics and antifungals (more about this on page 48).

▷ **Be careful of environmental mold.** Studies show that if you have a *Candida* colonization, you can become more prone to develop an environmental mold allergy. If you live in a building with prior water damage, it could elicit an immune system response if you are susceptible. Mold toxins in your home might also be contributing to SIBO, since they can affect bile production and tinker with the nervous system. Find a trustworthy environmental consultant in your area if you suspect mold is an issue in your home.

The Thyroid Thread & What Women Need to Know About SIBO

The vast majority of IBS and SIBO sufferers are women, and those numbers are on the rise. So, why are we ladies more susceptible to gut issues?

Medical science has historically treated men and women interchangeably, with studies primarily being performed on men, and the findings applied to women. In practice, however, women are not just smaller versions of the same model, but beings with a completely different operating system. Our finely calibrated hormonal cycles render us much more sensitive and prone to dysfunction. And of course, our body is also unable to be separated from the societal pressures lumped on top.

Here are some of the things that get in the way of our guts firing on all cylinders.

STRESS & LACK OF SLEEP

As caretakers of the human race, women take on a lot of stress in this world. We are constantly putting people (ahem, everyone) before ourselves. We are also more vulnerable to violence, which means we walk around on high alert without even realizing it. These might just sound like facts of life, but the result is a lot more stress. Stress that gets stored in our gut, reduces our stomach acid, disrupts our sleep cycles, and creates more hormone imbalances as a result. If we are stressed, our MMC doesn't work as well during our waking hours. If we aren't sleeping through the night, that housekeeper wave can't do its most thorough cleaning. The night shift is also the liver's time to shine, so impaired sleep can lead to more toxins and excess hormones floating around the body. Which leads us to big issue number 2...

ESTROGEN DOMINANCE

One aspect of our microbiome that has a direct correlation to our hormone levels is something called the *estrobolome*. This collection of microbes' entire reason for being is to metabolize and eliminate estrogen. Regulating the proper amount of estrogen in circulation is a delicate dance, and our hormonal motherboard relies heavily on our ability to eliminate what's deemed excess. Too much estrogen in the body—either thanks to an inefficient liver, growth hormones in the animals we eat, foreign chemicals that mimic estrogen in the body, a disrupted microbiome, or simply not pooping every day—can cause a cascade of problems in our gut. It can affect our ability to convert thyroid hormones. It can promote yeast overgrowth. But perhaps most notably for SIBO, estrogen dominance puts you at higher risk of losing your gallbladder. If you have gallbladder dysfunction and you don't make bile acid, you're missing one important line of defense for neutralizing unwanted bacteria in your small intestine.

HORMONAL BIRTH CONTROL

This may seem like a specific bone to pick, but the reality is that one of the most pervasive forms of excess estrogen comes in a pill many of us take every day. As Dr. Jolene Brighten discusses in her fabulous book, *Beyond the Pill*, hormonal birth control can lead to leaky gut, yeast overgrowth (candida), decreased microbial diversity, and altered gut motility, which can then lead to SIBO. With an estimated 16 percent of women aged fifteen through forty-four taking hormonal birth control pills, it's more important than ever to understand how oral contraceptives can affect the gut. Research has shown that beyond smoking, the use of oral contraceptives is perhaps the most consistent environmental risk factor for Crohn's disease, especially if used long term. The "why" is still partially unknown, but researchers speculate that out-of-whack immune function, changes in beneficial gut flora, and increased intestinal permeability (leaky gut) are contributing factors.

HYPOTHYROIDISM

To convert your inactive thyroid hormone (T4) to its active form (T3), you need to have a healthy gut and a high-functioning liver. But you also need T3 for your gut to function optimally. Which is why Hashimoto's and SIBO can become a vicious cycle.

Without adequate thyroid hormone, your stomach's parietal cells will not make enough HCl or intrinsic factor, which is the only way you absorb your vitamin B12. If you don't absorb your B12, the MMC can't function. As a result, two of the symptoms most commonly associated with hypothyroidism are constipation and brain fog. If you're not pooping every day, you're not getting your excess estrogen out. Constipation and estrogen dominance can lead to SIBO and further thyroid dysfunction.

As if that wasn't enough, without adequate thyroid hormone, your pancreas won't be able to make sufficient digestive enzymes, and your gallbladder won't be able to contract and secrete bile into your small intestine. Without that bile, you won't absorb your fat-soluble vitamins. This will make you nutrient deficient, leading to an even greater risk of food poisoning, and an increased likelihood of more SIBO.

↓

Hypothyroidism = Not enough T3 > Low stomach acid + Low B12 > Slowed motility = SIBO

SIBO = Nutrient deficiencies + inflammation > Difficulty converting thyroid hormone > Not enough T3 = Hypothyroidism

☞ Tips & Takeaways

▷ **If you have SIBO, get your thyroid levels tested.** As you can see, this vicious cycle works in both directions. If your gut is struggling, a simple thyroid hormone replacement drug could help give you a leg up and improve your nutrient balance. For more tips on how to boost your thyroid through lifestyle changes, consider picking up a copy of my book *The Wellness Project*, or visit my blog at www.FeedMePhoebe.com.

▷ **Track your menstrual cycle along with your GI symptoms.** For some of us women, a gut issue might not be to blame for our symptoms. Rather, they might just be side effects of what's going on with our hormones. Many women will experience an increase in GI issues during menstruation as our body flushes out excess estrogen. If you have estrogen dominance, these symptoms could be amplified. Pay attention to when in your cycle things flare up. You'll notice there is a space for this on the Symptom and Activity Tracker Worksheet (page 300).

▷ **Clean up your personal care products.** Your bathroom cabinet is the source of many environmental toxins, including endocrine-disrupting chemicals called xenoestrogens. These substances mimic sex hormones in the body and can cause a host of reproductive issues, hormone imbalances, and other conditions—not to mention exacerbate any endocrine issues (e.g., Hashimoto's, PCOS, or endometriosis) that already exist. If we paid half as much mind to how many of these chemicals we put on our skin as we do the food in our body, we would have a much easier time healing our gut issues. Switch to natural household cleaners, nontoxic beauty essentials, and unscented candles.

▷ **Travel smart.** If you're thyroid-challenged or have been diagnosed with post-infectious IBS, being at increased risk of food poisoning means traveling prepared. See page 53 for recommendations on supplements to take with you if you're eating street meat or going abroad to certain high-risk countries and eating street meat there. Or consider doing neither of those things until you get your thyroid and gut back on track.

▷ **You'll have to rethink SIBO treatment if you're pregnant.** I've seen many women with a history of digestive woes begin to panic when they get pregnant. They start thinking, *What will happen when my organs are crushed even further by a rapidly expanding melon in my abdomen? How will I solve my SIBO without being able to take certain herbs? And how the heck will I even poop every day without my usual infusion of coffee?* I posed many of these questions to Dr. Aviva Romm, a midwife, functional medicine all-star, and overall champion of women's health. She reassured me that while motility issues and constipation may persist, the whole immune system tends to die down while women are pregnant and she's rarely seen SIBO be a big issue. Since you cannot use herbal antimicrobials or things like Iberogast, her advice was to lean on diet for support. Ginger, up to 1 gram a day, is a powerful motility agent, and chamomile tea can calm your gut. A low-FODMAP diet is also always there as a tool if you need to reduce gas.

The SIBO Amigo Digest: 10 Investigation Rules of Thumb

1
SIBO is a sign that something in your digestive system has gone wrong, not a disease in and of itself.

2
You must uncover your root cause— the *reason* the bacteria are overgrowing. Often there are several.

3
A defective migrating motor complex (MMC) or structural issue are the two biggest drivers of SIBO.

4
Food poisoning is one of the most common root causes of a defective MMC.

5
Don't let breath testing be the only metric of diagnosis or barometer of progress.

6
Figuring out what type of organisms are overgrowing will help you choose the right treatment.

7
SIBO might seem like a light at the end of the tunnel, but don't let it blind you. Rule out other GI issues or food intolerances.

8
SIBO is the easiest thing to find. That doesn't mean it's the only issue.

9
Yeast and fungal overgrowths commonly overlap with SIBO and are not as easy to test for.

10
Estrogen dominance, thyroid conditions, and other hormonal imbalances might be part of your cycle of SIBO.

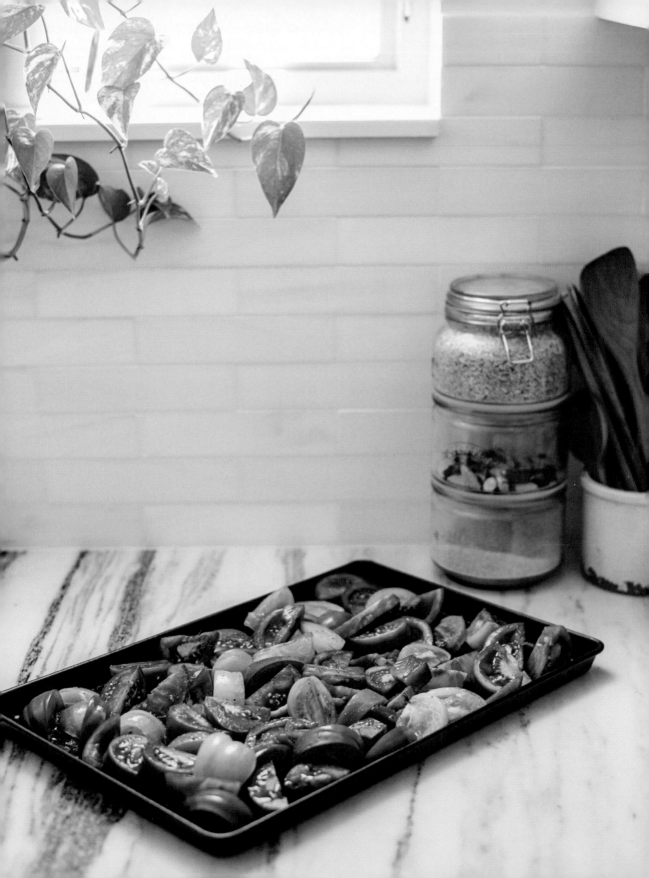

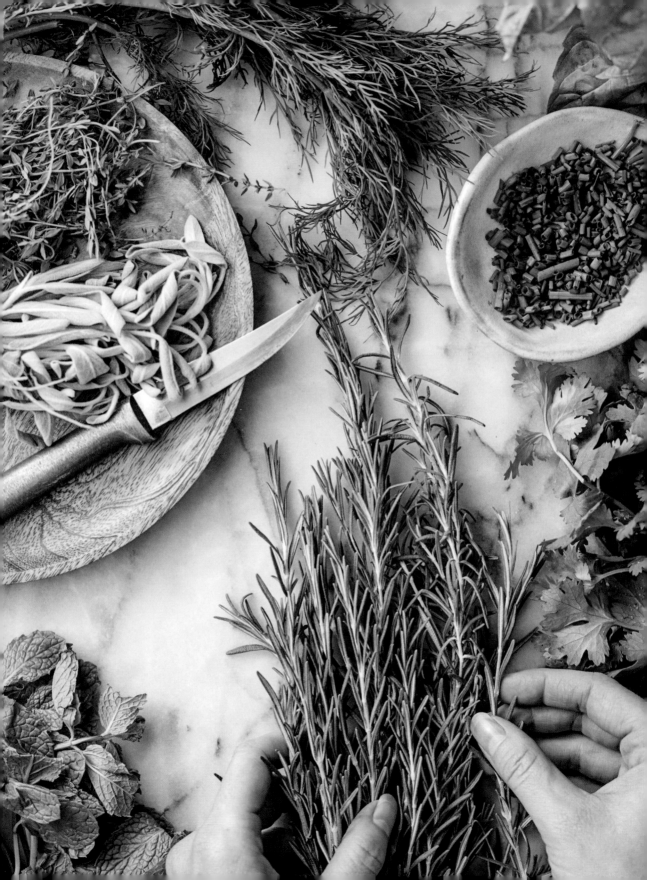

Chapter Two

CLEARING YOUR CRITTERS

Medications, Natural Treatments, and Integrative Therapies

DECIDING ON A TREATMENT PLAN can be one of the most stressful legs of SIBO recovery.

It certainly was for me, and I had a doctor telling me exactly what to do!

Part of the problem was belief: even after a few weeks of herbal anti-microbials—one of the three main treatment options, and the route my MD had chosen for me—my system still felt off. Perhaps even more so than when I had begun. My stomach continued to bulge, my bowels were poky. And despite these symptoms' having gotten slightly better, I feared that I would be joining the many desperate voices on the internet who needed multiple treatments to eradicate SIBO.

This SIBO-style paranoia seems to be common among sufferers. And for good reason. Treatment options are complicated and varied, and it often takes doctors a few tries to find the right mix to cover all the bacterial bases. And yet, having this diverse tool kit is necessary. While one tactic might work the first time, your bacteria can build up a resistance that makes subsequent rounds less effective. "I've seen every treatment work and I've seen every treatment fail," says Dr. Allison Siebecker, who has treated thousands of difficult SIBO cases in her practice.

As I waited for the results from my follow-up breath test, I planned for the worst-case scenario and diligently researched other avenues, debated which hodgepodge route I would try for the next round, and questioned whether I would ever end up desperate enough to get my meals in the form of a medical liquid (see "The Elemental Diet," page 44). Before my spiral causes you to spiral too, let me put a pin in your paranoia: It turns out mine was completely unfounded. My SIBO breath test came back negative. I was free to move on to the next stage of the process.

But my experience taught me two main takeaways that I hope you can consider before choosing your own SIBO treatment adventure. The first is that SIBO is not a life sentence. Although you will hear horror stories about multiple rounds and many relapses, plenty of cases, like mine, have straight-forward "one and done" outcomes. You just don't hear about them as much. SIBO specialists often are not the first stop and tend to see the most stubborn cases. Their advice, much of which I've synthesized in this section, is important to keep in your back pocket. But the totality of their toolbox is not necessary for the average person. The outlook is not as bleak as it may seem, especially if you take the time to uncover your root causes (see Chapter 1) and implement some of the big-picture lifestyle changes on page 101.

That said, my second piece of advice is: even simple cases benefit from playing the long game. You may beat SIBO on your first try, but you still might not feel 100 percent for quite some time. That's also completely normal. **Expecting overnight results is one of the biggest mistakes you can make going into SIBO treatment.** Even natural medications can disrupt your system and warrant a recovery in and of itself. **I'd recommend giving yourself a year to slowly get back up to speed and create your new normal.**

I know twelve months might seem like an eternity. But after spending a whole year on my health for *The Wellness Project*, I see how foolish I had been to expect deep, meaningful change to happen any quicker. Especially if your body has been battling chronic conditions, like SIBO, for a good portion of your life, healing takes time. The good news is, SIBO can become your own "wellness project"—the impetus to turn your life upside down and get healthier for the better. So many tools I test-drove during my year of health—such as sleep hygiene improvements and stress management habits—came up again and again as I was working on my SIBO plan of attack.

This chapter will encourage you to think broadly about your recovery and to be willing to try some modalities that you might have otherwise thought of as too woo-woo or unsubstantiated. Here, I lay out the three main approaches to killing your bacteria—antibiotics, herbs, and the elemental diet—and the many other supplement options for treating symptoms and preventing relapse. You'll also get an array of strategies for living with your microbiome in mind going forward, many of which are completely free and always there for you. Methods such as visceral manipulation (page 64), acupuncture, and other types of bodywork have been the secret weapons in so many people's SIBO stories. We also discuss data-backed ways to rewire your brain (e.g., hypnosis and neurofeedback) for when gut anxiety becomes a self-fulfilling prophecy (page 66). Finally, we get into some of the most confusing contradictions of SIBO treatment, including how probiotics and prebiotics can be part of your arsenal, on page 58.

Back to that thing I said before about belief. I can't stress enough how bad stress is for any chronic condition, even though chronic health conditions are some of the most stressful life forces on the planet. But one essential ingredient for SIBO treatment that's not discussed enough is optimism. As hard as it may seem, try to stay positive. Embrace the trial and error. And even if the road feels long, once you take the scenic route up Health Mountain, you'll be that much better equipped to guide others on the journey that lies ahead.

The "Kill Phase": A Three-Directional Road Map

Although some people will be able to shift their dysbiosis with just diet and supplements, the majority of SIBO patients will embark on at least one "kill phase." During this period of treatment, the goal is to eradicate unwanted bacteria from the small intestine. The main options for doing so fall into three categories: regular antibiotics, herbal antimicrobials, and the elemental diet.

The first thing that you should keep in mind when choosing a lane is that the most effective treatment differs depending on whether you have hydrogen- or methane-dominant SIBO (you can get a refresher about these on page 26). Regardless of whether you are going the herbal or antibiotic route, since methane-producing organisms don't operate the same way as most bacteria, the treatment protocol requires a second agent to target them specifically. The elemental diet, which is a pure and simple bacterial starvation technique, works for both types.

A breath test is an important prelude to treatment for two reasons: first, it will tell you which type of organisms you have overgrowing; and second, it will also give you valuable information about your gas levels. Each of the following treatments will bring your gases down, but some, such as the elemental diet, have a greater potential for accomplishing large reductions in one session. In other words, if you discover via your breath test that your gases peak at 90 ppm, you might be better served by choosing a treatment option that can reduce your gases by upward of 50 ppm versus one that would only accomplish 30 ppm and potentially require three rounds.

That said, choosing the right treatment also depends on your lifestyle and values. Some people want to go it slow and are willing to do multiple rounds. Others may be more attracted to the options with quicker courses and larger gas reduction potential. Maybe the most important thing for you is using "natural" ingredients. Maybe it's what's most affordable. Here, we'll explore some pros and cons to consider for each of the three main categories.

1. CONVENTIONAL ANTIBIOTICS

AVERAGE COURSE:	AVERAGE GAS REDUCTION:	Rx required by medical
2 weeks	30 ppm	professional

Several pharmaceutical antibiotics are commonly prescribed by medical professionals for SIBO.

Rifaximin (brand name: Xifaxan) has the best reputation of the group, even among naturopaths, as it's an antibiotic with "eubiotic effects." It specifically targets the small intestine and stays there to do its job rather than getting absorbed systemically. According to studies, the side effects are mild and the balance of flora in your stool is no worse than before taking it. In fact, it's been shown to improve beneficial bacteria populations in the large intestine. For those who are wary of antibiotics, especially what we said in Chapter 1 about their being a risk factor for SIBO, rifaximin doesn't fall into this category of ones to fear.

However, the biggest complaint about rifaximin is the cost. Out of pocket, one course can run you $600. It's important to check with your insurance provider if price is an issue, before going down this road with your practitioner, or see whether your pharmacy offers coupons.

Another problem with all pharma options in this category is that with repeat use, you increase the likelihood of becoming resistant. Meaning, it might be worth trying one round, but you don't want to get into a cycle of use. This is true of herbs to some extent as well.

For methane-dominant SIBO and those with constipation, rifaximin is less effective. To tackle the methanogens, additional antibiotics are required: neomycin or metronidazole. These medications *do* fall into the category of conventional antibiotics that kill indiscriminately. If you are methane-dominant and wish to proceed with rifaximin, you can also explore a hybrid herbal approach using an allicin supplement as your added ammo for methane. Although it has less data than the aforementioned antibiotics when combined with rifaximin, clinicians often use it with positive results. (See "Herbal Antimicrobials," which follows.)

Lastly, practitioners have reported that clinically the benefits of antibiotics top out after three weeks, so a two-week course is the sweet spot to discuss with your doctor.

2. HERBAL ANTIMICROBIALS

AVERAGE COURSE:	AVERAGE GAS REDUCTION:	Over the counter, but
4 weeks	30 ppm	professional guidance recommended

Naturopaths don't necessarily gravitate toward herbal options just because they're more "natural." Many do so because they've seen how effective they can be. Recently, one study proved what many clinicians have seen in their practice: that an herbal protocol can do the job just as well as rifaximin.

The downside: more pills, for longer, with the possibility of more side effects. Just because the substances are derived from plants doesn't mean they're benign. Especially with the compound formulas—brands with protocols that include many herbs in one capsule—because they are more broad-spectrum in nature, you might experience more intense symptoms of die-off (for more about die-off, see page 48). I certainly experienced discomfort and an increase in my GI symptoms while on the Biotics formula.

You can purchase these herbs without a prescription, but **I'd advise working with an educated practitioner to design your individual protocol and manage sensitivities**. Compound herbs, such as the two data-backed options that follow, often include antifungal and antiparasitic herbs, which might be beneficial if you suspect SIFO is part of your SIBO picture. But those who are extremely sensitive and expect to need several rounds of treatment will be better served by taking a combination of one to three individual herbs. If another round is needed, you'll be able to rotate some new players in and avoid building resistance.

For methane-dominant SIBO, allicin is the most effective herbal option to add to your protocol. Although it's derived from garlic, this strong antimicrobial doesn't contain the fibers and inulin (i.e., problematic FODMAP content) found in other parts of the clove that are known to be irritating to some guts. If you do react poorly to allicin, it might be a sign that hydrogen-sulfide gas is part of your SIBO picture, as this supplement is sulfuric.

Finally, though it is not the norm, some practitioners have found their patients are less symptomatic when using herbal tinctures instead of enteric-coated capsules. Tinctures essentially remove many of the volatile components that you find in essential oils, while preserving the anti-inflammatory properties of the whole plant, such as polyphenols. Those with a highly damaged gut might not be able to process capsules effectively enough to get the full efficacy of their contents. Liquids, such as teas or tinctures, are much easier to absorb and assimilate. If you are struggling with an herbal pill protocol, this is another avenue to discuss with your practitioner.

One of the most common questions I receive is when should you take your antimicrobial medications: with meals or on an empty stomach? Since herbs can often cause nausea, taking them with food will be the best option for some. Usually, practitioners advise taking herbs thirty minutes before a meal on an empty stomach, with food following soon thereafter. But it's important to see how you feel and to experiment—there's no right or wrong way.

Important note: Herbal solutions are not appropriate for women who are pregnant or are trying to conceive.

Data-backed compound herbal protocols:

- **METAGENICS:** Candibactin-AR + Candibactin-BR

- **BIOTICS:** FC Cidal + Dysbiocide

Single herbs:

- **OIL OF OREGANO:** This herb has been known as a longtime antifungal, antimicrobial, antiviral powerhouse.

- **BERBERINE HERBS:** Examples include goldenseal, Oregon grape, and barberry, among others. Many practitioners use one of these in conjunction with oil of oregano and neem for hydrogen-dominant SIBO. Berberine complexes are also available.

- **NEEM:** Neem is an Ayurvedic antimicrobial derived from a tropical evergreen tree. It is said to enhance the positive effects of berberine herbs.

- **ALLICIN:** This single-use herb has been found to be most effective for methane-dominant SIBO. It can be added to one of the compound protocols, rifaximin, or used in conjunction with berberine herbs and neem. The highest potency formula on the market is Allimed.

Note: When starting any course of herbs, be sure to check with your healthcare professional for any contraindications or side effects.

3. THE ELEMENTAL DIET

AVERAGE COURSE:	AVERAGE GAS REDUCTION:	Over the counter, but professional guidance recommended
2 weeks	50 to 70 ppm	

The elemental diet has the highest efficacy potential of any treatment for SIBO. And yet, it's often misused, misunderstood, and generally met with last-resort trepidation.

Contrary to its name, this approach is not really a diet; rather, an actual antimicrobial treatment. The protocol involves drinking a medical shake, made up of predigested micronutrients, for all your meals. The strategy has proven 85 percent effective at starving out bacteria while, on a purely elemental level, feeding the person. These liquid nutrients are in their most basic form so they assimilate immediately upon reaching the small intestine—high enough that bacteria never get a chance to feed off them. It's not recommended to take antibiotics or herbs during the elemental diet because the bacteria, without food sources, will essentially go into hibernation or die off on their own. The diet is suggested for fourteen days as a treatment, and some suggest retesting on the fifteenth day since you're already on the prep diet (see page 29). Others believe that you'll get a more realistic picture of where your gases stand if you wait until you're back on solid foods.

Those dealing with extremely high gases or on a very restrictive diet may actually find the elemental formula to be a relief. It can decrease gas as much as 70 parts per million in one two-week course. For those who are highly sensitive and still want to go the "natural" route, it offers an alternative to herbs, which sometimes irritate the system. There's also a positive financial component. Although the cost of a store-bought formula is more than herbal supplements, you have the savings of not spending money on meals.

In addition to SIBO treatment, the elemental formula is widely used in hospitals on GI patients—mostly those with IBD and celiac disease—whose digestive system needs to heal. Dr. Michael Ruscio, who's developed his own elemental formula, suggests that a more flexible approach to the elemental diet opens up a whole world of possibilities for SIBO patients with gut damage. If the idea of drinking your calories for two weeks straight seems unrealistic, the elemental diet can be used in therapeutic doses as a replacement for one or two meals a day or as a quick three-day reset for those experiencing symptom flare-ups. A more sporadic usage won't completely starve bacteria, but it will allow your gut to have a much-needed rest. Giving injured or inflamed intestines time to heal after SIBO, or even during, will only make them stronger and more capable of getting back on track.

One study found that after using the elemental diet, patients' gut microbiota looked healthier even though there was no fiber to feed beneficial bacteria. "If your immune system is kicking out all this inflammation in your gut, that poisons the milieu, and it makes the colony less healthy," says Dr. Ruscio. Giving the immune system time to die down is what gives the gut a chance to heal. (More about the immune system on page 17.)

Besides missing solid food, one of the biggest historical barriers for the elemental diet has been the taste. Some have likened homemade formulas to the flavor of envelope adhesive. Luckily, there have been some strides made on this front, Physicians' Elemental by Integrative Therapeutics and Dr. Ruscio's Elemental Formula being two of the better store-bought options.

As always, it's best to work with a medical professional, no matter what treatment you choose. A nutritionist can offer much-needed support coming off the diet and transitioning back to solid foods, per the advice that follows.

Navigating an Elemental Diet

Read the ingredient label. Not all formulas that claim to be elemental are so in practice. Scan the ingredient list to make sure that it doesn't include any fiber, full protein, or food ingredients. Some examples of things to avoid are: whey protein isolate, vegetable powder, and cocoa.

Sip it slowly. Elemental shakes are not meant to be downed in a few gulps. Since the formulas are made up of simple sugars, it's important for blood sugar balance to drink them very slowly over the course of an hour. Store in an insulated bottle and think of your consumption as an IV drip, adding more water if necessary. Sip through a reusable straw if you worry about what the simple sugars will do to your teeth.

Use it as an opportunity to do an elimination reintroduction. If you've been off high-FODMAP foods, you can use the period following the elemental diet (after you've successfully begun eating solid food again) to test certain ingredients. This can also be a tactic for testing allergens. See page 91 for more on elimination diet reintroductions and how to go about them.

Allow an adjustment period. Even though side effects from the elemental diet can be less dramatic than when using herbal antimicrobials, that doesn't mean there won't be any negative symptoms. Some adjustment period is normal. Going off solid foods can occasionally trigger flulike symptoms. If they persist after three days, it's probably an indication that you are intolerant of something in the elemental formula. You'll find more info on die-off symptoms and how to differentiate those from an intolerance on page 48.

Reintroduce solid foods carefully. The longer you do an elemental diet, the more gradual and cautious your food reintroduction should be. An easy way to ease back in is to do a hybrid application, whereby you continue the elemental diet for two meals a day and begin by transitioning to one solid meal. After a few days, you can slowly swap in an additional solid meal and eventually come fully off of the formula. For the transition, you want to focus on smaller, safer meals. Choose soft, cooked foods, such as steamed vegetables, soups, and broths. If you know you have a problem with high-FODMAP foods, reintroduce only low-FODMAP foods. See recipe suggestions in the Gut-Heal Bootcamp Menu on page 285.

Don't be discouraged by setbacks. Since you might see dramatic improvements on an elemental diet, readjusting to normal food might feel as though you've taken one step forward, two steps back. This is completely normal and not something that should cause anxiety. Just as your body needed time to adjust to the elemental formula, you need to have some patience with how it copes with solid food again afterward. Give your digestion one to three weeks to return to its new normal and understand that even if you were feeling 100 percent better on the formula, 80 percent better after reintroducing food is a huge victory.

SIBO "Kill Phase" Treatment Cheat Sheet

TREATMENT TYPE	RX	AVG. COURSE	AVG. GAS REDUCTION	AVG. COST	HYDROGEN (& SIBO-D)	METHANE (& SIBO-C)
Conventional antibiotics	Prescription required	2 weeks	30 ppm	$650 (w/o insurance)	rifaximin (Xifaxan)	& neomycin or metronidazole
Herbal antimicrobials	Over the counter	4 weeks	30 ppm	$175	**1–3 Individual herbs** Oil of oregano, berberine herbs, neem OR **Compound formulas** Biotics FC Cidal + Dysbiocide or Metagenics Candibactin-AR + BR	& allicin
Elemental diet	Over the counter	2 weeks	50–70 ppm	$400	**DIY formula** OR **Store-bought formula** Elemental Heal by Dr. Ruscio, Physician's Elemental by Integrative Therapeutics, or other	

Managing Symptoms and Side Effects: Inside Your SIBO Medicine Cabinet

"I just started my SIBO treatment and I'm feeling so much worse."

This is an email or comment I've received hundreds of times. The roller-coaster ride of IBS symptoms can drive a person crazy, especially as they ebb and flow during more proactive periods of your journey. Although these symptoms at the beginning of treatment are the norm in many cases, it's important to tease out whether you're reacting to the treatment itself, the process of bacteria dying, or simply trigger foods in your diet that you have yet to uncover.

Herxheimer reaction, colloquially referred to as "die-off," is what happens when either bacteria or fungi die and spill their endotoxins. The bacteria that tend to be present in SIBO, such as *Klebsiella* and *E. coli*, have lipopolysaccharide (LPS) in their cell walls. This molecule is one of the most potent triggers of inflammation, depression, and anxiety. In many ways, this toxin released in death is more harmful to your body than the bacteria was when it was alive.

If your liver isn't functioning properly or you have severe leaky gut (which, as discussed on page 23, is very common with SIBO), your body will experience these effects much more aggressively. Some have described the experience as feeling as if they are coming down with the flu—extreme fatigue, brain fog, aches, pains, and irritability. Constipation and bloating are also common. And if you're constipated to begin with and not eliminating properly, you will also be more susceptible to die-off. It all comes down to your detoxification threshold and ability. We'll talk more about how diet can help with die-off on page 89.

Adding a binder, such as charcoal or bentonite clay, can assist in ushering the toxins out of your system more efficiently, as can taking something to alleviate constipation. Reducing your dose and going slowly can also ease the transition. If none of these tactics moves the needle, the second possibility is you're reacting to something in the treatment itself. Nausea can be common with berberine-containing herbs. If symptoms continue past a couple of days, this is likely the case.

Luckily, a whole arsenal of over-the-counter remedies may relieve your symptoms before, during, or after treatment. Some of these can improve your outcomes with antibiotics or antimicrobials. Others are important for giving the digestive process a leg up and preventing relapse. And many are often necessary to ease a flare-up. This list may seem overwhelming, so remember that it is not an "all of the above" suggestion, but tools to pick and choose from as needed. You can refer to page 54 for a cheat sheet.

INCREASING EFFICACY OF ANTIMICROBIALS

Biofilm disruptors: Opportunistic bacteria and fungi can be tricky creatures to tackle directly with antibiotics. This is due in part to an adaptive tactic whereupon a whole community of organisms will join together into a colony that shares nutrients and is enveloped by a physical barrier called a biofilm. Think of this biofilm as a highly functional medieval city wall that can prevent immune cells from detecting the bacteria and antibiotics from targeting it. Since the surface area of our small intestine is larger than a football field, it offers plenty of nooks and crannies for bacteria and fungi to band together and begin building a shantytown. Areas of the intestinal wall that no longer have mucus to protect it are the most vulnerable to biofilms forming. According to the National Institutes of Health, the vast majority of human bacterial infections involve biofilm. One of the most notorious biofilms comes in the form of slimy plaque on your teeth! In fact, many people refer to biofilms in the gut as "digestive plaque." To make antimicrobials more effective during SIBO treatment, many integrative practitioners will add an agent that helps dismantle the biofilm itself. Several enzymes and minerals have good data for tackling biofilms. Some you might already have in your medicine cabinet include N-acetylcysteine (NAC), N-acetyl-glucosamine (NAG), and monolaurin. Some practitioners recommend compound commercial products formulated specifically to disrupt biofilm. More on those in the Resources section (page 303). Certain probiotics have also been known to inhibit the formation of biofilms; more on those are on page 58. Lastly, certain ingredients can be added to your diet to help with biofilms: apple cider vinegar, turmeric, and coconut oil. Garlic is also a powerful biofilm buster, but those with SIBO may benefit from taking an allicin supplement, since eating whole cloves can cause symptoms.

Bile acids: Another aid that has been studied alongside rifaximin and shown to increase efficacy is bile acids. While the habitat of the large intestine is primarily water, the small intestine, on the other hand, is filled with bile. Although the mechanics aren't yet known, one study showed that adding more bile acids during treatment helped rifaximin absorb better. They may also help weaken the bacterial cell membrane. Ox bile in particular is a great addition to your medicine cabinet as it can also help those with fat malabsorption better process their meals.

Partially hydrolyzed guar gum (PHGG): This prebiotic fiber has been shown in study after study to improve outcomes for a variety of IBS symptoms. We will get more into the efficacies on page 60. Most notable for your treatment plan is one study that found that adding PHGG to rifaximin improved SIBO eradication from 65 to 85 percent.

MANAGING PAIN, GAS, BLOATING & BOWEL ISSUES

Peppermint oil: Much of the abdominal pain caused by SIBO is due to your muscles' contracting against trapped gas. Peppermint oil has been studied extensively, particularly for relieving abdominal pain in IBS patients. It acts as a smooth muscle relaxant, and has the added benefit of being antibacterial (a plus for hydrogen-dominant SIBO). Peppermint can be brewed as a strong tea, taken as a tincture, or rubbed directly on the abdomen if using an essential oil. The most common vehicle is enteric-coated peppermint oil pills, which are best for reaching pain in the midabdomen. Peppermint is not ideal for those with acid reflux issues.

Activated charcoal: Charcoal is an extremely effective binding agent, working well for any unwanted junk, be it a toxin, bad bacteria, or virus. It's particularly useful for those with SIBO since it absorbs gas, thereby reducing abdominal pain and improving both diarrhea and constipation. It's also a good addition if you're experiencing symptoms of die-off, as the charcoal can help bind to some of the toxins your bacteria produce and eliminate them. An important note is that charcoal binds to everything, so make sure to take it two hours apart from any medication, supplement, or meal if you still want to benefit from its efficacy or nutrients.

Iberogast: These herbal drops are extremely popular as an adjunct to SIBO treatment. They were designed to treat gastritis, stomach pain, abdominal bloating, gas, nausea, and heartburn. It's fast-acting for relaxing abdominal muscles and moving gas out if taken with meals. It's also thought of as a prokinetic, helping to move food through your system if taken at bedtime, which can be helpful for those with constipation.

Important note: This herbal remedy is NOT appropriate for women who are pregnant or are trying to conceive.

Atrantil: Although it hasn't been studied specifically for SIBO, this herbal therapy was designed to limit the effects of methane gas in the gut. In one randomized trial, 91 percent of IBS patients reported relief from bloating and 77 percent had improved constipation. Many methane SIBO or IBS-C patients keep Atrantil in their medicine cabinet to relieve symptoms.

Magnesium oxide or citrate: In addition to being an essential mineral, magnesium can be helpful for constipation as it pulls water into the gut and functions as a mild laxative. Best practices are to take it before bed on an empty stomach. Since it's also a muscle relaxant and generally calming for the body, it's been known to promote a better night's sleep as well.

Ginger: One of the best fighters of nausea is good old-fashioned ginger. You can make yourself a fresh tea (Happy Tummy Digestive Tea, page 158) or seek it out in capsule, tincture, or chew form. Ginger is also a natural prokinetic (more about these on page 53), so it can help stimulate your motility.

SIBO Diet: Changing the food you eat is one of the most data-backed approaches for dealing with IBS symptoms. For a list of options, see Chapter 3. And, of course, the recipes in this book exist to help you put whatever food choices you decide on into practice.

Full-spectrum hemp oil: CBD oil, along with new research on how the endocannabinoid system works, has been on the rise over the past few years. We're still learning how the mechanisms work in the body, but it's clear that high-quality hemp products can be a huge asset in your medicine cabinet for managing IBS issues, activating the immune system, and reducing inflammation in the gut. "You can think of CBD as an adaptogen," says Chloe Weber, a Chinese herbalist and founder of Radical Roots. "If you need more energy, it gives you more energy. If you need more sleep, it'll help you sleep. It brings the body and the brain into homeostasis at the most basic level." Weber recommends finding oils that contain the whole plant rather than a CBD isolate. Hemp is very mineral rich and research indicates that the whole (which includes small nonpsychoactive doses of THC) is greater than the parts. Full-spectrum hemp also includes CBG, which is one of the cannabinoids that's been shown in research to be most effective for IBS, repairing tight junctions, and improving leaky gut. Some of these positive effects on the gut are thanks to how these cannabinoids affect the brain, regulating vagal tone and improving anxiety in many users. For best use, place the oil under the tongue and hold there for thirty seconds before swallowing. Full-spectrum hemp oil isn't a fast-acting medicine for a flare-up like many of these other supplements; rather, it's something you can take every day to regulate your symptoms and reduce your likelihood of having one.

IMPROVING DIGESTIVE FUNCTION

Digestive enzymes: High-potency enzymes can digest foods three times faster than if your system was left to its own devices, especially if those devices (such as your pancreas) have fallen down on the job. Adding these supplements won't give your gut a break in the same way as the predigested ingredients in the elemental diet. But they can be very helpful if you don't have the proper nutrient stores to ensure that stomach acid, liver bile, and pancreatic enzymes are being produced in high enough supply. As a reminder, when food isn't broken down properly prior (or upon arrival) to the small intestine, it gives unwanted bacteria a robust food source.

Betane HCl: If you suspect low stomach acid might be one of your underlying causes, fixing it can be a huge part of ongoing prevention. A meta-analysis of proton pump inhibitor use, which decreases stomach acid, showed that people taking these medications were much more likely to develop SIBO. Also, not having enough stomach acid makes you that much more susceptible to food poisoning, and food poisoning is one of the primary causes of SIBO. Ironically, low stomach acid is one of the reasons that some (not all) people have symptoms of reflux. When your stomach senses low levels of acid, it leads to relaxation of the lower esophageal sphincter, allowing that backsplash to take place. You can experiment with the right dose by doing an HCl test: take one pill right before a meal, increasing with an additional pill at subsequent meals until you feel any reflux symptoms. That should give you an indicator of how many it will take to reach a normal level without going overboard.

Apple cider vinegar (ACV): Another method to stimulate stomach acid prior to a meal is to drink 1 tablespoon of ACV or freshly squeezed lemon juice in 8 ounces of water before eating. This has also been shown in studies to improve insulin sensitivity in carb-heavy meals, so potentially helpful for those with blood sugar issues. If you're worried about your tooth enamel, sip it through a straw. This is also not the best ingredient for those who suspect a yeast overgrowth or histamine intolerance.

HEALING LEAKY GUT

We are deeply reliant on the intestinal wall's ability to discriminate properly between what should and shouldn't pass through. The keepers of this barrier are tight junction proteins, and they are responsible for making sure migrants have the right passport for entry. When the lining of the small intestine becomes damaged, the result is an increased permeability. Meaning, the fine-mesh sieve formerly in place now allows larger particles through.

Unwanted bacteria in the small intestine is one of the many things that can increase this permeability, also known as leaky gut. Once in the bloodstream, foreign organisms (e.g., bacteria) or food particles can fire up the immune system, creating systemic inflammation. Reducing inflammation in the gut relies in part on quieting the immune system. And an essential way to do this is to improve the integrity of your intestinal wall. Although removing unwanted bacteria via SIBO treatment is half the battle, there are other supplements that support repair of the tight junctions.

L-glutamine: The amino acid L-glutamine is one of the most well-recognized supplements for healing leaky gut. You can buy it in pill or powder form, but if your gut is in bad shape, start with the latter. It's also abundant in many foods, particularly in cabbage. Adding a daily shot of cabbage or kraut juice to your recovery plan is another tactic, as long as hydrogen-sulfide SIBO isn't suspected.

Collagen: The reason that bone broth is such a salve to the intestinal wall is due in part to its wealth of collagen, a web of potent amino acids. These are the big workhorses for rebuilding tissue and fortifying your hair, nails, and teeth. You can add powdered collagen to your morning tea (or my Golden Glow Latte, page 157), soups, smoothies, and baked goods. Or simply make one of the homemade broth recipes on page 140 and sip a cup as part of your morning or evening routine. Avoid collagen powders or long-cooked broths if you have a histamine intolerance.

Colostrum: This compound in breast milk prepares the baby's gut for receiving good bacteria and helps it transition from highly permeable to a functioning closed ecosystem. Studies have shown that colostrum improves outcomes for certain IBS symptoms, such as bloating, and it's used by many as added ammo for healing leaky gut.

Zinc carnosine: The primary benefit of zinc carnosine is as a powerhouse for cell repair. It travels directly to damaged tissue and lowers local inflammation in the process. In particular, studies have found it to have a beneficial impact on gut mucus, improving symptoms of IBD and IBS.

Vitamin D: Many studies have demonstrated the effect of vitamin D on intestinal barrier function. It's important to use a supplement that also contains vitamin K because it works in tandem with D. Another thing to keep in mind is that vitamin D is fat-soluble. If you have a history of autoimmune issues or have noticed fatty deposits in your stool, you would benefit from taking ox bile or another bile salt to make sure you're reaping the benefits of your vitamin D.

Saccharomyces boulardii: This beneficial yeast is a commonly used probiotic for traveler's diarrhea, and has also racked up compelling evidence for its capability to preserve and restore intestinal barrier function. Even practitioners who are wary to advise probiotic use during SIBO treatment sometimes recommend taking *S. boulardii*, since it can maintain gut balance but doesn't run the risk of overgrowing in the small bowel. More about probiotics and SIBO on page 58.

Curcumin: As you'll read on page 117, color is a great indication of a food's anti-inflammatory power. Because of this, turmeric is a long-hailed spice for healing. Curcumin, the main compound in turmeric, is specifically helpful for leaky gut because it encourages glands on the surface of your intestines to regenerate. The pills are commercially available in concentrated therapeutic quantities. Adding turmeric to food also works!

PREVENTING FOOD POISONING ON THE ROAD

The *SIBO Made Simple* travel kit: If you've been diagnosed with post-infectious IBS or you are traveling to a place where risk of parasites runs high (Central America, Southeast Asia, India, and other developing nations), it's important to fortify your digestive system every way possible. The first option is to take small doses of an antimicrobial, such as **oil of oregano**, while you're away. If you can afford it, Dr. Mark Pimentel recommends carrying rifaximin and taking a low dose (½ pill) with meals. It's also increasingly important to take **HCl and digestive enzymes**, to ensure that your stomach acid and bile are in full flow and ready to take down any foreign invader. If it agrees with you, a probiotic (such as those recommended on page 58) will also be useful for keeping your immune system in fighting shape. **Spore-based probiotics** are best for travel, since they don't require refrigeration (see page 59). Finally, make sure you pack an arsenal in case symptoms arise: charcoal can help mitigate the damage of ongoing food poisoning; **Iberogast or ginger chews** can calm your stomach and act as a prokinetic; **curcumin** can fight the inflammation.

GENERAL SIBO PREVENTION: Getting Your MMC Moving

As you may remember from Chapter 1, one of the biggest underlying problems that contributes to SIBO is a screwy, slowed migrating motor complex (MMC). Luckily, there are several easy changes you can make to your diet to help your digestive system catch up and keep your MMC running smoothly (we will talk about these on page 102). Although lifestyle changes can make a big difference, there is always the possibility that you might need pharmaceutical intervention or the assistance of extra supplementation. Those who fall in the post-infectious IBS camp—especially those with stubborn, highly elevated levels of anti-vinculin—may need to explore an ongoing prokinetic to prevent SIBO from relapsing until those antibodies have a chance to clear. SIBO commonly relapses within two weeks of initial treatment, especially if the root cause has not been addressed. The prokinetic options that follow are the best way to stimulate the MMC to prevent another accumulation of bacteria.

Prescription prokinetics: Particularly those who are hypothyroid, or have other conditions that limit motility, may benefit from a prescription prokinetic, such as low-dose naltrexone, prucalopride, or erythromycin. These medications are often implemented after the first round of SIBO treatment for ongoing support and prevention.

Natural prokinetics: Natural prokinetic options include herbal formulas with high concentrations of ginger (1,000 mg). Ghee and coconut oil—healthy fats that grease the wheels of your digestive tract—are also thought of as natural prokinetics, though they don't stimulate contractions of the MMC in the same way as the prescription meds just discussed. If you're suffering from constipation during treatment, you're better off turning toward options with laxative properties, such as magnesium citrate or oxide.

SIBO Medicine Cabinet Cheat Sheet

	SUPPLEMENT	MAIN USES	VEHICLE	NOTES
Die-off	Activated charcoal	Die-off, diarrhea, bloating, abdominal pain, travel prevention	Capsule	Make sure to take 2 hours before or after any other medications so they don't become ineffective.
	Bentonite clay	Die-off, diarrhea, bloating, travel prevention	Powder	Some people mix this with applesauce. It's also a base for a great natural DIY face mask!
Biofilm (Antimicrobial)	N-acetylcysteine (NAC)	Biofilm buster, detox support, immune support	Capsule	NAC is important for replenishing the most powerful antioxidant in your body, glutathione.
	Monolaurin	Biofilm buster, antimicrobial, immune support, travel prevention	Capsule	Because monolaurin is antiviral and antibacterial, it's also a good option for your travel prevention pack.
	Allicin	Biofilm buster, antimicrobial, immune support, travel prevention	Capsule or tablet	One of the main herbs in SIBO treatment, but can also be used therapeutically in a travel prevention pack.

	SUPPLEMENT	MAIN USES	VEHICLE	NOTES
Antimicrobial	Oil of oregano	Antimicrobial, immune support, travel prevention	Essential oil or capsule	One of the main herbs in SIBO treatment, but can also be used therapeutically in a travel prevention pack or if feeling the onset of food poisoning.
Digestive support	Elemental diet formula	IBS symptoms, digestive support	Powder	One of the main treatments for SIBO, but can also be used therapeutically as a meal replacement to give your gut time to heal during periods of intense GI symptoms.
	Digestive enzymes	Malabsorption, digestive support, low stomach acid, travel prevention	Tablet	Most SIBO Amigos could benefit from adding into their daily routine. Take 15 minutes before a meal for best results. Some brands also include Betane HCl and pepsin in the formula.
	Ox bile	Fat malabsorption, digestive support, antimicrobial efficacy	Capsule	Those with gallbladder issues will benefit. One study found that this digestive enzyme can improve the efficacy of rifaximin.
	Betane HCl	Digestive support, low stomach acid	Capsule or tablet	Experiment with dose by doing an HCl test: take one pill right before a meal, increasing with subsequent meals until you feel any reflux symptoms.
IBS symptoms	Peppermint oil	Abdominal pain, IBS symptoms, antimicrobial	Capsule, tea, tincture, or essential oil	Peppermint essential oil can help alleviate headaches if rubbed into the temples. Peppermint taken orally is NOT ideal for those with acid reflux issues.
	Iberogast	Gas, abdominal pain, bloating, digestive support, prokinetic	Tincture	NOT appropriate for women who are pregnant or are trying to conceive

	SUPPLEMENT	MAIN USES	VEHICLE	NOTES
IBS symptoms	Atrantil	Gas, abdominal pain, bloating, constipation, antimicrobial	Capsule	Designed to limit the effects of methane gas and reduce methanogens, but has only been validated for reducing symptoms.
	Magnesium oxide or citrate	Constipation, muscle relaxant, sleep support	Capsule or powder	If you're looking to get things moving, take it before bed on an empty stomach. It will also help your sleep cycle.
	Ginger	Nausea, immune support, prokinetic	Capsule, tincture, tea, or chew	Take high dose (1,000 mg) for prokinetic effects. Strong ginger candies or chews are another great option for your travel prevention pack.
Leaky gut	Full-spectrum hemp oil	IBS symptoms, immune support, anxiety, leaky gut, inflammation	Oil or edible	Using the whole plant (versus CBD isolate) means you will get CBG, which is one of the cannabinoids that's most effective for IBS. Place oil under the tongue for 30 seconds before swallowing, for best results.
	L-glutamine	Leaky gut, immune support	Capsule or powder	May be irritating for someone with histamine or mast cell issues.
	Collagen	Leaky gut	Powder	Add it to your morning tea, soups, or baked goods. Not suitable for people with histamine intolerance.
	Colostrum/ immunoglobulins	Leaky gut, immune support, IBS symptoms	Capsule	Colostrum contains immunoglobulins known to stimulate the immune system. EnteraGam is another immunoglobulin that's prescription only, but powerful for IBS-D symptoms.

	SUPPLEMENT	MAIN USES	VEHICLE	NOTES
Leaky gut	Zinc carnosine	Leaky gut, immune support, IBS symptoms, inflammation	Capsule	Supports small intestinal mucosal integrity and inhibits inflammatory responses in *H. pylori* infection.
	Vitamin D₃	Leaky gut, immune support	Liquid	Look for brands that combine with K. Take D in the morning—not afternoon or evening—so as to not disrupt your sleep cycle.
	Curcumin	Leaky gut, inflammation, immune support, travel prevention	Capsule	The anti-inflammatory compound in turmeric, which can be added to your spice rack, i.e., the kitchen medicine cabinet!
Prebiotic	*Saccharomyces boulardii*	Diarrhea, leaky gut, immune support, travel prevention	Capsule	This beneficial yeast needs to be stored in the refrigerator. Those with SIFO or yeast overgrowth need not fear this probiotic.
	Soil-based probiotic	Immune support, travel prevention	Capsule	Soil-based probiotics are shelf-stable, which makes them the best option for travel.
	Lactobacillus and *Bifidobacterium* blend probiotic	Antimicrobial, immune support, travel prevention	Capsule or tablet	The DSM17938 strain of *Lactobacillus reuteri* was specifically studied for its antimicrobial power. Those with motility issues should proceed with caution with blends.
	Partially hydrolyzed guar gum (PHGG)	Antimicrobial efficacy, IBS symptoms	Powder	A successful addition to treatment for both hydrogen- and methane-dominant SIBO. Improved the efficacy of rifaximin in one study. May be irritating for someone with histamine or mast cell issues.

Probiotic and Prebiotic Protocols:
A Management Misnomer

Probiotics and prebiotics get a bad rap in the SIBO community. The common assumption with the former is that adding more bacteria to the mix wouldn't be helpful for someone with SIBO. Bad motility might mean those bugs hang out too long in the small intestine and potentially join the ranks. And since certain prebiotic fibers are public enemy number one on a low-FODMAP diet, wouldn't people react just as badly to those fibers in supplement form?

The reality is a lot more nuanced.

Let's start with probiotics, since you probably already have a bottle of them in your medicine cabinet. Over the last five years, probiotic supplements have skyrocketed into a highly lucrative global industry. Many brands promise to deliver billions of organisms to your colon, along with any number of health benefits from weight loss to reduced risk of heart disease. However, one of the general misconceptions about probiotics is that these bottled bugs join your existing bacteria and take up permanent residence in the gut.

Rather, probiotic bacteria are transient visitors that allow the immune system to fine-tune its response to more dangerous microbes. In a roundabout way, this does encourage more beneficial bugs to thrive and increase in population. As we discussed in Chapter 1, you cannot have a happy gut without a calm, responsible immune system. But more notably, **different probiotic strains have specific actions as they pass through your system**. Some are antimicrobial agents. Others can improve gut transit time and stimulate the MMC, much like a prokinetic. The key, especially when it comes to SIBO, is to drill down and match the appropriate bacterial strains with the desired action.

"If we're talking about reducing the numbers of excessive microbes, we're after probiotic agents that have demonstrated antimicrobial activity against the microbes that are most commonly present in SIBO," says Dr. Jason Hawrelak, who did his PhD thesis on the role of dysbiosis in irritable bowel syndrome and is now a highly sought-after probiotic researcher, educator, and clinician.

One particular strain Hawrelak uses in his practice is the **DSM17938 strain of *Lactobacillus reuteri***, which was recently studied to see whether it could prevent SIBO development in patients taking proton pump inhibitors (PPIs). Use of PPIs puts you at a significant risk of SIBO—1.71 times more likely than the average person, according to a 2017 meta-analysis published in the *Journal of Gastroenterology*. The theory is, when your stomach acid is being suppressed, you miss a vital step in the digestive process that reduces the chances of bacteria making their way to your small intestine. In this study, 56 percent of the children taking PPIs developed SIBO, whereas only 6 percent of those taking PPIs along with this particular strain of *Lactobacillus reuteri* developed SIBO.

What makes this probiotic strain so effective is its capacity to produce an antimicrobial compound that's incredibly effective against *E. coli*, *Klebsiella*, and other bugs commonly found in SIBO. In other words, the probiotic seems to effectively do stomach acid's job of killing off unwanted critters entering the body in the absence of it.

For those who are prone to food poisoning or have underlying causes that might put them in a similar risk group, certain probiotic strains could be a game changer for preventing chronic SIBO. Similarly, other probiotic strains that increase motility could provide an essential action for those who tend toward constipation.

Unfortunately, this is a complicated equation and most practitioners are not well versed enough in the particulars of probiotics to be able to lean on them as a de facto prescription. And most people don't work with practitioners at all when it comes to probiotics, which some practitioners, such as Hawrelak, say can cause some sufferers to run into trouble.

Still, meta-analyses of research over the last fifty years using probiotics in the treatment of IBS show mostly positive outcomes for shifting symptoms. If SIBO is indeed the underlying cause of the majority of IBS cases, it seems silly to discount probiotics as a possible avenue for treatment, managing GI symptoms, or prevention.

That said, most SIBO-specific practitioners don't recommend dabbling in probiotics until after a round of treatment (e.g., one of the antimicrobial options on page 41) to rebuild the bacterial integrity of the large intestine. Since everyone's microbiota is more unique than a fingerprint, it may take some trial and error to find the combination of probiotics that agrees with you. Most probiotics fit within one of the following three groupings, and if you find you get a negative reaction it is likely due to the type (soil versus *Lacto-Bifido*) rather than the specific brand.

It's easiest to start with one of the following categories and layer from there to avoid an adverse reaction that you can't get to the bottom of. Those who tolerate a variety can work their way up to all three.

Lactobacillus and ***Bifidobacterium*** **blends:** Both *Lactobacillus* and *Bifidobacterium* strains are widely studied for their treatment of various infectious and inflammatory conditions. Most commercial probiotics on the market offer combinations of these strains. However, when bacteria are present in the small intestine, they are often one of these species, which is why some practitioners avoid using *Lacto-Bifido* blend probiotics during treatment and often turn to one of the next two afterward.

Soil-based probiotics: Spore-forming microorganisms that populate our soil used to have a much wider presence in our own digestive system. Since our food supply (and lives) have become increasingly sanitized and devoid of natural probiotic power, supplementing with these organisms becomes an even more necessary pursuit. Soil-based probiotics are incredibly sturdy and able to survive a trip through your stomach acid. They are also heat resistant, so don't need refrigeration. This is particularly convenient for travel and preventing food poisoning on the road.

Saccharomyces boulardii: As we discussed briefly on page 52, this beneficial yeast is an all-around powerhouse for IBS, immune deficiency, leaky gut, and traveler's diarrhea. Even those with candida or yeast overgrowth need not fear it. It's also been specifically studied and seen to decrease hydrogen gas in pediatric SIBO sufferers. If either of the two other groups of probiotics don't agree with you, *S. boulardii* is worth a try.

PREBIOTICS: Fibers That Don't Need to Be Feared

One of the resounding pieces of wisdom on gut health that I have come across is that probiotics can only do so much if your diet isn't laying the necessary groundwork. A helpful analogy is likening probiotics to expensive fertilizer. It's not going to do your garden any good if you don't remember to water the plants.

Prebiotics are the water in this scenario and thought to be the most effective food for your gut garden. These selectively fermented fibers encourage the growth of beneficial bacteria (the flowers, if you will) in your large intestine, which can then suppress the expansion of more inflammatory species (the weeds).

Different prebiotic fibers feed different microbes. Which means certain prebiotics might cause more symptoms in SIBO patients than in others. Examples of prebiotic compounds are: lactulose (yes, the substance that's part of your breath test), galacto-oligosaccharides and fructooligosaccharides (i.e., GOS and fructans, which you might recognize from the FODMAP acronym), and partially hydrolyzed guar gum (PHGG). Some include acacia fiber and beta-glucans on that list, as well as certain resistant starches, which have a similar efficacy, albeit with less research attached.

The prebiotic that seems to have more beneficial effects for SIBO sufferers than not is PHGG. Dr. Hawrelak did a systematic review of all the studies that looked at the use of PHGG in patients with IBS. The analysis showed an overall reduction in symptoms, including bloating, diarrhea, and constipation. It was clear that the prebiotic fiber itself dramatically improved quality of life by shifting the underlying ecosystem of the gut.

For SIBO patients in particular, a compelling study was done that compared the efficacy of rifaximin in eradicating SIBO when PHGG was added to the antibiotic dose. Although the rifaximin alone cleared the overgrowth in 62 percent of one group, it was 87 percent effective in the group taking both rifaximin and PHGG.

One of the reasons PHGG works so well for SIBO sufferers is that it is a food source primarily for butyrate-producing bacteria. Butyrate can inhibit the growth of the main organism that's responsible for methane overproduction. More butyrate-producing bacteria can also improve hypersensitivity in the colon, paving the way for a higher tolerance of all gas-producing prebiotic foods.

In his practice, Dr. Hawrelak has seen PHGG be a successful addition to treatment for both hydrogen- and methane-dominant SIBO. And although a small subset of people might not react well to the prebiotic fiber, he's found it's tolerated by most of his SIBO patients.

For those who are wary of kill protocols that blast the bugs away and want to address dysbiosis on a more macro level, trying prebiotics is an easy first step. Soluble fiber supplements are also a useful follow-up to treatment to heal leaky gut and reduce inflammation, especially if your gut isn't yet strong enough to lean on a heavily plant-based diet to accomplish the same goals.

☞ Tips & Takeaways

▷ **PHGG is a low-risk, high-reward supplement.** Across the landscape of gut science, there's a lot of evidence for using prebiotics to increase populations of anti-inflammatory gut-healing species. Nothing comes close in the probiotic realm. PHGG is a fairly user-friendly way to experiment as a layperson without too many adverse effects, and might be both a boon to your doctor's treatment plan or your "maintenance" period afterward. Make sure what you buy is partially hydrolyzed and not just plain guar gum, as it is a totally different product.

▷ **Not sure you have SIBO? Try a probiotic first.** Many people skip the breath test and jump right into a SIBO kill protocol. Per rules of thumb #7 and #8 in Chapter 1, just because your IBS symptoms might sound like SIBO, doesn't mean you have SIBO. Before you start killing off beneficial gut flora, it might be worth trying one or more types of the probiotics suggested here. If they make you worse, that could mean SIBO is likely. If they make you better, then you've just saved yourself a lot of time and money, and your good bacteria, from unnecessary destruction.

▷ **Space out probiotics from herbal antimicrobials.** Dr. Hawrelak often uses probiotics in tandem with herbal treatments, making sure to space the doses a few hours apart from one another. For example, probiotics can be taken at lunch and before bedtime, whereas herbal antimicrobials are consumed at breakfast and dinner. Again, he is using highly specific strains, not your average over-the-counter probiotic. If you do go the route of taking probiotics in tandem with treatment, make sure you work with a practitioner who has done their homework.

▷ **Probiotic effects are fleeting.** The most important thing to keep in mind with probiotics is that their effects are short-lived. They're not permanent residents. If you begin taking a probiotic strain to help improve motility or constipation, when you stop taking it, you stop getting that benefit.

▷ **Give yourself a waiting period after antimicrobials.** The most common application of probiotics is after antibiotic or antimicrobial treatment. A recent study out of Israel (that wasn't specific to SIBO) suggests that probiotic usage is most beneficial if you wait four weeks after antibiotics to begin the reseeding process. For SIBO Amigos, this waiting period might also give you a chance to retest and establish the outcome before proceeding down the probiotics path.

Structural Treatments: Bodywork Techniques to Give Your Intestines a Boost

About nine months after my negative SIBO breath test, I had a setback like no other.

It took the better part of a year, but after months of baby steps, I was finally eating most plants. My bowels were working like clockwork, thanks in part to a prokinetic, low-dose naltrexone. On a trip to Paris over the holidays, I felt confident enough to eat with abandon and only suffered the consequences (seriously) during one emergency bathroom-bound occasion. These flare-ups happened infrequently enough that I wasn't overly concerned. All in all, it seemed as though I was living the recovery dream.

That was, until I returned stateside. Almost immediately, my system started to have a meltdown. I was back home, back to my routines. And after weeks of eating butter as a major food group, I was happy to be cooking my usual (semi-low-FODMAP) comfort food and getting my ass in gear at daily Pilates classes. It seemed like all of my choices were virtuous on paper—certainly more so than my wine- and macaron-fueled behavior of the previous week—and yet, there I was every afternoon huddled in the fetal position, deep in the vicious cycle of diarrhea-constipation.

What had happened? Was the stress of being back at work throwing my whole gut off? Did I unknowingly get a parasite overseas? Or was I just one of those people with chronic SIBO that had somehow been spared a relapse for a few months?

Many people in a similar boat may have never found out the answer to that question. And I wouldn't have either, had it not been for a bodyworker that I saw for some unrelated lower back pain. What she told me was that my vagus nerve was completely compressed. All those front-body crunches, thanks to my new Pilates routine, had thrown off my alignment in a way that was preventing my body from dipping seamlessly in and out of rest-and-digest mode. On top of that, I had created so much rigidity and tightness that my intestines were being impeded even further. And I'm sure postvacation stress certainly didn't help matters...

Even after everything I'd learned about SIBO, I didn't think structural issues were part of my root cause list, nor did I think they were something that could just materialize without a traumatic event. But the experience reminded me that **what we do with our body physically can help and it can also hurt**. Some of us have been forced into surgeries that forever changed our fascia. Others are simply sensitive enough that even small shifts to the core can disrupt our whole line of digestive fire.

To dig myself out of the physical rut I'd gotten myself into on the Pilates reformer, I began seeing a visceral manipulation specialist, who works the internal cavities of the body with small, gentle movements. On the table, it felt as though my bodyworker was barely moving her hands, her touch so targeted and slight. But within hours of the session, I felt like a new person. The next morning, I was back to my old self, as if none of the recent gastro misery had ever happened. It felt like witchcraft.

I continued seeing this practitioner once a month into the spring. She was able to peel back the layers of my body in ways that no one had before. We worked on physical traumas from decades earlier—such as a bad horseback-riding fall that severely bruised my tailbone—things I barely remembered, but my body was still holding on to.

After I did this work, I was never the same. I could finally eat bigger quantities of FODMAPs with impunity. I was moving through the world freer. It seemed to be the missing piece that created the new normal I had been after for over a year.

It was also a reminder that SIBO is not just an infection to fight with bug-blasting herbs. It's a sign that something inside your body is not working correctly. The kill protocols that we discuss in this chapter do not address structural issues that could make SIBO a revolving door for you (more about these root causes on page 17). Those who have had surgical interventions for endometriosis, a cesarean, hysterectomy, appendectomy, or another type of abdominal surgery, or simply have had a car accident, broken a bone, or taken a fall that you've never fully recovered from: body-work could be the difference between healing your digestive system and staying in pain for the rest of your life.

All healing needs to be a part of a whole picture, and for each person, that looks different. You could do it through bodywork, through energetic work, through diet. There are so many ways that we can find an "in" and discover what our body answers to. I'm telling you this part of my story because I didn't think that "in" for me would include someone gently putting their hands on my abdomen. And yet, visceral manipulation was one of the most impactful treatments I tried. The following are some ideas for how you can find and invest in your own brand of physical therapy.

☞ Tips & Takeaways

▷ **Move your body (gently) as much as possible.** For more subtle injuries or alignment issues, rehab can sometimes be as easy as adding more movement to your day. Stretching, yin yoga, qigong, tai chi, and Pilates are very effective at creating range of motion. Yoga in particular is an evidence-based therapy for gastrointestinal disorders like SIBO. This might be as much because of the mental release a yoga habit reinforces (more on this in the next section) as the release for a stuck body part.

▷ **Focused, moderate movement can never harm.** That's a different story from the hyped-up New York City Pilates regimen I was on! Often, we are better served by going at our own pace in a self-study at home than pushing ourselves to the beat of a group. "I would say a decent portion of my practice are very, very in-shape people that really work out and work out hard," says Dr. Jason Wysocki, a naturopathic physician and structural integration practitioner. "Sometimes they need to take a break as we're working together. Certain types of exercise, specifically abdominal crunches, could actually make things worse."

▷ **Rehab your fascia after surgery.** A lot of structure in the body relies on this thing called fascia. It interweaves with bones and muscles, separates nerves and blood vessels. If you've ever stuffed a chicken breast, you might have noticed the clear, sticky layers separating the skin and flesh. That's fascia. As our movements change or our body heals from injury, fascia can become adhered in a problematic way, like misplaced networks of plastic wrap. Some people will feel this as dysfunction in their muscles or bones. Others will simply notice that there is some part of their body not moving as it used to. In SIBO cases, the most common form of adhesions are abdominal, when fascia wraps around the intestines and doesn't allow them to work correctly. Studies have shown that even a minor abdominal surgery can cause adhesions, and breath tests were often abnormal after that. Although many of these operations are vital and shouldn't be feared, getting some type of visceral work afterward is important for preventing GI issues down the road. Many different fields of medicine can help: acupuncture, cupping, craniosacral therapy, or one of the following modalities—anything that brings the body's movement and energy to a particular area has the potential to work through an adhesion.

▷ **See a visceral manipulation specialist.** Simply stated, visceral manipulation is moving the omentum, the fat layer that covers our vital digestive organs. A practitioner who specializes in this type of bodywork will use their hands very gently to move what is stuck. This type of bodywork can also help realign the vagus nerve, which regulates the parasympathetic nervous system. Improving vagus nerve function helps with a lot of digestive symptoms, such as bloating, burping, stomachaches, and constipation, not to mention neurologic symptoms. These tiny adjustments have a big impact on both a physical level but also on an emotional and energetic level.

▷ **Try structural integration.** Structural integration is a form of bodywork developed by Ida Rolf over the forty years of her medical practice. Her method involves ten sessions that slowly move through the layers of the body until each segment functions in harmony with its whole. "Its goal is to make your body freer and more adaptable to whatever may come its way, whether that be physical, mental, emotional, or spiritual," says Dr. Wysocki. "At its core, this is both corrective and preventative medicine at its finest." To find a practitioner, you can begin with the International Association of Structural Integrators or graduates of the Rolf Institute.

▷ **Heal brain injuries (TBI) through neurofeedback therapy.** Brain injuries occur more than any other disease and they are usually underreported in the moment. In fact, you may think this section doesn't apply to you, but if you've ever fallen off your bike, wiped out on the ski slopes, had a fender bender, head-butted a soccer ball, slipped on ice, or hurt your neck, this could be more relevant to your gut issues than you think. Since the brain is not snug within its cavity, you don't need to have actually hit your head; a brain can be just as easily damaged by whiplash or reverberations that cause it to slam against the skull. You also don't have to lose consciousness or even feel disoriented. It's now widely recognized that **we should not view brain injuries as isolated events, but as the beginning of a disease process**.

The functions of our brain and our nervous system have a vital impact on digestive health, and injury can easily lead to SIBO. The brain stem is where the autonomic nervous system resides. When that is disrupted, it can make our MMC less efficient. In one study of mice, researchers found that just a few weeks after a moderate head injury, there was a change in the mucus layer and reduced contractions in the small intestine.

If we just focus on killing bacteria, we miss an essential opportunity to get the whole system back online and the brain working again. One of the leading techniques for this recovery is the low-energy neurofeedback system (LENS), which is used by therapists to stimulate the brain by giving it information about its own performance. If this type of therapy is out of reach (insurance often won't cover it), there are also a handful of techniques you can use at home to activate the vagus nerve and reopen lines of communication in the central nervous system. More about these on page 67.

▷ **Consider that it's never just physical.** The body remembers not just physical pain, but emotional pain. Dealing with the spiritual or metaphysical takes a little bit more complexity than simply moving one's arm. But many people who have tried bodywork notice that viscerally moving an organ can also release some deep-seated emotional baggage. Tackling this side of the coin might require a therapist, counselor, or spiritual leader, or all of the above. Sometimes it might just come down to finding better tactics to manage stress. We will discuss in the next section how the emotional plays into the physical and how you can tailor your treatment plan accordingly.

Getting Your Head in the Game: Strategies to Manage Stress and Anxiety

The gut-brain axis is a two-way street. If the brain gets damaged, the gut gets damaged, and vice versa.

The gut is constantly sending signals up to the brain, and the brain is constantly sending signals down to the gut. In most people, this dialogue isn't very loud. We might not even notice it, except for the occasional butterflies in the stomach or an urge to run to the bathroom right before a big presentation. But in people with GI issues, that communication becomes dysregulated. The brain starts to interpret perfectly normal sensations from the gut as pain signals. As we discussed briefly in the last section, this often happens thanks to a breakdown in transmission from the vagus nerve.

One way our vagus nerve loses its ability to seamlessly move from fight-or-flight into rest-and-digest mode is through overuse of our stress response. So many aspects of our modern world create cues that prime us for anxiety. Even everyday noises—car horns sounding in the street, the app notifications you can't ever seem to turn off—can activate your sympathetic nervous system. When we're stressed or anxious, our heart rate increases, our breathing gets shorter and shallower, and our digestion and immune function get put on hold.

Stress can be extremely corrosive for the body, fueling a variety of the issues that are contributing factors to SIBO, including hormone imbalance, damaged gut flora, dehydration, and insomnia. There's even evidence that children with a history of trauma are more susceptible to bowel issues and impaired microbial diversity later in life.

Mild levels of anxiety can be adaptive—helping us prepare for the future, get jobs done, think ahead. It becomes more problematic when your day-to-day life becomes bogged down by fears of the unknown or things you can't control. This type of spiral can often happen to SIBO Amigos because of issues with the vagus nerve, lack of serotonin being produced in a damaged gut, or simply because the treatment becomes its own source of anxiety (we'll talk about overcoming SIBO diet food fears on page 99).

Of course, we can't undo past traumas. More often than not, we can't even eliminate the majority of our unconscious or subconscious stressors. But we *can* control our response to them. Because we are complicated emotional beings, relieving the mind of its tormentors is a profoundly individual process. For some, the solution might be exercising a couple times a week, for others many years of talk therapy. Don't underestimate the importance of having stillness in your life and ways to emotionally process things (e.g., journaling, float tanks, infrared saunas, massages, and other practices that help quiet the mind). Any type of daily ritual can help you tune into your nervous system.

☞ Tips & Takeaways

▷ **Use deep-belly breathing when you're anxious or stressed.** Anytime we're able to slow down our breathing, it can activate the parasympathetic (rest-and-digest) system. This helps with the digestive process by releasing our body's tension and urgency. Tune into your breath when you're feeling triggered, breathing in through your nose for about four seconds, feeling your belly rise, holding your breath for four seconds, and exhaling out through your mouth for six seconds, letting your belly fall. With this type of breathing, your diaphragm is activated, and it starts to internally massage your intestines. Chest breathing, on the other hand, tenses other muscles in your body, which further exacerbates digestive problems. This tool is always available to you, and it can work immediately.

▷ **Try hypnotherapy for IBS.** Studies that look at the effects of hypnotherapy on IBS have shown incredible results. Patients had over 80 percent reduction in symptoms with about six to ten sessions of hypnotherapy. This is evidence that GI symptoms can be controlled by directly dealing with the subconscious mind and enteric nervous system. For GI patients in particular, hypnosis can decrease the brain's awareness of pain in the gut. It can also target the anxiety and anticipation of having symptoms around meals. Hypnosis teaches you how to more deeply relax your body and corrects the way in which your brain is interpreting sensations from your gut (visceral hypersensitivity). There are two data-backed protocols, the North Carolina protocol and the Manchester protocol (see Resources for more info).

▷ **Find someone who practices cognitive behavioral therapy (CBT).** CBT is an evidence-based type of psychological therapy that's commonly used in medical settings. It helps people look at their unhelpful thought processes and come up with different default patterns. CBT can be an especially helpful technique for exploring food fears. If you're approaching your meals from a negative perspective, CBT can make you aware of the language you use around food and replace it with constructive self-talk. More tools for disordered eating and food fears are on page 99.

▷ **Start a meditation or yoga practice.** Across disciplines, meditation has been studied as a panacea for stress. Even the insurance company Blue Cross/Blue Shield discovered that meditators were cheaper to cover. Their data, which followed subjects for five years, found that those who practiced had 50 percent fewer hospital admissions compared to nonmeditators and controls. There were also fewer instances of cancer, heart attacks, and even car crashes. For IBS sufferers, meditation, yoga, and other relaxation techniques have been shown to be extremely effective for reducing symptoms and alleviating gut anxiety.

▷ **Get a good night's sleep.** Our circadian rhythm governs when we secrete hormones, and one of its main regulators is melatonin. The majority of our melatonin production happens in the small intestine, which can mean sleep cycles get disrupted for SIBO Amigos, making it even harder to create time under the sheets for repair and detoxification. A melatonin supplement two hours before bed can be a helpful aid. It's also important to refrain from eating too close to bedtime (more about this on page 105). In the morning, melatonin's counterpart is vitamin D. Supplementing with a liquid vitamin D or getting a good dose of natural sunlight in the morning suppresses our melatonin production and tells our digestive system it's time to start the day.

▷ **Create boundaries around your devices.** The constant stimulation from our smartphones puts more stress on our body than we could ever comprehend. But on a much more tangible level, we all know the feeling when our phone is buzzing or beeping nonstop with demands from others. Switch your email settings to fetch manually, turn off notifications, stop checking your feeds every five minutes, and designate time in the morning and evening for leaving your phone on airplane mode. Better yet, check your phone at the bedroom door. The blue light from our devices mimics cues from the sun that our body can misinterpret as a message to stay awake. Studies have shown that the length of exposure to blue light does matter—ten minutes is much less jarring to your melatonin production than an hour. F.lux is a fantastic app for your computer to turn off blue light after dark, and there are now plenty of night modes that do the equivalent on smartphones. Lastly, there's always a sexy pair of blue light–blocking glasses you can wear at night.

▷ **Rehab the vagus nerve.** Sing out, Louise! Yes, one of the many ways we can stimulate the vagus nerve is to sing, hum, laugh, yodel, chant, or gargle. When you activate the muscles in your throat, you stimulate the brain center that sends signals through the vagus nerve. Studies have also shown that deep-belly breathing, yoga, meditation, self-massage, and acupuncture have also been useful for improving vagal tone. The cadence of "om" and other chants in Kundalini yoga are particularly beneficial. Lastly, periodic exposure to cold is one of the most powerful and easiest ways to heal a wonky vagus nerve. A cold shower or cryotherapy causes us to immediately switch into fight-or-flight mode, regulate our breathing and, often, aggressively shiver. While it might sound counterintuitive, these things also allow us to better access the parasympathetic nervous system down the road. Think of it as the vagus nerve's equivalent of a defibrillator for your heart, shocking it back into high gear.

Getting Dirty: Rules of Greater Gut Health

The jury is still out on how the overall health of our microbiome contributes to SIBO. But we do know that many people with SIBO have other issues with dysbiosis that go beyond an overgrowth of bacteria in the small intestine.

Unfortunately, treatments for SIBO can further disrupt this balance, either by blasting bacteria away with broad-spectrum antibiotics or depriving the ecosystem of your large intestine some of its favorite fibers while on a highly restrictive diet. **We don't want one acute health issue to create bigger, long-term problems**. Which is why it's so important for the next stage of your recovery to understand what lifestyle factors make the biggest impact on your gut flora.

Having a diverse microbiome, meaning lots of different kinds of bacteria—and not too much of any particular kind—protects you in a lot of ways, not just from developing a condition like SIBO. Research has uncovered in the last few years that immune function, metabolic health (especially the ability to lose weight), and mental well-being are very much tied to the health of the bacteria in your large intestine.

Your immune system, in particular, wants to see a variety of different microbes—as diverse as the organisms on this earth. When it doesn't have that exposure, it can mean your relationship with compounds in the environment around you becomes more fraught. Our body has evolved with nature, and **we need to have tolerance inside to have tolerance to the outside world**.

Each person's microbiome is more unique than a fingerprint, so it may take several strategies to fill in the gaps and find your own sense of gut harmony.

☞ Tips & Takeaways

▷ **Only use broad-spectrum antibiotics when absolutely necessary.** Antibiotics can be lifesaving, but they can also be doled out for unnecessary short-term gains. The average American child takes one course of antibiotics a year, primarily for minor illnesses—relief from a sinus or ear infection, a temporary clearing of acne, the slaying of a stomach bug. Every time we use a broad-spectrum antibiotic, we wipe out a third of our gut bacteria in the large intestine. This impacts many functions, but most notably for SIBO patients, destroying butyrate-producing species means we are killing key drivers of our motility. The inflammation and nerve damage that results from antibiotic exposure can also cause a breakdown in the MMC. This is one of the reasons that antibiotic use is a big risk factor for SIBO. For those who get traveler's diarrhea (post-infectious IBS) and take antibiotics, it's a double whammy.

If it's a virus or bug you're fighting, engage your doctor in a respectful conversation around the following questions: Is the antibiotic treating an actual infection or is it preventative? What's the worst thing that would happen if I didn't take anything? If you decide to go forward with the prescribed meds, take a probiotic beginning four weeks afterward to make sure you're encouraging regrowth.

▷ **Only use proton pump inhibitors (PPIs) when absolutely necessary.** Antacids and proton pump inhibitors change the pH of the stomach, breaking down that first wall of defense against bacteria. People taking PPIs have a 750 percent increased risk of developing SIBO. Not everyone with reflux can come off of them, but some may be experiencing symptoms as a result of too *little* stomach acid. See page 51 for some tips on how to test your stomach acid level at home. See page 58 for advice on how certain probiotics when used with PPIs can reduce the risk of SIBO.

▷ **Avoid nonsteroidal anti-inflammatory drugs (NSAIDs).** These medications injure the intestinal lining, causing bacteria to translocate easier, and create a system-wide intolerance to your own beneficial organisms. Instead of taking something like Advil the next time you get injured, consider some of the natural pain-relief options on page 49. If you've been taking NSAIDs habitually, consider adding to your routine some of the leaky gut–repairing supplements discussed on page 56.

▷ **Don't sterilize your life.** Especially during childhood, when the microbiome is being colonized for the years to come, it's important not to scrub away all the organisms we come into contact with. Ditch the sanitizing wipes, antimicrobial soaps, harmful household cleaners, and chemical-ridden personal care products for the sake of your long-term immunity. Regular castile soap and warm water is all you need to protect yourself from the bad guys. It's quite literally an old wives' tale that bacteria-riddled sponges are going to infect your family. One study revealed that children who grew up in a household that used a sponge instead of the dishwasher were much less likely to suffer from allergies. And you should banish the bleach as well. Kids who live in environments where bleach is used regularly are more likely to have chronic respiratory infections and bronchitis. It could be the chemical, but more likely it's related to the microbial diversity that we need to stay healthy. Pets in the home also increase your microbial diversity and have been a predictor of reduced risk of illness in adult life. While having SIBO can make us ultra-fearful and vigilant about ridding our life of bacteria, eliminating our exposure entirely will only do more damage in the long term. Instead of becoming afraid of bacteria, remember that tackling the root cause of your SIBO will be your best bet going forward, not waging a war on microbes that we've thrived on since the dawn of time.

▷ **Eat some dirt.** Soil microbes have been shown to enhance mood, increase focus, improve cognition, and reduce anxiety. Instead of buying expensive probiotics, you can increase your exposure through light gardening or playing in the dirt and not being too vigilant about washing your hands. You don't have to live in a rural area or go off the grid to get that benefit; you could simply buy your vegetables at the farmers' market and not power-wash them when you get home. "In one teaspoon of soil there are as many organisms as there are people on the planet," says Dr. Maya Shetreat, a pediatric neurologist and author of *The Dirt Cure*. "You don't have to eat mouthfuls, just a few traces will do."

▷ **Spend time in nature.** Just getting out into nature is tremendously therapeutic for your mind and your microbiome. Plenty of data support how being outside improves your microbial diversity, vagal tone, and sleep. Even your cortisol levels drop and anticancer proteins go up. "Forest bathing" is a new concept that simply means immersing yourself in the beauty of the woods every once in a while. A hike works too!

▷ **Filter your water.** Unfortunately, the "live dirty" mantra doesn't apply to our water system. The regulations on public drinking water are woefully outdated, which means that under the Clean Water Act, rocket fuel additives and dry-cleaning solvents can still legally flow from our tap. Especially after the crisis in Flint, Michigan, people often talk about the risk of lead and other heavy metals—a by-product of aging pipes and infrastructure. The pharmaceuticals, though, are what I'm the wariest of. Although wastewater is treated before it makes its way to reservoirs, rivers, or lakes, and then again before it ends up back in the glasses of consumers, most treatment plants don't properly filter drug residue. Given the other tips, you might understand why avoiding small inoculations of antibiotics in your drinking water every day is so important. For the sake of our gut microbiome, it's also important to filter out harmful purifiers, such as chlorine; like bleach on your floors, these harsh chemicals kill delicate microbes on your skin and in your gut. Untreated well water can be equally problematic because of parasites and other opportunistic organisms. It's best to filter your water at home. I use a solid carbon block ten-stage water filter that attaches to the faucet. It requires a replacement filter only once a year, which makes it a more affordable and convenient option than a pitcher filter, whose cartridge needs replacing every two months. See Resources, page 303, for my recommendations.

▷ **Diversify your diet.** Adjusting your diet is one of the most profound ways to support or hurt your microbial diversity. This is important to remember as we segue into the food section, since diets like the low-FODMAP approach can negatively impact the balance of flora in the large intestine if used for an extended period of time. Ideally, the rules of greater gut health tell us that the more different types of plants we eat, the more diversity we will foster inside our body. **Work toward eating forty or more plant-based foods every week**. You don't have to eat large quantities. Especially if you're slowly reintroducing more variety, start with 1 tablespoon and go from there. Forty might seem like a lot, but all it takes is six different plants a day, two to three at each meal.

▷ **Add back fermented foods and fiber.** As we discuss in this chapter, probiotic and prebiotic foods are often feared during SIBO treatment, yet both have wide-reaching efficacies for improving gut health. We have better absorption of vitamins and minerals from foods that have gone through the fermentation process. Their impact, however, pales in comparison to eating more prebiotic fiber. Ideally, you will do both in tandem with such things as homemade Sauerkraut (page 165) as you begin expanding your diet. If you react poorly to fermented foods, it might be because of the histamine, yeast, or mold load. For this reason, you may notice a real change in your tolerance once SIBO or SIFO has been eradicated. But it's still important to go slowly. After my SIBO treatment, I began with 1 ounce of kombucha and slowly worked my way up to a full bottle over the course of a few weeks. If your gut is having trouble with plant fiber, you can first try supplementing with powders like PHGG (page 49).

▷ **Get a sense of your stool.** Practitioners can order comprehensive stool tests that look at the DNA in your poop to account not just for what species are present today, but also past exposures. A more user-friendly option is to go with one of the direct-to-consumer companies, such as Onegevity or Viome, which will sequence your stool and tell you how your microbiome is functioning. They also allow you to download the raw data so you can take it to a practitioner to interpret further and make dietary recommendations.

▷ **Use a stool to help your stool come out quicker.** If you're prone to constipation, simply changing the shape of your body while you're on the toilet can make a world of difference. We'd all be better off pooping as we did in the backcountry, squatting over an open hole in the ground with no stacks of *Us Weekly* magazines nearby. Luckily, this position can be re-created while still using your modern toilet. All you need is a set of small stools or a platform to raise your knees. This opens the colon and gets your intestines into the proper position for evacuation. Although my Squatty Potty looks like something that belongs in a nursing home, I've become addicted to it and can never go back.

The SIBO Amigo Digest: 10 Treatment Rules of Thumb

1
Don't expect to heal SIBO overnight. Give yourself a year to create your new normal.

2
There is no magic pill or silver bullet for SIBO—embrace the trial and error.

3
Herbs and antibiotics are not without side effects.

4
Toxins released by bacteria as they die can cause more symptoms than the bacteria themselves.

5
Recovery goes way beyond your "kill phase."

6
Don't let the stress of treating SIBO become a new impediment to healing.

7
You must address the physical or emotional wounds your body is still holding.

8
Progress is often one step forward, two steps back.

9
Don't oversanitize your life—get dirty and live with your whole microbiome in mind.

10
Preventative medicine is the best long-term medicine.

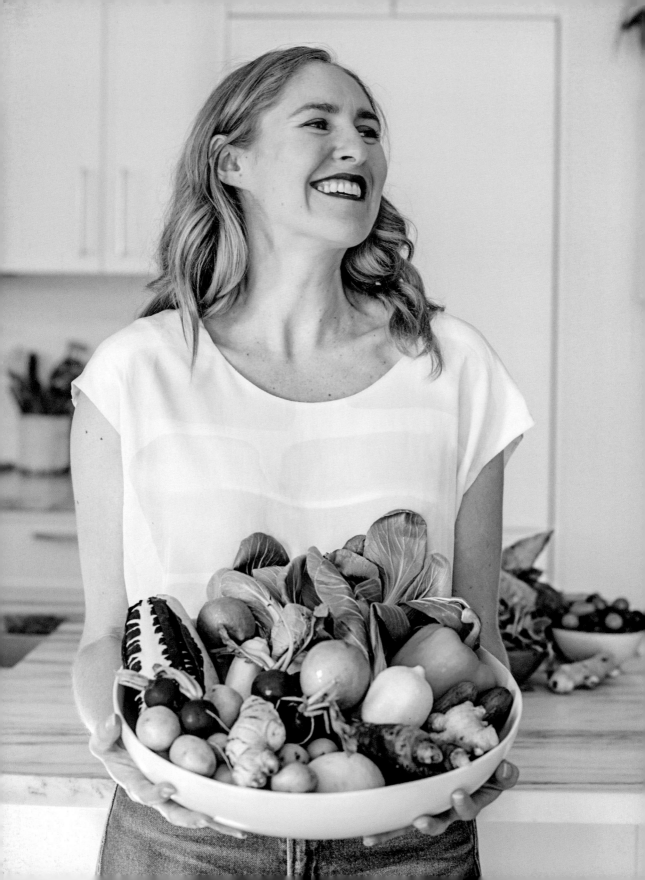

Chapter Three

THE DIET PLAN

SIBO Food Rules and Lifestyle Changes to Live By

FOOD IS AN ESSENTIAL PIECE of the SIBO puzzle, but it is not usually a cure in and of itself.

People often lump diet into a list of SIBO treatment options, when in fact it is not really a treatment at all. It is completely possible to overcome SIBO without making a single change to the way you eat. That said, as with any inflammatory condition, especially one that involves the digestive system, it's hard to problem-solve without also considering how what we're consuming is helping or hurting the overarching goal of a more balanced microbiome.

Although food alone might not always get rid of SIBO for good, there are other ways it can be used as medicine, especially while you wait for an official diagnosis. Certain diets can be tremendously effective at limiting the worst of your IBS symptoms. They do so by denying your critters their favorite delicacies and limiting the overgrowth. And also by giving your gut lining time to heal, reducing gas and inflammation, and, eventually, encouraging more beneficial bacteria to flourish in their true home, your large intestine.

There are numerous approaches for achieving any one of these goals. Many have been discovered through clinical trial and error, as unfortunately, **there is still no data-backed diet specifically for SIBO**. Nearly every practitioner I talked to, even those with their own original diet plans, emphasized that the approach differs for every patient.

Chapter 3 is your handbook for making the best food decisions for your own individual sensitivities and lifestyle needs. In the pages that follow, I've shared some of the most common diets that practitioners use for SIBO. The low-FODMAP approach is the most widely studied in relation to IBS symptoms, and we will do a deep dive on why it works so well on page 76. You'll also learn about the importance of uncovering your allergens (page 85), how to design your diet in tandem with your antimicrobials (page 89), and what to do if histamine plays a role in your sensitivities (page 95).

The biggest mistake people make with a SIBO diet is staying on it for too long. If the restrictiveness puts you off, rest assured that all of these diets are therapeutic and are not meant to be long term. If the restrictiveness attracts you, well, that is another sign that it might not be the best choice emotionally. We will talk more about food-fear pitfalls and how they can lead to disordered eating on page 99.

Ultimately, no matter what plan you begin with, **the goal is to get your gut to a place where you can eat as diverse an array of plants as possible**. Studies are very clear that a plant-based diet with colorful vegetables that include all the antioxidants under the rainbow (and all the FODMAPs), along with whole grains and healthy fats—what is commonly referred to as a Mediterranean diet—is the best thing for nurturing your good gut flora, supporting detoxification, and improving immune processes in the long term.

The key is getting there.

I like to think about SIBO food rules as a three-pronged process that could take up to a year, with the first prong being the most restrictive period:

- **PHASE 1, TREATMENT:** **rebalancing** the gut by reducing the overgrowth and starving unwanted critters, removing food triggers, and healing the gut lining. (2 months)

- **PHASE 2, REINTRODUCTION:** **retraining** your digestive system, discovering sensitivity levels, and slowly building food rules for the long term. (2–4 months)

- **PHASE 3, GUT GLORY:** **diversifying** your diet to feed your beneficial gut flora and living with your whole microbiome in mind. (6 months–forever)

Finally, if you were to ignore these phases altogether and throw all food rules out the window, I'd be okay with it so long as you applied the tips in the last section of this chapter. **So often we fixate unnecessarily on** *what* **we're eating, when the most profound impact on our digestion comes from** *how* **we're eating it.** You will avoid relapse and make your gut so much stronger by implementing the lifestyle suggestions on page 101.

Each of the following sections gives you a different layer of the onion (and explains why onions, in general, may be off-limits) for how to think about food as part of your recovery plan. In Part 2, we will get more into the specifics of how to put your new diet rules into practice in the kitchen.

The SIBO Diet Menu of Options

Most diets used for SIBO have a common thread: they reduce carbohydrates. Some, such as a traditional paleo approach, will remove grains and legumes. Others, such as those that focus on low-FODMAP ingredients, reduce the load of specific sugars, fibers, and starches. In doing so, you pare down the foods that are most likely to produce symptoms in someone with SIBO.

However, the idea that the fewer carbs you eat, the better you'll starve your bacteria, is a SIBO myth that leads to stress and disordered thinking around food. Even if you ate only meat and fat, you'd still be feeding bacteria—just different bacteria. These species might not produce irritating gases, but that doesn't mean they don't cause damage or inflammation in other ways.

It's important to understand that carbs are not the enemy of long-term gut health. Women, especially those of us in our childbearing years, need carbs to produce essential hormone reserves. We talk more about how to find the right balance in the "Careful Carbs" section on page 191. But it's important to keep in mind as you go through the following menu of options that, if you're a woman with hormone imbalances (hello, HashiPosse) or underweight, an ultra–low-carb diet may not be the best diet for you.

Lastly, whichever diet approach you choose, my advice would be to challenge the rules and be willing to make it your own. The recipes in this book are all labeled accordingly so that no matter what direction you decide on, you'll always be able to design a menu for it.

LOW-FODMAP (LF)

FODMAP is an acronym that represents various groups of carbohydrates that are easily fermentable and, often, difficult to digest. These carbs are found in all plants, but some foods contain higher concentrations than others. Created by a group of researchers at Monash University in Melbourne, Australia, the low-FODMAP diet's omissions include legumes, high-lactose dairy, wheat-based grains, high-fructose fruits and sweeteners, members of the allium family (garlic, shallot, onion), and other vegetables high in inulin (asparagus, artichokes). It's one of the harder elimination diets to eat out on, since it removes so many aromatics (garlic, onion) that make clean cuisine still taste amazing, and the list, which involves many healthful vegetables, is hard to keep track of. But it's also the most data-backed approach for reducing IBS symptoms, and therefore, one of the most popular routes for easing discomfort during or after SIBO treatment. Due to its prevalence, this diet also has far more online resources than the other more niche diets that follow, including the fantastic Monash App, which allows you to easily search ingredients to determine their FODMAP load. Since this is the approach I've adopted for the recipes in this book, we'll talk more about it in the next section (page 127).

SPECIFIC CARBOHYDRATE DIET (SCD)

This diet targets all foods that are more conventionally thought of as carbohydrates: sugars, grains, and starchy vegetables, such as potato. Unlike the low-FODMAP diet, it doesn't drill down into specific carbohydrate groups and might be slightly easier to follow since garlic, onion, and most green vegetables are allowed. It was originally designed for people dealing with inflammatory bowel diseases to give their gut a break, allowing only specific carbohydrates that require minimal digestive efforts. Since this diet wasn't created with SIBO or IBS in mind, and includes many high-FODMAP veggies, some might still feel symptoms on it. There have also been criticisms about the wording (*illegal* versus *legal*) as being highly triggering for anyone suffering from disordered eating.

SIBO-SPECIFIC FOOD GUIDE (SSFG)

Dr. Allison Siebecker developed an approach for highly sensitive SIBO patients that combines the two preceding diets, layering high-FODMAP vegetables (see page 83 for a list) on top of SCD's sugar-, starch-, and grain-free mantra. The hybrid approach starves bacteria and removes irritating grains to allow any gut permeability a chance to heal. The chart on her website is a helpful resource for seeing where these two diets differ and dovetail. This extremely low-carb approach is intended more for the tough cases, and may not be suitable for people who are underweight or with histories of disordered eating. It also should be noted that the stricter the diet, the more important it is to limit the period of time on it.

BI-PHASIC DIET (BPD)

In her practice in Australia, Dr. Nirala Jacobi began implementing the SIBO-specific food guide (SSFG) in phases to limit the most restrictive period to only a few weeks and give people more of a step-by-step for reintroducing foods. The bi-phasic diet begins with its strictest period prior to treatment, then adds back limited portions of rice and starchy vegetables as you begin antimicrobials. We will talk about the strategy of feeding versus starving bacteria during treatment on page 89. Dr. Jacobi has seen much clinical success with this approach. For those who crave a more fleshed-out protocol, her free download is a fantastic guide. That said, Dr. Jacobi created the diet for practitioners, and emphasizes that patients should work with a trained professional to guide them.

CEDARS-SINAI LOW-FERMENTATION DIET

Slightly less strict than the rest of the lot, this diet developed by Dr. Mark Pimentel is a fantastic option if your starting point looks more like the standard American diet (SAD). Dr. Pimentel is one of the leading researchers on SIBO and has used this diet as a second phase of his treatment protocol. The guidelines are similar to the low-FODMAP diet but written in simpler terms. The last line of the free handout is "sometimes it just feels good to be bad," which was written in conjunction with the recommendation to use grocery store cakes as a "cheat." This diet focuses less on limiting inflammation that's a result of SIBO, and more on unwanted bacteria. All the recipes in this book would fit the parameters.

PALEO (P)

A standard paleo approach will get you closer to the goal of eating a clean, anti-inflammatory diet that supports your overall gut health. It's also a good template for a basic elimination diet, as big allergens such as gluten, dairy, soy, and corn, are off the menu, which is not true of the low-FODMAP diet. By eliminating legumes (in addition to grains), it also removes the most potentially irritating member of the FODMAP family. Other than those big ingredient categories, the paleo approach allows every vegetable and protein. Since that includes potatoes and natural sweeteners like maple syrup and honey, it's slightly less low-carb than SCD. The paleo diet is also ubiquitous, which makes it easier to find options at the grocery store. But if you continue to have symptoms on a paleo diet, it might be worth eliminating high-FODMAP foods to see what else is irritating you.

AUTOIMMUNE PALEO (AIP)

Autoimmune paleo is an approach specifically designed for people with inflammatory conditions. In addition to eliminating gluten, dairy, corn, soy, and refined sugar, AIP also weeds out anything that could cross-react with your antibodies, including all grains, legumes, eggs, peanuts, nuts, seeds, nightshade vegetables, and gums. If you've been diagnosed with an auto-immune condition and are experiencing acute symptoms, or have very high antibody counts, a total reset like this one might be in order. Otherwise, there are more lenient options. The main con for those dealing with SIBO is that by eliminating nightshades (which are all low-FODMAP) on AIP, you're going to be more reliant on vegetables that are known to increase IBS symptoms.

THE KETOGENIC DIET (KETO)

The keto diet is similar to a paleo approach, but puts even more of an emphasis on eating fewer carbs and high quantities of fat. Ironically, the main efficacy is that it can help you burn fat more effectively. The name is derived from "ketones," which are small fuel molecules produced during a state of ketosis, where your body begins burning fat for fuel instead of carbs. To enter this state, you're supposed to eat about 75 percent fat, 20 percent protein, and 5 percent carbs, which means most fruit and starchy vegetables that are allowed on a paleo diet won't work. The good fats you get on a keto diet can encourage your intestinal cells to release a protein that reduces temporary bouts of inflammation. This all sounds well and good for SIBO sufferers; however, focusing on nonstarchy produce in paleo and keto diets also means more prebiotic fiber that is like (extremely healthy) fast food for the unwanted critters in your small intestine.

SIBO Diet Matrix

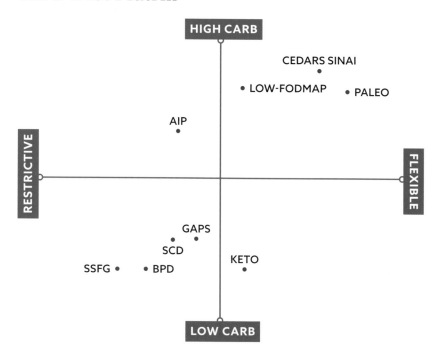

FODMAP WTF: Why Live Life Without Fermentable Carbs?

Since the low-FODMAP diet is one of the most common approaches to lessening IBS symptoms, and the recipes in this book fit within the framework, let's take a minute to get into the nitty-gritty of what eliminating fermentable carbs from your life actually looks like, and how this diet can affect your long-term gut health for better or for worse.

But first, I want to acknowledge why this diet can be so utterly bewildering.

I initially heard the acronym FODMAP back in 2015, when readers of my blog began writing in asking for solutions to this *Chopped* mystery box of a diet. I dutifully complied, putting together my cooking tips for making flavorful meals without garlic and onion (many of which I stand by today, and you can find on page 127), and compiling an encyclopedia of recipes on the web that fit the bill. But while I knew there was clearly a need (those posts remain some of my most popular to this day), I still didn't understand why this diet would help anyone with gut issues.

At the time, I was knee-deep in Hashimoto's-related health experiments and research, having just begun my official "year of health." I had been interviewing top-tier gut scientists, like Erica and Justin Sonnenburg, and burgeoning GI stars, like Dr. Robynne Chutkan. And their diet advice was all the same: eat mostly plants, preferably those rich in prebiotic fibers and resistant starches, such as dense legumes, nuts, and seeds. As I ticked off the "no" list for the low-FODMAP diet, what jumped out at me was that it perfectly matched my gut sensei's favorite foods. Artichoke, asparagus, and avocado. Leek, shallot, and garlic. Beans, beans, and more beans. WTF?

A year or so later, I found myself chatting about IBS with an old college friend during a wedding reception cocktail hour. As the head of gastroenterology at a hospital, he was presumably more used to talking intestines over gin and tonics than I was, and began going on about how excited he was about all the new data around the low-FODMAP diet. A recent study, he said, had found that those with non-celiac gluten insensitivity might actually be reacting to FODMAPs, not the gluten protein. And many of his patients were now finding relief by eliminating high-FODMAP foods.

It was surprising to me to hear a member of the mainstream medical establishment getting so excited about any diet as a potential prescription. Still, the incongruities nagged at me. "But, Dave," I said, "how do you reconcile this diet with the advice of all these other gut experts? And with the Blue Zone populations, who all eat beans, fermented foods, whole grains, and far more plants than animal protein? Don't you think this IBS population might only be feeling better because their guts are so imbalanced in the first place?"

Dave acknowledged that the questions were interesting, but then we were asked to find our seats for dinner, and I went off, by myself, to ponder them further for the next few months, until my own SIBO diagnosis brought on a cascade of aha moments and answers.

WHY DOES A LOW-FODMAP DIET HELP SIBO SYMPTOMS?

Although there are other explanations for why a low-FODMAP diet might work so well for people with IBS, an overgrowth of bacteria in the small intestine appeals to my common sense: If you have perfectly normal beneficial bacteria that have taken up residence too far up your intestinal tract, and you feed them their favorite foods (per my OG gut sensei's advice), it's only natural that the gas they produce would cause uncomfortable bloating, burping, and other irritabilities. It's also completely understandable that if you denied them these ingredients, those symptoms would lessen.

Of course, the microbiome is infinitely more complex than any reductive common sense reasoning allows for, and there are also plenty of other possibilities besides SIBO for why one individual might be sensitive to certain types of fiber. For many, it might be due to missing certain keystone bacterial species that industriously help break down those ingredients, or others that might offset their gas production.

"If you've lost all your butyrate-producing bacteria, you can eat all the burdock root in the world and it's just going to make you miserable," says Dr. Andrea McBeth, a microbiologist and founder of Flora Medicine. "And that's because you've lost all the bacteria that's going to help you break down beneficial inulin into butyrate." In other words: if you're someone who has eradicated your SIBO, but still struggles with lentils and onions, it might be because of bigger imbalances in your large intestine. (See "Rules of Greater Gut Health," page 68.)

Even if fiber is good for your microbiome in theory, forcing it on a gut that's not healthy or strong enough to handle it may only add insult to injury. In this sense, **the low-FODMAP diet follows the *Field of Dreams* model: if you build a healthy environment, healthy bacteria will come**. Sometimes the best method to do this is to focus on a diet that is lower in fiber, but anti-inflammatory. Studies have shown that the low-FODMAP diet not only reduces gas levels, but also improves gut permeability, inflammation, histamine dysregulation, and serotonin levels, 90 percent of which is produced in the digestive tract.

The takeaway: We all have different weaknesses that require different solutions, and we're only just beginning to hone in on what those exact avenues are. But the best way to heal SIBO and foster a better microbiome going forward is to choose a diet that's anti-inflammatory for your system.

WHAT ARE FODMAPS?

Now that we've established the why behind the low-FODMAP diet, let's talk about the what.

The first letter of the acronym stands for *fermentable*, meaning carbohydrates that create gas. The ODM and P are different types of these carbohydrates.

O stands for *oligosaccharides*, which hopefully is a word you will not need to throw around in casual conversation at a cocktail party. Its two main subcategories are *fructans* and *galacto-oligosaccharides*, which are types of prebiotic fibers that are found in such things as wheat, onion, garlic, and beans. This is the grouping that tends to give people the most trouble.

The D in FODMAP is a *disaccharide*, which just means a two-chain sugar. In the FODMAP realm, the most notable one is lactose. A sensitivity to lactose might be due to SIBO, meaning it's not permanent. Folks who are truly lactose-intolerant have lost the ability to make the enzyme that breaks down lactose. When extra lactose arrives in the colon, that's when a lot of GI symptoms arise. You might be able to parse out the difference for yourself simply by where your bloating is occurring—in the upper or lower abdomen—or by taking a supplement, such as Lactaid, to see whether it helps.

Then you have M, the *monosaccharides*. Single-chain fructose is found in many foods, but it's usually only problematic or causes symptoms when the ratio is much higher than glucose. High-fructose corn syrup, per its name, would be one of the biggest offenders. On the natural front, agave clocks in at around 90 percent fructose. Pure maple syrup is considered safe on a low-FODMAP diet, whereas honey is not. However, some argue that certain types of honey have lower fructose content and, therefore, are not as symptom-producing. One of the biggest differences between SIBO diet approaches is that SCD and the SIBO-specific food guide allow only clover honey, whereas low-FODMAP permits any low-fructose sweetener, including table sugar. Pure maple syrup and clover honey are used interchangeably in this book as the two preferred unrefined options. Examples of fruit with excess fructose can be found on page 83. Although fruit in general is an important part of a balanced diet, if you're limiting FODMAPs, the goal is to eat smaller quantities and prevent fructose malabsorption.

Finally, the P in FODMAPs stands for *polyols*; these are natural sugar alcohols that are found in a number of fruits and vegetables, from cauliflower to sweet potato to fruits that have a stone in them, such as apricots and plums. Polyols are also found in nature based artificial sweeteners, which are commonly malabsorbed. If you've noticed your stomach is upset after a powder probiotic or protein powder, it might be the xylitol or erythritol. Besides the bacteria feeding frenzy, the tricky part about these sugar alternatives is that they pull water into your gut and cause diarrhea, which becomes an even more likely outcome when consumed along with fructose. **Ideally, when on a healing diet, you'll avoid anything that sounds as if it was made in a lab**, which should deter you from any of these sugar alternatives ending in *-ol*.

HOW DOES A LOW-FODMAP DIET WORK?

FODMAPs are not a problem for everyone. Even though one in three people have fructose malabsorption, a much smaller percentage of them will experience IBS symptoms as a result. The issues arise when your intestines are already damaged and extremely sensitive, or when excess bacteria have taken up residence to feast off these poorly digested carbohydrates.

The primary goal of the low-FODMAP diet is twofold: first, to remove irritating, hard-to-digest ingredients to allow your gut time to repair; and second, to help starve out any unwanted bacteria in the small intestine and make you more comfortable in the process. As we discussed in the last section, diet alone is not usually enough to clear SIBO, but some people with milder imbalances may find that a low-FODMAP stint will get them on the right track without needing additional medical interventions.

Lastly, a strategic reintroduction of high-FODMAP ingredients will help you determine which foods are causing you the most issues. Some people may discover they are malabsorbing fructose, in which case, they've just uncovered a potential underlying cause of their SIBO. For others, eradicating SIBO might mean a shift in food sensitivities. They might now be able to eat high-fructose foods (in moderation) without issue once the bacteria are gone, whereas before this treatment, those ingredients caused symptoms. In other words, **FODMAP sensitivity changes over time** and after the initial strict trial period, your goal should be to consistently retest your tolerances.

☞ Tips & Takeaways

▷ **FODMAPs are quantity specific.** Although the recipes in this book are designed to be low-FODMAP, you may see some ingredients from the chart on page 83 in my dishes. Fear not, as long as you follow the serving guidelines, they are in small enough amounts to be safe. We all have individual sensitivities, however, so always listen to your body.

▷ **You are not allergic to FODMAPs.** These carbohydrates are the building blocks of most plant-based foods. Rather, you may be sensitive to certain types. People are rarely intolerant of the entire acronym. The goal of the elimination diet is to find out which are your biggest triggers (and at what amounts), so you can moderate accordingly.

▷ **Many people feel better with just a few eliminations.** If the laundry list of foods and quantities is overwhelming, start with just the big guns on the high-FODMAP chart. For many people, onions and legumes tend to be the hardest to tolerate. "I really try not to get my patients on an overly micromanaged diet," says Kate Scarlata, a registered dietitian and author of *The Low-FODMAP Diet Step by Step*. "If you're throwing onion and garlic into everything and you have bagels each day for lunch, we can remove the onion, garlic and bagels and you're probably going to feel remarkably better. It's not a FODMAP-free diet, we're just taking it down from where you were and if you need to tweak along the way, you tweak along the way."

▷ **If you don't react, don't restrict.** If you find you're not sensitive to something on the high-FODMAP chart, there's no point in not eating it. Diversity! Individuality! Embrace it in life and in your diet.

▷ **GOS ingredients have a two-day time lapse.** With garlic, onion, and legumes, you may not notice symptoms until the next day. They have a slower transit time, so pay attention to your symptoms for a few days before ruling out a problem.

▷ **Don't stay on a low-FODMAP diet for more than two months.** This is exceedingly important, as research indicates that eliminating high-FODMAP foods for the long term can damage the balance of flora in your large intestine. Remember that the goal of any elimination diet is to mine for information about your body, and the only way to do that is to reintroduce without fear.

▷ **It might not be the FODMAPs.** Another benefit of a low-FODMAP diet is that you will be eating less gluten, dairy, soy, and packaged foods in general. If you feel better on the diet, it could be because of reducing or eliminating one of these allergens. It could also be because you're cooking more and eating less junky restaurant oils. Which is all to say: don't use the diet as a source of protection, but instead use what you've learned to change your lifestyle for the long term. It's also my advice to do a regular elimination diet if you've never done one (more on this in the next section).

High-FODMAP Food Chart

FODMAP NAME	TYPE OF CARBOHYDRATE	FOODS THAT CONTAIN THE MOST OF THEM	
Fermentable **O**ligosaccharides	Fructans Galacto-oligosacchararides (GOS)	Artichokes Asparagus Beans Beets Brussels sprouts Cabbage Cashews Celery Chickpeas Currants Dates Figs	Garlic Grapefruit Leeks Lentils Onions Peas Pistachios Prunes Rye Wheat Barley Other non-GF grains
Disaccharides	Sucrose Maltose Lactose	**Dairy products:** Soft cheeses Milk Regular yogurt	
Monosaccharides	Glucose Fructose Galactose	Apples Pears Nectarines Peaches Plums Mangoes	Watermelon Sugar snap peas High-fructose corn syrup Honey Agave
Polyols (sugar alcohols)	Mannitol Sorbitol Xylitol Maltitol Isomalt	Avocados Sweet potato Cauliflower Snow peas Watermelon Mushrooms	Blackberries Cherries Prunes Artificial sweeteners that end in *-itol*

For a list of medium-FODMAP foods that are quantity-specific and need to be eaten in moderation, see page 130.

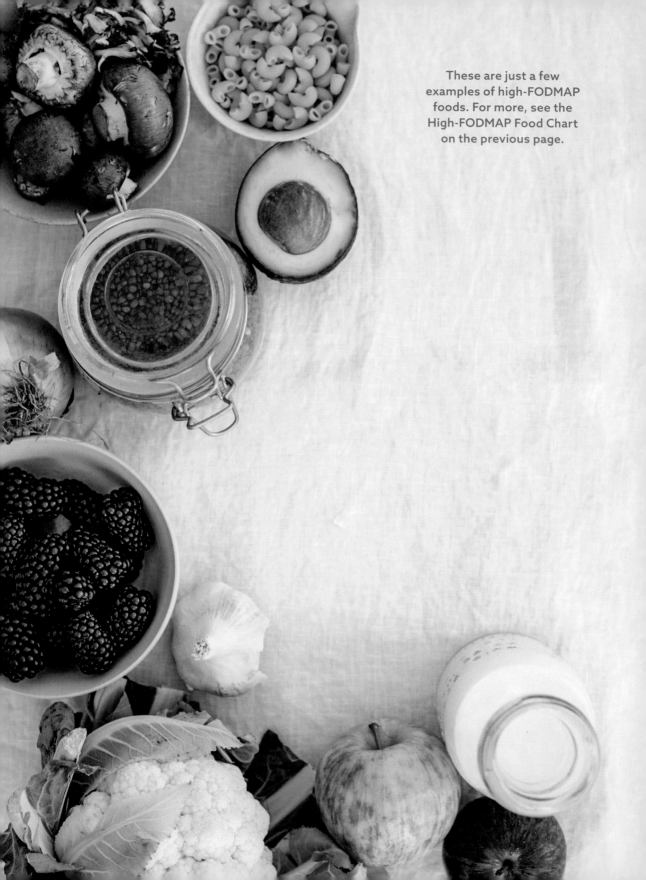

These are just a few examples of high-FODMAP foods. For more, see the High-FODMAP Food Chart on the previous page.

Identifying Allergens: Elimination Diet 101

One of the good things about SIBO—and there are a *few* good things, I swear—is that it may be the first time you've considered changing your diet.

Awareness around the low-FODMAP approach means those changes are often drastic. Although largely positive if executed properly, one downside is that you risk skipping over other potential diet culprits that are not just making you sick, but adding to your SIBO root causes.

One of the most common sources of chronic inflammation—i.e., your immune system getting all hot and bothered—is a hidden food sensitivity. Mysterious headaches, hair loss, anxiety, depression, fatigue, acid reflux, muscle soreness, allergies, acne, rashes—name a symptom, and chances are a shift in diet can help alleviate it. Name an autoimmune disease, and chances are there's also an ingredient that your immune system no longer likes (see page 22 for a refresher on the cycle of autoimmunity, leaky gut, and food sensitivities).

Eight years ago, when I was suffering from many of these symptoms, I finally got to the bottom of my food triggers. I had been diagnosed with Hashimoto's a few years earlier, but stubbornly continued to plow through everyday life unmedicated, until my best friend and most trusted colleague—my gut!—decided to turn on me.

My physician did bloodwork to test for food sensitivities, and while we waited for results to come back, he put me on a basic elimination diet plan, knowing that seeing the changes in how I felt would be the biggest indicator of what to do going forward. For three weeks, I cut out soy, corn, dairy, eggs, nuts, and wheat. And once that agony came to a close, it was clear that gluten was the big culprit.

Had I read more about my condition—an autoimmune thyroid disease—before my health really took a nosedive, I might have learned that gluten is a big cause of inflammation for people with Hashimoto's because the gluten protein looks very similar to the thyroid protein—another case of molecular mimicry. But even if I had, the knowledge on the page would have been far less convincing than the health renaissance I experienced after gluten was removed. And, more important, how sick I feel now when I eat it.

Since so many people with SIBO have autoimmune diseases, **a proper elimination diet might be an equally important step toward overhauling your health as reducing FODMAPs.**

WHY DO FOOD SENSITIVITIES CAUSE LEAKY GUT, AND VICE VERSA?

FODMAPs are not allergens in the traditional sense (just poorly digested foods). Those of us who react to problematic food groups—such as gluten, corn, soy, peanuts, tree nuts, and dairy—often do so thanks to our immune system.

Let's take dairy, for example. If you're sensitive to dairy products, it might be that you don't play well with the carbohydrate lactose because of a bacterial overgrowth. It could also be a straightforward intolerance that has nothing to do with SIBO: your body doesn't produce the enzyme to break down lactose. Then, there's a third possibility that has nothing to do with lactose at all: your immune system has mistaken the proteins in dairy—whey and casein—as foreign invaders.

When we are consistently eating foods that our body thinks are bad guys, it leaves our immune cells in a constant state of hyperactivity. The fog of ongoing war makes it harder to pinpoint an acute reaction to what we're eating; the symptoms aren't as severe because our baseline "normal" may already include said symptoms. This is why an elimination diet is so important for finding the culprits.

Remember what happens when our immune cells begin storming our small intestine with pitchforks? Does this sound like anything you read about in Chapter 1?

Over time, low-grade food sensitivities can have a similar impact on your intestinal wall as a more violent case of food poisoning. Although a foreign invader, such as *E. coli*, may warrant a larger fleet called to arms—more endotoxins sprayed, more of your own nerve cells damaged in the process—if your body thinks soy is a bad guy, it's going to use similar tools to get rid of it.

Unlike a pathogen, soy doesn't have its own defenses and is not interested in staying for good, so there might be less damage to your gut in the moment. But if you're eating small amounts of soy every day, your immune system is going to be in a constant state of attack. And the damaged intestinal wall may never get time to recover and regenerate. This process in and of itself puts you at a higher risk for SIBO.

Although there's no data linking food sensitivities and SIBO, we can look to celiac disease as an example. Those with celiac experience an autoimmune reaction when exposed to the gluten protein that denigrates the villi in their small intestine. There is also a high prevalence of SIBO in celiac patients, especially those who continue to have symptoms even after being on a gluten-free diet. We don't have a clear explanation of the mechanism as we do in post-infectious IBS, but it's clear that in the fog of war of celiac disease, something can happen that seems to trigger SIBO.

On the flip side, parasites, SIBO, or other imbalances in the gut can also be the root cause of immune system–fueled food sensitivities.

As we discussed in Chapter 1, bacteria in your small intestine releasing gas and eating their way through your mucous membrane, contributes to leaky gut. These bacteria then breach the intestinal wall, eventually making their way into the bloodstream, where our central immune system gets involved and begins attacking. Food sensitivities can result from this inflammation, as our overworked immune system begins unraveling and attacking indiscriminately.

If reactions go on for too long, eventually, the immune system can become completely dysfunctional. Our T regulator cells stop working due

Food sensitivity = Eat an everyday ingredient > Body sees it as a foreign invader > Immune system attacks > Leaky gut + Intestinal wall damage > Possible impaired motility = SIBO

SIBO = Bacteria damage intestinal wall > Leaky gut > Systemic inflammation > Heightened immune activity > Loss of tolerance = More food sensitivities

(See page 23 for how this flow chart connects to autoimmune disease.)

to chronic exposure, and we develop a loss of tolerance to various food groups or our own tissue. Whether SIBO caused your autoimmunity, or autoimmunity contributed to your SIBO, **immunity dysregulation, food sensitivities, and SIBO go hand in hand**. This is especially true if you've confirmed one of the root causes of your SIBO was food poisoning and you showed high levels of anti-vinculin antibodies on the IBS Smart Test. **It's going to be an uphill battle healing your gut without first calling off the dogs and allowing your immune system to calm down.**

There are many ways to skin that fish: by removing SIBO first, or tackling the immunity aspect with an elimination diet. Either way, **the role of food sensitivities as a vicious cycle for SIBO is one of the underappreciated truths that doesn't get enough airtime when talking about SIBO diets**, which mostly revolve around eliminating ingredients that feed your bacteria.

Everyone with SIBO should at some point rule out the big allergens.

A BIG ELIMINATION DIET DISCLAIMER: FIRST, CHECK FOR CELIAC

Although the only medical prescription is a gluten-free diet, celiac disease (CD) is not just a simple food allergy. It's a potentially life-threatening condition that can make you much more likely to develop certain cancers and subsequent autoimmune diseases if left unchecked. The majority of sufferers are "silent celiacs" who don't exhibit any gut or IBS symptoms, which is one of the many reasons why CD is often missed. The confirmatory procedure for celiac disease is either a blood test to look for antibodies, or an endoscopy that can give you a sense of how damaged your intestines are. The only caveat? **You have to be eating gluten at the time of either test to get a true diagnosis.** The recommended dose is the equivalent of one to four slices of bread a day for at least six weeks. "It is medically negligent to put someone on a gluten-free diet without first testing for celiac disease," says Dr. Lisa Shaver, a gastroenterologist who specializes in treating CD.

Since nearly every SIBO approach listed on pages 76–78 by default eliminates most gluten, it's very important to first rule out celiac disease before taking out gluten as part of an elimination diet. And since SIBO occurs in 20 percent of celiac patients, having SIBO in and of itself is reason enough to want to eliminate CD as an underlying cause.

HOW DOES A TRADITIONAL ELIMINATION DIET WORK DIFFERENTLY THAN A LOW-FODMAP DIET?

Remember the main goal of a low-FODMAP elimination diet? It's to give the gut time to heal, starve out bacteria by removing their food sources, and in the process, reduce your symptoms. With a traditional elimination diet that targets allergens, **the most important aim is for your immune system response to recede, which will in turn allow huge healing potential for the gut**.

Like any overworked army, once your antibodies have had that rest period, they are that much more capable of attacking invaders with all their might. This is why an elimination diet works so well: at the end of the exclusion period, you add back foods one at a time, leaving a few days in between. On test day, you have a heaping helping of the ingredient in question so you'll get a really clear read on how your body reacts to it. On the flip side, the reintroduction of FODMAPs is all about finding the quantity you tolerate, beginning small and working your way up to find the cliff of intolerance. **With a low-FODMAP diet, you don't have to be perfect.** A slipup doesn't have many lasting effects beyond your digestion cycle. **With a traditional elimination diet, however, you want to be strict about your omissions so any antibodies have twenty-one full days to clear.**

An important part of either elimination diet is tracking symptoms. This also goes for the week before you start, so you can establish your baseline. **Keep a journal and write down any changes in how you feel**—not just IBS symptoms, but changes in your skin, energy levels, and mood. I created the Symptom and Activity Tracker (page 300) for this exact purpose.

WHAT FOODS ARE EXCLUDED ON A REGULAR ELIMINATION DIET?

You can design an elimination diet around any combination of omissions, but most people find it's easiest to start with the heavy hitters: gluten, dairy, corn, and soy. Luckily, these are all taken care of for the most part in the recipes in this book. (Just make sure you rule out celiac disease before fully removing gluten, per page 87.)

Other protocols include even more allergens: eggs, tree nuts, peanuts, shellfish, fish, seeds, pulses/legumes, citrus fruits, nightshade vegetables (tomatoes, peppers, potatoes, and eggplant), and grains.

Some people also choose to cut out alcohol, caffeine, and refined sugar so that you're not adding any extra insult (more about this on page 122). If you omit sugar, it essentially forces you to avoid all packaged, processed foods (since 80 percent of supermarket-aisle foods contain added sugar). The soy and corn omissions translate to no fried foods, either, since most restaurants use soy or corn oils. The macro intention: to **make your diet as clean and simple as possible**.

Finally, there is a theory that many food allergies are actually being caused by glyphosate, the main chemical in the pesticide Roundup, which damages the tight junctions in the gut. When you reduce gluten and grains, you're actually reducing your exposure to Roundup. To take this healing concept a step further, try to eat organic as much as possible to avoid harmful pesticides.

HOW DOES THIS FACTOR INTO SIBO TREATMENT?

You won't find much information on protocols that combine an allergen elimination diet with a SIBO treatment protocol, but you can easily design your own two-prong approach. **Just choose which allergens you want to avoid and make sure you have twenty-one days free of them**. Those who go the route of the SIBO-specific food guide or bi-phasic diet will naturally remove many of these major allergens. They aren't meant to be low-allergy diets, but they happen to be low-allergy diets. You will just need to structure your reintroduction around both allergen groups and FODMAP groups according to the guidelines on pages 91–93.

If you've already done an elimination diet at some point recently, your work is done. However, if you suspect SIBO was an issue for you at the time of your elimination diet, it might be worth reintroducing problem ingredients after your SIBO is gone, to see whether there are any changes. Once your leaky gut heals, it's possible that the systemic immune reaction that was causing your body to attack unsuspecting food particles has righted itself. You shed your intestinal lining every 48 to 72 hours, so your body is constantly changing and renewing.

If the idea of a low-FODMAP diet is too intense and your doctor has recommended "feeding" your bacteria during treatment, it could be an opportunity to do an allergen elimination diet first before messing around with FODMAPs. We talk more about how diet can be paired with antimicrobials and the varying approaches to feeding versus starving your bacteria in the next section.

Feast or Famine: How to Make Your Treatment and Diet Work in Tandem

One of the most frequent *SIBO Made Simple* podcast listener questions I've received revolves around the timing of treatment and diet. Is it better to feed the bacteria while on herbal or conventional antimicrobials by eating normally, or to starve them with a low-FODMAP approach?

The first school of thought is held by Dr. Mark Pimentel and is the approach he uses in his SIBO research at Cedars-Sinai. The idea is that by denying the bacteria in your small intestine their main food sources, some of them may be starved, but more likely they will just go dormant. This hibernation doesn't serve you if you're on a treatment protocol that's intended to kill as many bacteria as possible. His recommendation is to eat normally while on antimicrobials, then transition to a low-FODMAP diet once the treatment is over, to give the gut a chance to heal and help clear any lingering bacteria.

The main pushback for this argument is that it leaves patients with no immediate relief, and often will contribute to more intense symptoms during treatment due to the phenomenon of die-off. As you learned in Chapter 2, this is your body's reaction to when bacteria or fungi die and spill their endotoxins. For these reasons, Dr. Nirala Jacobi pioneered a phased approach that begins with an extremely restrictive diet, then introduces antimicrobials during Phase 2 as your diet expands to include more carbohydrates.

In the bi-phasic diet, Phase 1 is divided between two subphases: restricted and semi-restricted. While Dr. Jacobi waits for test results, her goal is to get symptoms down as much as possible and to allow the gut to heal. If the test results are positive, she moves straight into Phase 2 of the diet, which adds back some grains and larger quantities of high-FODMAP vegetables, so that you promote some bacterial activity while you kill them. Each phase lasts about six to eight weeks, but oftentimes the restricted phase can be as short as two weeks.

The biggest benefit that Dr. Jacobi has seen with this approach is lessening the effects of die-off. Although diet alone doesn't usually clear SIBO completely, it can help shift the bacteria populations in the right direction, meaning fewer endotoxins spilled once the battle begins. More important, by eliminating grains and other possible allergens, you've taken bigger steps toward healing leaky gut and reducing inflammation. In her practice, people that have been on Phase 1 of the diet for two to four weeks do not have as many issues while on herbal antimicrobials as do people who didn't do the diet.

Some practitioners have offered a third approach that provides a bit of a hybrid: wait to start a low-FODMAP diet a week into treatment, knowing that it will take some time to get the hang of it and be 100 percent compliant. Other doctors, including my own, simply advise applying the low-FODMAP diet in looser strokes during treatment, knowing that any slipups will help coax bacteria back into action.

Here's the sweet spot I found: I was at my strictest at the beginning of treatment, when I assumed die-off would be at its most intense. I tried to follow the low-FODMAP diet as much as possible; went completely sugar-, alcohol-, and caffeine-free; and focused on whole grains over refined carbs. At the halfway mark, I began loosening my grip, eating out at restaurants and allowing myself the occasional condiment or sauce that I knew probably had garlic or onion in it. This allowed me to (a) have a more flexible stress-free social life; (b) keep my bacteria on their toes, even if it meant a small setback in my symptoms; and (c) frame slipups as helping rather than hurting treatment.

Although this timing tango seems to be a source of stress in and of itself for many people, from my research, I feel confident saying there's no right or wrong way. As with all these diet options, **it's best to choose the rules that fit best within the real-world circumstances of your life**. Luckily, the impact of diet on the gut can be incredibly fast-acting. If you are experiencing bad die-off, you have the ability to change course at any time and layer in diet to aid you.

Onward: Reintroduction & Retraining Your Digestive System

Before you start celebrating the end of your restrictive SIBO diet and dive face-first into a tub of ice cream, press Pause. **What happens afterward might be even more important than during.** This is when you get all the valuable information that will help you design a path forward and rebuild your gut for the long term. Don't blow it all over a bowl of creamy dessert.

Your reintroduction could last anywhere from three weeks to several months, depending on what you eliminated during your SIBO diet and how slowly you choose to ease back in. Everyone does it a little bit differently, all with the same goal in mind. If you are extremely sensitive, be cautious. But it's also important to approach the reintroduction without fear. For more ways to get yourself in the right mindset, read the tips on page 100.

Finally, depending on whether you are testing FODMAPs or big allergens in a traditional elimination diet, you will go about the reintroduction slightly differently. The following tips are for navigating both options.

INSTRUCTIONS FOR A TRADITIONAL ELIMINATION DIET:
Gluten, Dairy, Soy, Corn & Other Allergens

① **Plan to reintroduce during a "typical" day.** It's better to schedule your testing days when life isn't too crazy and you can be relatively in control of your environment or schedule. Doing it while traveling or during a heavy period of stress at work may throw off your reactivity levels.

② **Avoid other irritants on testing day.** Potential triggers, such as caffeine, alcohol, and sugar, should be omitted on reintroduction days, so you don't muddy the waters.

③ **Start with either the ingredient you missed the most, or the one that you were best about eliminating.** I know that might sound like two opposites. But here's the thing: if you slipped up on dairy during Week 2, you want to wait to reintroduce it to make up for that slip...even if you're dying to have it back. Remember, our goal is to have at least twenty-one days fully free of the item in question. Look back over your Symptom and Activity Tracker and circle the days where you might have "cheated."

④ **Make a schedule for your reintroduction.** Choose one item for each test day, followed by at least three days of downtime in between for your immune system to calm down if there's a reaction. For example: dairy on Monday, gluten on Friday, soy on the following Tuesday. Or you can go slow and simply choose one food each week. You can use the Elimination Diet Reintroduction Worksheet (page 299) as a template.

⑤ **Eat the reintroduced foods in their purest form.** For dairy, that might be whole milk (NOT ice cream). For gluten, that might be plain pasta (NOT sandwich bread with a million additives). For soy, that might be whole edamame (NOT teriyaki sauce).

⑥ **On test day, have a heaping helping of the food in question for breakfast.** Do so with as few other variables as possible. For example, pasta with olive oil and salt, not pasta with tomato sauce. Otherwise, you won't know whether you're reacting to the wheat or the nightshades.

⑦ **Log the results.** Notice every aspect of your wellness, not just digestion. Are you feeling groggy, anxious, or as though you're having trouble concentrating? Are your joints achy? Is your skin covered in zits or hives? These are all signs of a reaction that you don't want. It doesn't necessarily mean you can't eat these ingredients ever again. You'll just be doing so with full awareness as to the risks. Of course, if your reaction is to immediately vomit or run to the bathroom with diarrhea, then you may want to consider that you have a serious food sensitivity and try cutting that food out of your life. The Symptom and Activity Tracker Worksheet on page 300 can be helpful for tracking progress.

⑧ **A little bloating is not a failed test.** As is the case for a FODMAP reintroduction, a few gas bubbles or a little bloating does not mean you didn't pass. Sometimes, those mild symptoms may be a result of not having eaten something in a while. It's great information, but not a hard line you can never cross again. You're looking for dramatic, debilitating reactions: an IBS-like flare-up that includes the onset of diarrhea, severe constipation, pain, cramping, joint pain, headaches, or dramatic reduction in quality of life—extreme fatigue, hives, breakouts, and so on. **Since a diverse, varied diet is such a boon to our gut bacteria overall, we have to keep the bar high for taking an ingredient out permanently.**

MODIFICATIONS FOR A LOW-FODMAP ELIMINATION DIET

Since people aren't allergic to FODMAPs, your reactions will most likely depend on quantity. Unlike with the food groups in a traditional elimination diet, you're going to be reintroducing in smaller portions of high-FODMAP ingredients to begin with and increasing them over time until you discover your limit. The good news is that most people find they can successfully reintroduce plenty of FODMAP groups in moderation and create a diet with a lot more variety. Here are some additional things to keep in mind.

① **Test one subgroup at a time.** Remember, food can affect you for up to 48 hours. So, just as with the regular elimination diet, as you reintroduce foods, keep a record in your journal and make sure to space out each new FODMAP group introduction by at least two days. See sample schedule on page 94.

② **Stay on a low-FODMAP diet throughout the testing period.** Whereas in the classic elimination diet scenario, you can go back to eating an ingredient after you've successfully tested it, since FODMAPs are quantity specific and can add up during one meal, it's best to continue to eliminate high-FODMAP foods until you have finished testing all of the FODMAP groups. For example, even if you pass the fructose test with mango, don't start adding mango back into your everyday meals just yet.

③ **Start small and gradually test larger quantities.** One method is to dedicate an entire week to one ingredient, starting with a low dose, followed by a rest day. If there is no reaction or minimal symptoms, continue with a medium dose the following day. If you experience a bad reaction at any point, don't test further and give yourself until the following week to try a new group. You can also test doses on consecutive days, but leave more room when testing the fructan/GOS group, because these ingredients take longer to work their way through your system.

④ **Eat test foods as you would in daily life with meals.** Food works synergistically in the body, and we very rarely eat or drink things completely in isolation. Protein will enhance fructose absorption. Sometimes, fat can slow things down. For example, if you're testing lactose, start with ½ cup of milk with breakfast. On Day 2, change that to 1 cup of milk. If you would never drink more than a cup of milk in one sitting, there is no need to continue to increase your portions.

⑤ **Keep at it: every few months, retest.** Your microbiome is constantly changing. Something that maybe you didn't tolerate on test day may be able to be brought back in once your gut has healed further. Be willing to constantly explore, increase quantities, and work your way toward eating 8 to 10 cups of vegetables per day. It takes a little time after getting a knee brace off before you can run; the same is true of reintroducing certain FODMAPs—consider the slow reintroduction your food physical therapy!

⑥ **What if it's not FODMAPs?** If you can't seem to identify your triggers through a regular elimination diet or a low-FODMAP elimination, it's possible that you're reacting to either yeast- and mold-containing foods or high-histamine foods. These ingredients are mostly allowed in both scenarios, and would require an additional elimination experiment to weed out. We'll talk about histamines in the next chapter. See page 30 for guidance on yeast.

FODMAP SAMPLE SCHEDULE A

MONDAY: Low dose
TUESDAY: Rest
WEDNESDAY: Medium dose
THURSDAY: Rest
FRIDAY: High dose
WEEKEND: Rest

FODMAP SAMPLE SCHEDULE B

MONDAY: Low dose
TUESDAY: Medium dose
WEDNESDAY: High dose
THURSDAY–SUNDAY: Rest

FODMAP SAMPLE REINTRODUCTION CHART

WEEK 1: FRUCTOSE

Dose:

- 1 teaspoon honey, 1 tablespoon honey, 3 tablespoons honey
- OR ¼ medium mango, ½ medium mango, 1 medium mango

WEEK 2: SORBITOL

Dose:

- 3 blackberries, 6 blackberries, 9 blackberries
- OR ¼ avocado, ½ avocado, 1 avocado

WEEK 3: MANNITOL

Dose:

- ¼ portobello mushroom, ½ portobello mushroom, 1 portobello mushroom
- OR ½ cup cooked cauliflower rice, 1 cup cooked cauliflower rice, 1½ cups cooked cauliflower rice

WEEK 4: LACTOSE

Dose:

- ½ cup (4 oz) organic whole milk, 1 cup (8 oz) organic whole milk, 1½ cups (12 oz) organic whole milk

WEEK 5: FRUCTAN GRAINS (WHEAT)

Dose:

- ½ cup cooked elbow pasta, 1 cup cooked elbow pasta, 1½ cups cooked elbow pasta
- OR ¼ cup cooked barley, ½ cup cooked barley, 1 cup cooked barley

WEEKS 6 + 7: FRUCTAN VEGETABLES (TEST BOTH OF THE FOLLOWING SEPARATELY, 1 WEEK APART)

Dose:

- ¼ garlic clove, ½ garlic clove, 1 garlic clove
- OR 1 tablespoon cooked diced onion, 2 tablespoons cooked diced onion, ¼ cup cooked diced onion

WEEK 8: GALACTANS (GOS)

Dose:

- ¼ cup cooked chickpeas, lentils, or black beans; ½ cup cooked chickpeas, lentils, or black beans; 1 cup cooked chickpeas, lentils, or black beans

WEEK 9: FRUCTOSE + SORBITOL (ONLY IF YOU PASSED BOTH INDIVIDUAL FODMAP TESTS)

Dose:

- ¼ apple or pear, ½ apple or pear, 1 apple or pear

The Hurdles of Histamine

Your main exposure to the concept of histamine probably involves a television ad for seasonal allergies. It's true that excess histamine can cause a stuffy nose, itchy eyes, and all those other symptoms that indicate spring is in the air. But it also has many other vital functions in the body and is not always the enemy.

Histamine regulates about ten different systems. It's a neurotransmitter that's part of our central nervous system. We use it to build stomach acid for digestion, create estrogen to regulate our hormones, and increase mucus within our respiratory tract. Our body is constantly producing histamine to aid in these functions, and conversely, it is also producing enzymes to break it down so that the levels never become out of balance.

One way we can experience a surge in histamine is if an allergen enters the body (e.g., pollen or pet dander), which triggers histamine to release and communicate to our immune system that an offender is coming through. It's part of a normal inflammatory response as a means to protect you. The second way our levels of histamine rise is through certain foods we eat that carry their own histamine. In this section, we'll look at the role SIBO plays in causing our histamine levels to get out of control and how to offset the effects with diet.

SYMPTOMS OF HISTAMINE DYSREGULATION

When there's too much histamine in circulation, whether due to not having enough enzymes to break it down properly, or because we are ingesting too many high-histamine foods, the various functions it supports will go haywire. In addition to the classic allergy symptoms, signs of histamine levels being too high are hives, itchy skin, increased hormonal swings around menstruation, asthma, heartburn, and IBS symptoms. Although these inflammatory responses may not seem connected, the common thread of this narrative is histamine.

Histamine is also a major part of our sleep cycle. It's very neuroexcitatory, and can cause an increase in anxiety or wakefulness in the middle of the night. Hence why Benadryl is so effective as a sleep aid, and why those with allergies may need it for more than just stopping up their stuffy nose.

Over-the-counter medications are very effective at limiting histamine symptoms. They work by blocking histamine receptors from doing their job and triggering a reaction. However, they can also disrupt other normal, vital histamine functions in the process. Although we may not experience the misery of having too much histamine, it also means that the histamine we actually need isn't able to do its chores. If you're always blocking those receptors, you're going to see a certain level of deficiency in terms of your ability to regulate blood circulation, estrogen, and digestion, among other things.

WHY DOES SIBO LEAD TO HISTAMINE INTOLERANCE?

You can develop histamine intolerance for many reasons besides a bacterial overgrowth, but there are a few ways that the aftermath of SIBO can make it harder for your body to produce the necessary enzyme—diamine oxidase, also known as DAO—that breaks down histamine.

DAO is made in the intestinal wall, right at the tip of our microvilli. General inflammation, leaky gut, and the gases that are produced by unwanted bacteria can impair our ability to produce it. Depending on the types of bacteria in your small intestine, they can also produce their own histamine. You can see how adding more histamine to the fire, while also hurting your enzyme reserves to break it down, can cause an imbalance.

By reducing the overgrowth, oftentimes, histamine issues regulate. There's even research showing that just a low-FODMAP diet can reduce serum histamines. For others, though, a low-FODMAP diet used to limit SIBO symptoms might cause other histamine-related issues. When you're reducing the variety of vegetables and carbs you can eat, inevitably you're going to lean more heavily on some low-FODMAP foods on the yes list, such as tomatoes, eggplant, spinach, and eggs, all of which are either high-histamine or histamine-liberating foods.

SIBO = Bacteria increase histamine levels > Damage intestinal wall > Impair DAO production > Histamine enters the bloodstream > Systemic inflammation = Histamine intolerance

"When you're not producing as much DAO and you increase the level of dietary histamines, it's like drinking liquid histamine," says Heidi Turner, a registered dietitian who has become a seasoned histamine expert in her nutrition practice. "It can trigger an immune response which creates even more inflammation in the gut, and even more IBS symptoms. If leaky gut is an issue, that histamine can then recirculate in your system and cause many of the other typical symptoms like rashes, anxiety, and sleep disruption."

Cue another SIBO vicious cycle.

If you're experiencing symptoms of histamine intolerance, this is where changing your diet to limit the amount of histamine coming into the plant is going to be your best bet for turning things around.

WHAT IS A LOW-HISTAMINE DIET?

Although there are a few tests that can tell you where your histamine levels stand—one for histamines in your urine, another to check the DAO circulating in your bloodstream—the quickest, cheapest, and most effective way to see whether you have an intolerance is to simply remove high-histamine foods from your diet for a week and see how you feel.

Fermented and aged foods, such as wine, vinegar, Asian condiments (fish sauce, soy sauce), sauerkraut, kombucha, yogurt, and hard cheeses are the biggest culprits, as they build histamine through bacterial fermentation. If you notice wine, beer, or cider makes you feel terrible, but tequila or vodka is no problem, that's a good indicator that the histamines are to blame, not the alcohol content. Although for many people, fermented foods are an important part of building better gut health, those with SIBO often have the histamine issue to contend with.

Other vegetables, such as tomatoes, avocados, eggplant, and spinach contain their own natural histamine. Then, there are histamine-liberating foods, such as eggs, citrus, bananas, and nuts. They don't necessarily contain histamine, but they can trigger more histamine to be released in the body. Finally, certain drinks, such as alcohol and caffeinated teas, can inhibit DAO from doing its job of breaking down histamine. For a full list of foods to avoid on a low-histamine diet, see page 295.

If reducing histamine on top of FODMAPs sounds like there are very few foods left on the table, you're right. Luckily, Turner has partnered with Dr. Jacobi to create a low-histamine bi-phasic diet that removes *fermentable* carbs and *fermented foods*. Turner reports that as long as you're also tackling the root cause (potentially, SIBO or SIFO), you should be able to reverse histamine intolerance in just a week or two by removing a few of the big offenders.

☞ Tips & Takeaways

▷ **Start by eliminating the big guns.** Turner recommends that you remove fermented beverages (wine, beer, cider, kombucha) and fermented foods as the first wave. Tomato sauce, canned foods, and cured meats should be the second. If you're extremely sensitive and still experiencing symptoms after a week, reduce the high-histamine and histamine-liberating foods listed on page 295.

▷ **Find your threshold.** Similar to the low-FODMAP diet, a low-histamine diet is about reducing, not eliminating. The more histamine that you consume, the closer you're going to get to your own personal limit. Take a look at your diet to see what your usual dose is. If you're eating eggs for breakfast every day, followed by a spinach salad for lunch and pasta with tomato sauce and a glass of red wine for dinner, it's possible you can make smaller changes to reduce the overall load without having to strictly eliminate all histamine-containing ingredients.

▷ **Keep things fresh.** As food ages, the histamine content increases. For example, fresh tomatoes (especially cherry tomatoes) have much less histamine than tomato sauce and are often tolerated in smaller amounts. Try to eat as many fresh whole foods as possible, as opposed to canned, especially when it comes to animal proteins. Smoked salmon, canned tuna, and cured meats are going to be higher on the histamine front.

▷ **Opt for quicker cooking times.** One healing food that can be problematic for histamine intolerance is bone broth. Since it's simmered over low heat for many hours, bacteria can form. More collagen is also coaxed from the bones, which can exacerbate histamine symptoms. Focus on dishes with quicker cooking times versus all-day soups and stews. Cook your broth for

2 hours max per the guidelines on page 142. Instant Pots and pressure cookers are great tools for histamine peeps. The slow cooker is not your friend.

▷ **Keep temperatures very hot or very cold.** For people with really severe histamine intolerance, leftovers can be tricky. As soon as you're done cooking, transfer your food to individual containers, let cool for a few minutes, and place directly in the freezer, to stop bacterial development. Keeping temperatures high works too—you're just trying to get out of the middle zones where bacteria formation is most active.

▷ **Try an elemental diet.** This approach can be very effective for ridding your intestines of SIBO *and* limiting histamines in the process. Not only are you giving your gut time to rest, but you're also eliminating all histamine from food. The diet consists of nutrients at their simplest form, so everything gets absorbed quickly. More about this on page 44.

▷ **Carry a back-pocket remedy for your triggers.** If you know you're going to have a histamine-heavy meal, there are a few supplements that can help in a pinch. Turner recommends Zeolite as a binder for histamines, in the same vein as activated charcoal or bentonite clay, which could also work. Keep these limited to emergency situations so you don't risk disrupting other important histamine functions. Consult your health practitioner for the proper dosage.

▷ **Consider candida.** If your SIBO has been cleared and you're still experiencing signs of histamine intolerance, another potential underlying culprit is candida or fungal overgrowth (SIFO). The endotoxins that are produced by candida die-off have to be detoxified through a similar pathway that histamine goes through. If your antimicrobials include antifungals, and you become much more sensitive to histamine, that could be candida at play. See page 31 for tips on how to differentiate whether it's the yeast or mold in foods versus the histamine that's bothering you.

▷ **Consider mast cell activation syndrome (MCAS).** Mast cell activation syndrome only got an official diagnosis code a few years ago, and yet it is a condition that explains so much about what goes wrong with the immune system and how that dysfunction can lead to chronic inflammation. Histamine intolerance might be a low-level by-product of MCAS. Beth O'Hara, founder of the website and medical practice MastCell360, points to the development of symptoms as soon as you eat or smell food—such as flushing, swelling in hands or feet, or allergies—as specific signs of MCAS. Sensitivity to environmental toxins, such as fragrance, could also mean MCAS. If you suspect this could be at play along with histamine intolerance, be wary of certain SIBO kill protocol herbs and supplements, such as clove, guar gum, and L-glutamine, as they can exacerbate symptoms.

▷ **Look at other lifestyle areas.** If your SIBO and SIFO are gone, your diet is low in histamine, and you're still experiencing symptoms, it's time to step back and look at all of the other pieces. Stress has been shown to impact histamine production significantly. Start a meditation practice or use everyday breathing exercises, such as those on page 66. Regulating sleep and anxiety is a critical part of our healing process, especially with histamine dysregulation.

For a list of foods to avoid on a low-histamine diet, see page 295.

Fearing Food & Disordered Eating in the Face of SIBO

For all the positive progress a SIBO diet can afford us in limiting IBS symptoms and beginning to overcome our overgrowth, there's also a shadow side to these highly restrictive food plans.

In more extreme cases, this might translate to the development of disordered eating or the reigniting of past food fears. But at its most basic, a SIBO healing plan lays a minefield when it comes to your mindset around food.

As someone who has made her livelihood from cooking for others and has the spirit of an omnivore, delving into the lists of off-limits foods when I was first diagnosed was deeply crushing. The first few weeks, my meals left me feeling deprived. I isolated myself from friends because I feared being "that girl" asking for a plain chicken breast with steamed vegetables on the side instead of sharing with the table. I came very close to succumbing to a bomb of self-pity and letting it destroy me.

That may sound like hyperbole, but any practitioner will tell you: anxiety, stress, resentment, fear, obsessiveness, perfectionism, control—these are all things that can torpedo your healing journey before it even starts.

Luckily, it didn't take me long to turn lemons into low-FODMAP, refined sugar–free lemonade. Instead of wallowing in the unfairness of it all—the feeling that my health journey was a never-ending maze of torture—I used my day job as a silver lining and dove headfirst into creating recipes that would make myself and others feel excited to sit down and eat. But these mental pitfalls are waiting for all of us, and I was certainly not immune.

Self-pity is one side of the coin. On the other side, obsession awaits—and that's an equally unhealthy place to find yourself on a SIBO diet. Because food is one of the few things we can control as a patient—and many of us have been through years of experiencing symptoms that were so out of our control—when we are given a printout of one of the diets on page 78, we can become fixated on food, turning it into something that needs to be constantly questioned instead of savored.

If our focus going into a meal is around killing our critters instead of embracing our healing, it ends up turning self-care into self-harm. As you learned in Chapter 2, the gut-brain axis is a powerful superhighway. Stress is far more corrosive than FODMAPs. And letting anxiety about a recurrence of symptoms get in the way of your reintroduction period does dual damage to the health of your microbiome, which many studies show can be depleted from increased stress levels *and* long-term use of the low-FODMAP diet.

If you fear beginning a SIBO diet plan, or fear slowly getting off one, I've included some tips on overcoming food anxiety, shifting your mindset around mealtime, and embracing the abundance of food on your plate.

☞ Tips & Takeaways

▷ **Don't expect a gold star for your recovery.** "SIBO sufferers are traditionally more of a type A personality," says author and SIBO health coach Rebecca Coomes. "We are really driven; we're perfectionists; we're often quite stressed. We deal with anxiety. We really want to be the best at our recovery, and we want to do things the quickest we can do them, when in reality, we need to allow our bodies the time to heal." Check your perfectionism and don't rush the process; otherwise, you're setting yourself up for failure when your body takes longer than your preconceived timetable. There's no such thing as getting an A+ in SIBO.

▷ **One meal that causes symptoms will not set you back to SIBO.** Remember, diet on its own did not cause your SIBO, and diet alone will not be the reason it relapses. If you've reintroduced something that is making you feel ill repeatedly every time you eat it, tune into those messages, and consider taking a breather from that food. But don't let an initial fear of bloating, gas, and other symptoms be a reason for not expanding your diet. Fearing relapse can become a self-fulfilling prophecy through stress, not food.

▷ **Food reactivity is not a life sentence.** Just because you can't eat something today does not mean you won't be able to eat it in the future. So many SIBO sufferers whittle themselves down to five foods without being open to their body's ability to change. Conversely, many of us mourn the intolerance discoveries after an elimination diet. Commit yourself to the concept that your gut is constantly evolving and your diet will need to evolve with it.

▷ **Your strict diet is always waiting for you as a reset.** If your gut is feeling troubled for more than a few days, a low-FODMAP or SIBO-specific diet is a great way to reset. This is another reason not to stress about any symptoms experienced along the way on your road to diversifying. If you're suffering, just dial back the FODMAPs for a couple of meals and see whether that returns you to normal. A day or two of the elemental diet (page 44) is another reset tactic.

▷ **Say affirmations before meals.** If you keep telling yourself you're going to react to foods, you will react. Especially during reintroductions, remind yourself before you eat that what's on your plate is nourishing. Visualize the food going into your mouth before even taking the first bite and experience it feeding your cells. Another simple tweak to your self-talk is repeating, "I am safe. I am satisfied"—or any similar mantra that resonates. Remember that you and your body are playing on the same team, and shift your language to reflect that.

▷ **Get an inner balance device.** Dr. Jacobi recommends a product by HeartMath, which measures your heart rate variability. She tells patients to log the data two minutes before meals to see whether you are in fight-or-flight or rest-and-digest mode when faced with food. You are much less likely to react to an ingredient when in the latter. If not, even more reason to focus on the tips on this page (and breathing techniques on page 66) to retrain your nervous system.

▷ **Avoid the rabbit hole of online negativity.** Especially when you're first diagnosed, it can be easy to fall into research obsessive mode. I know, because I did it myself. You go onto every blog, every Facebook group. You listen to every podcast. The internet is an amazing place for finding information on SIBO. But there's also a lot of fear-related messaging, especially in support groups where people are often quick to share the negative and add to your sense of doom. "There comes a point when you need to cut yourself off from outside voices and tune into your own experience," says Coomes. Your SIBO is very different from somebody else's SIBO. Empowering yourself with information (e.g., picking up this book!) is one thing, but if you're lying in bed at night dwelling on what you've read or heard, then perhaps it's time to take an information vacation and just be.

▷ **Use a "gratipad" or happiness jar.** Before bed, write down three things that you're grateful for or made you happy that day. It can be on a pad, or if that feels like too big of a commitment, Coomes recommends a happiness jar to her clients. She uses different colored sticky notes so by the end of the year, you've got this really brightly colored jar of things that made you happy.

▷ **Focus on what you can have, not what you can't.** Print out a list of the foods you'll feel best eating, and put it on the fridge so you can fill your kitchen with these options. Make the challenge into an opportunity to get more creative in the kitchen. There's plenty of ammunition in this book!

▷ **Celebrate small victories.** Don't make your goal to get 100 percent better; 80 or even 60 percent is a fantastic improvement and a wonderful place to be.

Beyond Diet:
SIBO Lifestyle Changes That Last

There is a difference between controlling symptoms and actually clearing your bacteria. It often takes a more complex approach than diet alone to do the latter and prevent SIBO from recurring. If you have a malfunction of the migrating motor complex, too little stomach acid, or structural impediments, such as scar tissue from abdominal surgeries, just eliminating FODMAPs won't cover all your bases.

In fact, with SIBO, the ingredients in your meals are often less important than *how* you're eating them. In this section, we are going to focus on the small changes that not only are going to help your GI system function properly again but will be essential for preventing relapse. These practices are basically free and always available to you.

The following habit tweaks and rules of thumb, many of which revolve around the ways you approach your meals, can be game changers for some of these contributing issues—perhaps even more so than the carb count on your plate.

GIVE YOUR DIGESTIVE SYSTEM DOWNTIME BETWEEN MEALS.

If you've got one foot in the door of the wellness world, then you've probably heard of intermittent fasting. The idea is to go for an extended period of time without eating, usually at least twelve hours and up to sixteen. In today's culture, that has translated to skipping breakfast and fasting from roughly 9:00 p.m. until lunchtime the next day.

However, this is not exactly how intermittent fasting was meant to be applied—rather, we'd be better off eating according to our circadian rhythm. Meaning dinners before sundown and breakfast after sunrise. "Our cells actually have circadian clocks in them," says Dr. Amy Shah. "In the evening hours when the sun is down, our digestion is not functioning at optimal speeds because those genes are turned off. Part of the reason people get acid reflux or have issues with SIBO and IBS later in the evenings is because of this internal circadian clock."

If this sounds hard and complicated given the constraints of modern life—don't worry. You can start with a much simpler formula. **Meal spacing has a similar end goal**, in that it gives your intestines ample time after meals to get the job done, but relies on shorter fasting windows. As you learned in Chapter 1, **our migrating motor complex (MMC) only kicks in during a fasting state of ninety minutes or more**. That means if you're someone who's prone to snacking, even if it's a healthy snack, such as a handful of nuts every hour, your MMC isn't able to fully clean up after your meal. This can contribute to bigger issues, like SIBO, but it can also just make your whole digestive system less efficient.

If you're feeding yourself nutritious, well-balanced meals—meaning plates packed with vegetables, healthy fats and protein, and free of hidden sugars—on a regular schedule, you shouldn't be facing the types of food cravings that drive snacking. If you find that you feel starving two hours after lunch, it's time to reconsider what you're eating for those meals. Perhaps you're not having a large or filling enough lunch. Perhaps you have bigger fish to fry when it comes to balancing your blood sugar. Use your SIBO protocol as a time to reboot how you look at mealtime and find foods that keep you fuller for longer.

☞ Tips & Takeaways

▷ **Have two or three substantial, filling meals and don't snack in between.** Water, tea, or bone broth is fine, but no solid foods.

▷ **Make sure there are at least four to five hours between these meals.** If you can get all of them in before sundown, even better.

CHOOSE COOKED, PUREED FOODS OVER RAW FOODS.

You've probably heard a lot of mixed messages from raw foodists over the years who have beaten it into your head that the longer a food is cooked for, the less nutrients it will have when it makes it to your plate. But here's the thing they don't tell you: If your digestive system is a hot mess, you're not going to be able to extract those nutrients anyway. Your food is literally being flushed down the toilet...and it's not uncommon to see it there.

When our system feels inflamed or stagnant, we don't want to stress our gut out even more by giving it a mountain of woody, dense kale to process. Instead, we want to do the work of breaking down our food before it makes its way into our gut, so that it doesn't have to.

Cold foods slow down the digestive process, whereas warm, cooked foods tend to be easier on your GI tract. If your gut is extra distressed, consider choosing pureed foods over solids throughout the day to give your digestive system an even more restorative break. There are some great anti-inflammatory soups and stews in this book to get you going (such as my Orange Remedy Soup on page 217 or Warming Root Vegetable Chicken Tagine with Chard, page 233). At the same time, you will also see plenty of raw salads, since again, our ultimate goal is diversity. You may not be ready for those at the beginning of your healing process, but eventually you'll be able to handle more fiber and roughage.

☞ Tips & Takeaways

▷ **Eat cooked foods.** Especially in the morning, if you've been drinking smoothies or eating something straight from the fridge, try first sipping on something warm, such as an herbal tea or hot water with lemon, to wake up your system.

▷ **Break your foods down further by pureeing or mashing.** Seeding and removing tough skin from vegetables may be helpful for those with a very damaged gut, whether you eat your vegetables raw or cooked.

▷ **See recipe suggestions in the Gut-Heal Bootcamp Menu on page 285** for some easy-to-digest, warming foods in this book.

CHEW YOUR DAMN FOOD.

Getting back to "primal" behaviors does not mean buying a beef jerky that's seasoned with coconut aminos. It means using the tools that have been available to us since the dawn of humanity (fire, teeth), and putting our body to work in the way it was designed to be used. Which brings us to an often-overlooked part of the digestive process: CHEWING.

Yes, chewing. What is meant to happen many, many times between mouthfuls if only you weren't so distracted by the emails you're writing on your lunch break. If you're swallowing your food whole, it really doesn't matter how many grass-fed meats or plants are on your plate, because you're going to have a harder time extracting the nutrients. When we chew, the enzymes in our saliva begin the digestive process, working with our teeth to break down whole foods into usable parts.

☞ Tips & Takeaways

▷ **Instead of counting bites, try to make sure that whatever is in your mouth becomes liquid before swallowing.** This will feel like it's taking an excruciating amount of time and may even be a little off-putting. But go with it. Don't be afraid to be the last one finished at a group meal—make that your GOAL!

▷ **Put your fork down between bites.** Force yourself to be fully finished with what's in your mouth before you even begin scavenging your plate for the next bite.

▷ **For at least one meal (but preferably all of them!), make sure there are absolutely no distractions.** No emails. No TV. No books. Just you and your plate and your thoughts. This also will have a wonderful effect on your mental well-being and whole nervous system.

REV UP YOUR STOMACH ACID BEFORE MEALS.

Pep-themed pills that promise to relieve your heartburn, reflux, and gut pain by suppressing your natural juices have given stomach acid a bad rap. These ads perpetuate a huge misconception that our digestive juices are something to be feared, when in fact the presence of these conditions is sometimes a result of...dum dum dum...a LACK of stomach acid.

We get into this in Chapter 1, because one of those downstream conditions caused by low stomach acid is a bacterial overgrowth in your small intestine. Your stomach acid is the first leg of the labyrinth for killing unwanted bacteria. Just like your saliva, it's there for a reason, and that reason involves a vital part of maintaining gut health. Since pathogens mainly come into our body through the nose and mouth, it's only sensible that our gut would have a powerful antimicrobial substance in place to neutralize unwanted visitors before they have the chance to take up residence in our vulnerable small intestine.

"If you don't have hydrochloric acid and you don't get the party started up top, then nothing works right downstream," says Dr. Jolene Brighten. "Stomach acid actually helps your gallbladder and your pancreas function more optimally. We need to leverage what your body was designed to do so that bacteria stay in the large intestine." Without stomach acid, those bugs don't get killed. Without time spent in a fasting state between meals, our MMC doesn't properly move those critters into the large intestine. And without chewing our food, more large particles end up in our small intestine to give these bugs a consistent food source. It's a domino effect.

☞ Tips & Takeaways

▷ **Most SIBO Amigos will benefit from a digestive enzyme or HCl supplement taken before meals.** More about this on page 55.

▷ **In lieu of pills, you can also opt to drink 1 tablespoon of cider vinegar or freshly squeezed lemon juice diluted in 8 ounces of water before meals.** Either of these acidic substances will signal to your digestive system that food is on the way, and it's time to prepare more stomach acid to greet it. It's an especially great practice for when you're traveling and may be more susceptible to foreign pathogens. Of course, folks who have GERD, are histamine intolerant, or suspect a yeast overgrowth should skip this.

▷ **If you're taking antacids and proton pump inhibitors, talk to your doctor about weaning off of them, as PPIs in particular are a huge risk factor for SIBO (for all the above reasons).** Or look into taking a probiotic with it, per page 58.

DON'T EAT TOO CLOSE TO BEDTIME.

Our body is not great at multitasking. Meaning, if you're trying to digest food while at the same time shutting down certain motor functions for sleep, both your rest and your digestion are going to be impaired. It's better to get all of that food moved through your system before going horizontal (when gravity is not on your side) and before your body starts spending energy on other things. This is especially important if you have a history of SIBO, because you don't want all of that undigested food sitting in your small intestine overnight.

Per our circadian rhythm, digestion slows down between 10:00 p.m. and 2:00 a.m. If you're eating dinner at 9:00 p.m., you're still going to be in the process of digesting it by ten o'clock. It's also worth noting that our digestion gets weaker as the day goes on.

DRINK LOTS OF WATER IN BETWEEN MEALS.

Regardless of whether you're SIBO-C or SIBO-D, staying well hydrated is hugely important for making sure your digestive system runs on schedule, and if you're prone to the latter, replenishing some of the vital liquids you might be losing down the toilet.

Think about your body's appetite for water in the same way as food. Just because you've had a big breakfast doesn't mean you're not going to be hungry again by dinnertime. Drinking a quart of water at the beginning of the day and then going dry for the rest is the same concept. What we don't need in a given moment gets flushed down the toilet, and our cells' thirst returns shortly thereafter, regardless of whether we can recognize it.

Think about having three good "water meals" a day: one 16-ounce glass before breakfast, repeated before lunch and also dinner. It's good to have these "water meals" outside of your actual meals. To maximize retention, you're supposed to stop drinking thirty minutes before eating and wait an hour after you're done to drink more. Passing up water during a meal also helps with digestion. Water dilutes the natural enzymes in your saliva that help break down food and has a similar effect when it reaches your other digestive organs. Wine is metabolized differently, so the same rules don't apply. (Phew.)

▷ **Put a pitcher or water bottle on your desk.** This not only helps you measure your daily intake, but it's also a powerful reminder to drink. **The rule of thumb is half your body weight in ounces daily.** If you don't want to count, you can get a container that holds your quota.

▷ **Avoid carbonated beverages.** Soda water is a noted enemy of IBS sufferers because of the increase in laxative effects, bloating, and gas. Since carbonation can travel, those air bubbles might be responsible for carrying bacteria from one part of your gut to another.

WEAR LOOSER CLOTHES.

Okay, okay. Not everyone wants to wear a muumuu to work. But perhaps during your treatment phase, it's worth giving your gut a break from the Spanx, high-waisted jeans, and other modern corsets. As we've learned, structural problems—meaning anything that constricts our organs and gives them less room to do their job—is a precursor to SIBO. See what happens to your digestion when you give your insides a little room to breathe.

SIBO Amigos, pay attention not just to what you're eating at meals that causes symptoms, but also to what you're *wearing*.

☞ Tips & Takeaways

▷ **Avoid garments that press up on the abdomen or restrict movement for your digestive organs.**

▷ **Bras that are extremely tight around the ribs could be another source of reflux.**

EAT LIKE A PREGNANT PERSON.

If you have a history of SIBO, you likely have a history of food poisoning. This can make you more prone to future bouts of food poisoning, and thus, the vicious cycle of SIBO. While some of the earlier tips will make sure that your digestive system is functioning properly, even with stomach acid in place to kill foreign pathogens, we want to avoid exposure to potentially harmful critters.

If you're going to be traveling to a foreign country or eating at a questionably hygienic establishment, see page 53 for some supplements to have in your arsenal. But on a daily basis, you can avoid foods that are high risk for unwanted pathogens by eating like a pregnant person. Depending on who you ask, these foods include raw seafood, deli meats, and unpasteurized cheeses. You may not want to order your steak blue or your seared salmon pink. And you may not want to eat Fourth of July potato salad that has been sitting on a counter all day, as this is one of the most common incidents of salmonella.

👉 Tips & Takeaways

▷ **Avoid foods that are high risk for opportunistic bacteria, such as raw meat and seafood, cured meats, and unpasteurized cheeses.**

▷ **Travel sensibly in high-risk countries: Avoid raw vegetables rinsed in tap water and fruits you can't peel, drink bottled water, and skip ice in your drinks.** Consider taking an antimicrobial along, just in case as a form of prevention.

KEEP YOUR MOUTH CLEAN.

Your mouth is the trailhead of your digestive tract and the primary entrance for bacteria. Many studies have linked poor oral health to disrupted gut health, and vice versa. If you're not doing an adequate job of keeping bacteria levels at bay, that bacteria can migrate to the gut and throw off your ecosystem and immune function.

Gingivitis may be the canary in the coal mine for systemic inflammation. When our gums bleed, bacteria can access the circulatory system, crossing the blood-brain barrier, and create so many more problems than just for your teeth. "Leaky mouth" is a new term that illustrates that issue. One study in mice with Alzheimer's showed notable levels of oral bacteria in their brain. Bacterial toxins in the mouth can also influence insulin resistance by causing the brain to no longer recognize sugar regulation.

Mercury fillings are another issue that's raised many red flags in recent years. In addition to the possibility that the toxin can pass directly to the brain stem, mercury ingestion has been associated with the destruction of intestinal flora and a higher risk of pathogenic infection.

👉 Tips & Takeaways

▷ **Take stock of the history of your mouth.** Root canals, fillings, dead teeth incubating bacteria, infections, and oral surgeries could be an essential connection to a history of gut imbalance.

▷ **Floss and brush your teeth daily.** Also, brush your tongue and use a folic acid or probiotic swish. Avoid mouthwashes with a lot of alcohol, which is used as a preservative and doesn't actually do an adequate job of killing bacteria. On the contrary, it actually dries out your mouth, which provides a better environment for bacteria to flourish.

▷ **Get amalgams removed by a biological dentist.** Highly toxic materials, such as mercury, have no place in your mouth and only contaminate the river that flows from it.

The SIBO Amigo Digest: 10 Diet Rules of Thumb

1
Diet did not cause your SIBO, and any "cheats" or reintroductions will not cause your SIBO to return.

2
Figuring out your allergens and food triggers is more important than starving bacteria.

3
FODMAPs are not allergens; they are poorly digested carbs found in all plants.

4
Staying on a restrictive diet for more than a few months is harmful for your overall gut health.

5
What you eat is not as important as HOW you eat it.

6
Don't let your diet be the enemy of your inner and outer worlds.

7
If you don't react to an ingredient, EAT IT!

8
Consume a diverse array of plants; it is the most important factor for good gut health.

9
Fearing relapse can become a self-fulfilling prophesy through stress, not food.

10
Be gentle with yourself. All SIBO food rules are able to be broken.

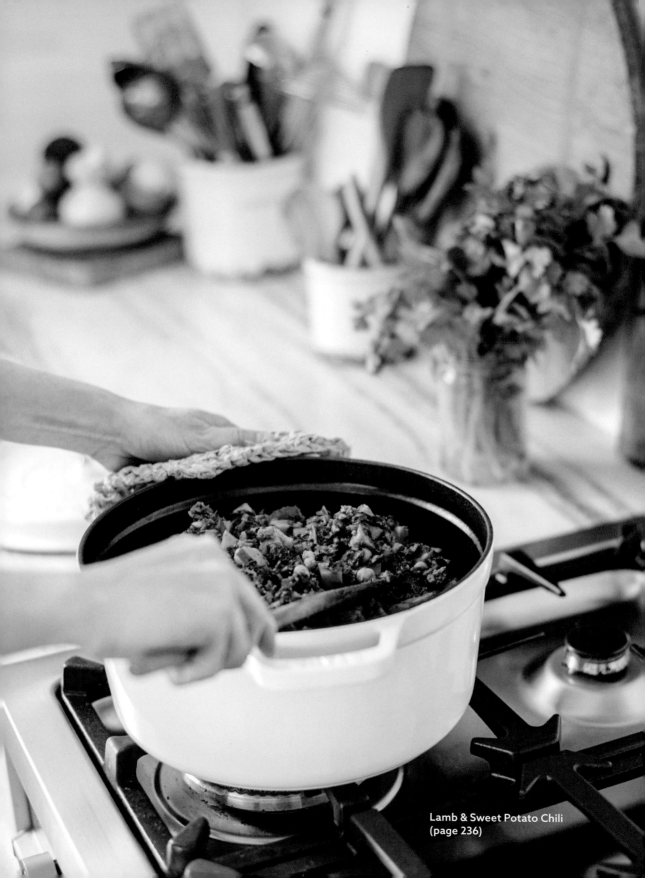

Lamb & Sweet Potato Chili
(page 236)

Part Two

PUTTING YOUR SIBO DIET INTO PRACTICE

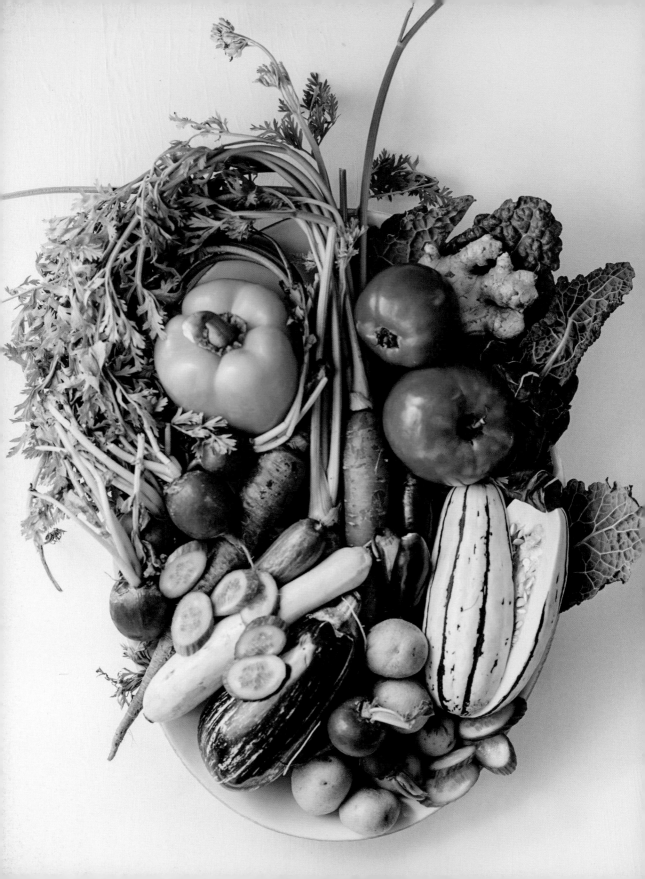

Chapter Four

• • •

GET COOKING

Stocking Your Kitchen Medicine Cabinet

———

FIGURING OUT YOUR FOOD RULES is all well and good, but a restrictive diet is impossible to maintain unless you know how to actually put that food on the table.

The kitchen is where you will have your come-to-Jesus moments of your SIBO diet. For many, eschewing some of your most-used ingredients will force you to learn a new way of cooking. For others, this may be the first time you roll up your sleeves to do more than boil water. No matter where you're at, this book should help make your time—and, at first, there will definitely be more of it than usual—in the kitchen as fun, painless, and delicious as possible.

Cooking is not an exact science (despite what many chefs will tell you), and the tips in this section provide a great jumping-off point for you to find variety even in the most hopeless dietary place. **If you're thinking "there's nothing I can eat in this book," you're simply not using it properly.** One of the silver linings of SIBO is the creativity it can spark in the kitchen.

Reading through this section will help alleviate any confusion about how to tackle the recipes in Chapter 5 To get you closer to the point where you can "freestyle," I've included plenty of tips for how to make low-FODMAP meals taste fantastic (page 127). On page 117, we'll also talk more about why specific foods are so beneficial for healing, and why others may be getting in your way. And finally, since you'll be adapting these recipes to your individual needs, I've included a troubleshooting section for ingredients in this book that some people may find irritating and how to work around them.

Lastly, you'll notice that I do not include a set meal plan—at least not in the traditional sense. Despite reading countless health books that include dish-by-dish, meal-by-meal guidance, I've never been able to fully stick to one. And frankly, for many people, yours truly included, seeing those charts, with not just two, but often four different recipes to prep for the day, makes my chest tighten with anxiety.

Spending every free hour at night making your food, and eating each anti-inflammatory, perfectly designed meal in a dark house by yourself, is not the key to healing. It is how your diet begins doing more harm than good. Treating SIBO can already feel like a full-time job that leaves very little room for actually living. **My hope for you is that the cooking piece can become a source of joy, rather than a chore you can never fully keep up with.** And my biggest advice for achieving this is to make the majority of your meals over the weekend. Some people call this meal prep. I call it batch cooking. And it's how I've organized your meal plan suggestions on page 285. There, you'll find recipe bundles that are perfect for making in one or two cooking sessions. There's also a whole section with tips on how to make cooking into a sustainable habit through meal prep on page 131.

Remember that there are always small ways you can tip the scale and rebalance your experience toward healthy hedonism. Maybe it's a favorite podcast or playlist blasting while you chop, a pretty notepad to write your shopping list on, or a new kitchen gadget that sparks joy. Whatever it is, my biggest commandment for you is to **make your kitchen a place where you truly want to spend time**.

Your food will taste better for it, even without the onion, I promise.

How to Use the Recipes in This Book

The dishes in Chapter 5 are organized by type—vegetable sides and salads, soups and stews, and main courses that include poultry, meat, and seafood. If you are plant-based, don't worry. Over half of the recipes in this book are vegetarian, and many more can be adapted to be so. Although some grains and potatoes play supporting roles in other dishes, I've kept the starch-heavy recipes in their own "Careful Carbs" section so that those taking on a more restrictive approach can skip or moderate accordingly.

Unlike most cookbooks, there is no typical breakfast, snack, or dessert section here. But you'll find a handful of options that fit the bill in "Foundational Dishes" (page 139), where I've put together some back-pocket staples for drinks, bites, sauces, and condiments. This is also where you'll find many subrecipes in the book, such as homemade Gut-Building Broth, Four Ways (page 140). Since meal spacing is such an important part of SIBO recovery (as explained on page 102), many people avoid snacking. Contrary to what you might believe, breakfast also is often not the most important meal of the day. On page 123, we talk a little bit more about why reducing your sugar intake is such a vital part of restoring your digestive system to its peak strength. If you want to keep breakfast in your life, any of the savory recipes in this book would be a big improvement to the usual muffin, pancake, or bowl of sugary cereal, though it might take some getting used to. I've included some back-pocket breakfast ideas on page 129, if you need them.

Each recipe includes a dietary key with labels for some of the more popular SIBO dietary approaches that we lay out on page 116. **The recipes in this book are all soy-optional and completely free of gluten, corn, refined sugar, and dairy**, with the exception of 24-Hour Yogurt (page 163) and ghee. Hence, you will not see notations for these restrictions. Often, a recipe can be tweaked, and where applicable, I've included some recommendations on how to modify to suit your needs.

Since so many diets, such as the low-FODMAP approach, are portion-specific, it's important to **note the servings listed for each recipe**. Exceeding those portions in one sitting may put you over your FODMAP threshold and cause some symptoms. It's something to pay attention to, not become maniacal about. To help you better understand certain medium-FODMAP ingredients and how their portion sizes matter, I've included a guide on page 130. If a recipe doesn't list a specific limit, it means you can enjoy unlimited quantities without worry.

Finally, in each recipe, you'll also see a section called **"Onward."** This is where I've offered a variation that incorporates one ingredient you may be reintroducing to your diet at some point on your SIBO journey. If you already eat said ingredient, feel free to incorporate it from the get-go. Otherwise, this will provide a simple road map for how you can begin adding higher-FODMAP foods to your recipes. The quantities I specify are on the lower end, so as to ease you back into incorporating these ingredients with minimal reaction. Cross-reference page 91's full, step-by-step reintroduction for more guidance.

RECIPE DIETARY RESTRICTION KEY

For more information on some of these special diets, see page 75. You can also find additional lists and resources in the Appendix on page 303.

LF	→ Low-FODMAP (for a list of foods to avoid, see page 83)
SCD	→ Specific carbohydrate diet
SSFG	→ SIBO-specific food guide
BPD1R	→ Bi-phasic diet, Phase 1—Restricted
BPD1	→ Bi-phasic diet, Phase 1—Semi-restricted
BPD2	→ Bi-phasic diet, Phase 2
P	→ Paleo
V	→ Vegetarian / plant-based
SF	→ No added sugar
HI	→ Low-histamine (for a list of foods to avoid, see page 295)
YC	→ Yeast- & candida-friendly (for a list of foods to avoid, see page 296)
HS	→ Hydrogen sulfide–friendly (for a list of foods to avoid, see page 297)

Healthy Hedonism and Hero Ingredients

As you learned in Chapter 3, there's so much more to a SIBO diet than starving your bacteria by removing their favorite carbs. **Your healing relies on what you add, not just what you take away.** And keeping that abundance mindset is one of the key ways to find *healthy hedonism* while cooking for SIBO.

As a reminder, the official definition of this motto of mine is to **balance the things that nourish your body with the things that feed your spirit.** One of the mistakes many people make while treating SIBO is forgetting about the nourishment factor. And yet, finding ways to add more "good" to your plate is also one of the key ways to find more joy in your meals.

You can easily eat a low-FODMAP diet or a SIBO-specific diet and still not be eating an anti-inflammatory diet. As people reduce their plate to a handful of things they don't react to, they are also reducing their nutrients. If you follow these guidelines, you will be adding ingredients to your meals that ensure your body has the resources to heal. Keep these basic tenets in the back of your mind when it becomes too preoccupied by the killing concept. The kitchen is where you will negotiate between these two sometimes opposing aims.

BASIC ANTI-INFLAMMATORY PRINCIPLES

Eat the rainbow. Intense hues in fruits and vegetables usually indicate a high level of antioxidants, which limit inflammation. Plus, steering clear of members of anything in the beige family will help you weed out dairy, bleached carbs, and other processed things that agitate the gut. If you add as many colors to your plate as possible, you'll also be hedging your bets on the nutrient front and getting a wide array. Diversity on your plate translates to diversity in your large intestine's gut flora, as different critters eat different things. And as we know, keeping these beneficial bugs happy and in their rightful home has a big impact on the health of your immune cells.

Make your meals 50 percent vegetables. You probably didn't need me to tell you that. But it's the common takeaway from pretty much every anti-inflammatory diet. Ideally, this will mean less room on your plate for simple carbs and animal protein. But even if you're choosing to indulge, have a small plate of greens as a starter before your steak frites. Colorful antioxidant-rich veggies alkalize your stomach in advance of more inflammatory choices. And the more different plants you can pack into that real estate, the better. If your gut isn't yet in salad shape, there are plenty of ways to get your veggies in puree form (see the "Soups & Stews" section, page 215).

Balance your blood sugar. Your liver is one of the underappreciated allies of your digestive system. It processes everything—both emotionally and physically—that we put in our body. This scrappy organ also manages the storage of sugar and its conversion into energy, produces a vast reservoir of your body's proteins, regulates hormones, and cleans your blood. When your liver is constantly modulating the sugar piece, it doesn't have as much power for all these other necessary chores. For SIBO people, that means a less efficient job eliminating toxins produced during bacterial die-off. Including fiber is one of the key ways to slow down sugar absorption and give your liver time to catch up. Although fiber tends to be shunned on a SIBO diet, it serves an important role in your overall health. Try to avoid consuming refined carbs, such as white rice, sweet juices, or dishes with high volumes of sugar (natural or otherwise) on an empty stomach without the presence of any plant fiber to modulate your blood sugar (unless, of course, you're prepping for a breath test!).

Be careful with carbs. You have to walk a fine line with carbs when healing from SIBO. Too many, you're feeding your bacteria and experiencing symptoms. Too few, for women especially, you might find your energy levels plummet and your stress hormones increase. Women in their childbearing years need carbs to build their hormone reserves and often don't do well on ultra-low-carb diets. But choosing the right carbs for you will take some experimenting. Refined carbs without added fiber (e.g., white rice or processed gluten-free pasta) can present issues for your insulin levels, as they're more quickly converted into sugar. On the other hand, whole grains, such as brown rice and quinoa, which have their own built-in fiber, can be irritating to some peoples' gut as they heal. You'll have to find that sweet spot yourself, which might just be a matter of adding a bundle of steamed chard to your spaghetti (see Shrimp Spaghetti with Cherry Tomato Puttanesca, page 279).

Mind your ratios of macronutrients (carbs, fiber, protein, fat). If you're balancing your plate with grains, protein, veggies, and healthy fats, often the portion control for each quadrant gets taken care of. Our macronutrients work together in tandem, and it's usually when one bucket gets elevated (be it with FODMAPs, animal products, or starches) that we run into trouble. If you have too much fiber, your stomach is not going to empty as well. If you have too much fat, that can cause distension. The recipes in this book, with the exception of those that aim to be lower-carb, try to balance each of these prongs within the context of one recipe.

Avoid insult. Sadly, many ingredients in our modern food system add insult to gut injury (and I'm not talking FODMAPs, which are completely natural parts of plants). Although my *healthy hedonism* mantra is to always focus on the good rather than the bad, it's important to be aware of your own food triggers (per page 85) and avoid added chemicals and toxins that might be overloading your liver and contributing to leaky gut. I've included a list of things to monitor, later in this chapter, but the more pervasive irritants are pesticides in our produce and antibiotics in the animals we eat. Make sure to print out a list of the Dirty Dozen and Clean 15 (the produce most and least likely to contain harmful pesticides, available at ewg.org) when you go shopping and buy organic as much as possible when it matters.

Just because it's "healthy" doesn't mean it's healthy for you. As always, if your food is ending up unprocessed in the toilet or causing you to double over in pain, it doesn't matter how many colors were on your plate or whether your liver is happy. You're not going to be reaping the rewards of what you're eating. Remember that the aforementioned principles are an end goal. You may not be there yet, but every day that you heal your gut is another opportunity to work slowly toward that perfect anti-inflammatory home-cooked meal. Listen to your body. It's all a balancing act.

SIBO AMIGO HERO INGREDIENTS & HOW TO USE THEM

Leafy greens. Spinach, kale, arugula, watercress, collards, and other greens are packed with nutrients like folate, vitamins A, C, and K. They are also powerful detoxifiers that support your liver during times of stress, which SIBO antimicrobial treatment falls under. While many people can't handle mounds of raw woody kale, there are plenty of recipes in this book where you can get the benefits of leafy greens with less work for your gut, such as Green Detox Soup (page 218), Green Immunity Smoothie (page 160), and Nutty Steamed Greens (page 184). As you heal, you may even be able to handle the Marinated Kale with Roasted Fennel, Parsnips, and Sunflower Seeds (page 187), which is partially broken down, thanks to freshly squeezed lemon juice.

Healthy fats. Extra-virgin olive oil, coconut oil, avocado oil, and grass-fed ghee are all fantastic ways to reap the rewards of fat as a macronutrient— balancing your hormones, healing leaky gut, greasing the wheels of your intestines. Ghee, in particular, is a clarified butter that's lactose-free and popular in Ayurvedic cooking for digestive healing. Avoid soybean, palm, peanut, corn, and miscellaneous vegetable oils, which are highly processed and bad for your heart health. Also, use your fats without compromising their burning point, which changes the makeup of the oil. Olive oil is best for low heat and raw preparations, whereas ghee, coconut, avocado, and grapeseed oil can stand up to high temperatures needed for searing meats and stir-frying vegetables.

High-quality lean meats and poultry. The risk of low-carb diets is that they force you to eat more animal protein. If you are watching your grocery budget, this can sometimes cause you to compromise quality in favor of quantity. Buy organic, grass-fed, and free-range whenever possible. You read about how antibiotic use puts you at a higher risk for SIBO in Chapter 2. Well, 80 percent of antibiotics in this country are used for livestock, which trickles down to the gut of the people who eat them. This book focuses on leaner cuts of red meat, since fat malabsorption is an issue for many SIBO sufferers, but tends to favor dark meat poultry for its ability to stay moist. I still consider this a lean protein. Try to avoid highly processed products such as conventional salami, bologna, and deli meats, which have been classified by the World Health Organization as carcinogens. You'll find some bacon and prosciutto here and there (because, hedonism), but make sure to buy paleo varieties without added sugar, nitrates, or other additives.

Wild, low-mercury seafood. The best species for omega-3s, low mercury, and minimal environmental impact are mollusks (clams, mussels, oysters, scallops), and smaller oily fish, such as sardines and anchovies. Those with histamine issues will have to be careful with this grouping, but others will benefit from their richness in zinc, selenium, iodine, and other thyroid-supporting nutrients. Wild salmon is also worth the premium—just look at that scarlet color! Try to avoid eating large amounts of high-mercury fish, such as tuna and swordfish. And if you do, add cilantro! It's a chelating agent that will help your body better remove the toxin.

Colorful vegetables. Per anti-inflammatory principle #1, we can't let a low-FODMAP or SIBO diet make us afraid of plants, because we will be losing out on so much more than we'll gain. Especially as your gut heals and diet expands, take advantage of all the varieties. In this book, you'll find plenty of ways to add color to your plate with red and orange peppers, carrots, eggplant, radicchio, cucumber, bok choy, radishes, squash, and zucchini, among others. You'll also see modified portions of broccoli, green beans, fennel, sweet potato, and red cabbage (the medium-FODMAP items on page 130).

Ginger. As you read in Chapter 2, high doses of ginger can be used as a prokinetic, and as a back-pocket remedy for bloating, nausea, and general IBS woes. Eating the root, as you'll do in many of the Asian-inspired recipes in this book, also offers a panacea of benefits beyond gut issues. Ginger is an Ayurvedic all-star ingredient with a long list of medicinal uses, including as a therapy for colds, cramps, and muscle soreness. Try Gingery Stir-Fried Collards and Quinoa (page 196), Carrot-Ginger Dressing (page 181), or Turmeric-Ginger Stewed Eggplant (page 185).

Fresh lemon and lime juice. Lemon juice, in general, is one of nature's secret weapons. Its antiseptic nature acts as a solvent for toxins, and though it makes zero sense on paper, when added to water, becomes an alkaline solution, instead of acidic. Starting the day with an alkaline drink rather than something acidic, such as coffee, helps your liver flush all the junk it accumulated overnight when it was doing double duty cleaning your blood. Before meals, freshly squeezed lemon juice in water can also help stimulate stomach acid production, which is a key part of the digestive process. These recipes use lemon and lime juice as the primary source of acid, since it tends to be better tolerated by those with histamine issues, and because, especially with raw food, it can act as a backup antimicrobial.

Digestive spices. Cumin, coriander, ground ginger, fennel seeds, and cinnamon all have properties that aid in digestion in some capacity. Many of the recipes that are inspired by Indian and Middle Eastern cultures—such as Warming Root Vegetable Chicken Tagine with Chard (page 233), Brown Rice Kitchari (page 192), and Mild and Creamy Butterless Butter Chicken (page 255)—pack a big punch with these spices.

Pink Himalayan or Celtic sea salt. Like fat, salt has gotten a bad rap in the age of processed foods, despite the fact that it's an essential nutrient. Salt is in the makeup of virtually all our bodily fluids, which means we're constantly losing it in the form of sweat, urine, and tears. Choose unprocessed options, such as pink Himalayan or Celtic sea salt, to maintain the beneficial mineral content, which aids in absorption and supports electrolyte balance. The recipes in this book were all developed with sea salt, so if using kosher, you may have to adjust the quantities as it tends to be less potent.

Fresh herbs. Although it's hard to ramp up to the same concentration as what's in your herbal supplements, you'll still benefit from eating your herbs. Adding plenty of antimicrobial varieties, such as oregano, rosemary, and basil, along with powerful detoxifiers, such as cilantro, parsley, and basil, is a good move. You'll notice that most recipes are served with a garnish of fresh herbs at the end and that many sauces, such as Green Harissa (page 170), Creamy Cilantro-Jalapeño Ranch (page 145), and Three-Herb Chimichurri (page 256) use them as the base.

Fermented foods. Most people will wait until the second phase of their SIBO recovery to begin adding back fermented foods, as those with histamine or yeast issues might react prior to SIBO's being eradicated. The probiotic live cultures in these foods are what make them one of the traditional gut health all-star ingredients. Things like sauerkraut and kimchi cross-train your gut by giving your immune system a retuning, and at the same time feeding your existing gut flora the prebiotic fibers they crave, what's known in the vitamin aisle as a "symbiotic." Of course, those with SIBO need to make sure that they're not fanning the flames of their overgrowth and derailing their gut-repairing process. Use your judgment for when these foods are appropriate to reincorporate for you, and then try adding small amounts of Coconut Kefir (page 167), Sauerkraut (page 165), and 24-Hour Yogurt (page 163) to the meals in this book. You will also see some suggestions throughout in the "Onward" sections. Fermented dairy, in particular, was associated in several studies with beneficial shifts in the microbiome. If you've established in an elimination diet that dairy isn't an issue for you, supplementing these recipes with yogurt could be part of your healing strategy post-SIBO to rebuild gut flora. Also, drinking fermented cabbage juice—even just an ounce a day—will also help with gut healing, thanks to all the amino acids (see page 122 for more about the benefits of cabbage).

Sprouted grains. Until about a hundred years ago, humans harvested their grains and left them in the field until they were ready to process. With this exposure to the weather, at least some of the grain would begin to sprout. Skipping that essential step may be one of the reasons that we are unable to digest grains as well as we used to. The sprouting process increases the bio-availability of some vitamins (notably B vitamins, such as folate, and vitamin C), and can often be less irritating to those with sensitivities to grain proteins. Although the recipes in this book don't specifically call for sprouted varieties, those who are sensitive to grains may get a leg up by seeking out pre-sprouted store-bought options or by sprouting whole grains themselves at home before cooking. The process is simple, but takes a little forethought: start with a whole grain (such as brown rice, with bran and germ intact), soak it in room-temperature water overnight, and drain before using. Although they are not fully sprouted at this stage, these soaked grains often require less liquid to cook and are easier for your body to break down.

GUT-HEALING HERO INGREDIENTS

Collagen. Drinking bone broth is a great addition during every phase of the SIBO process as it's packed with amino acids and collagen that help heal the lining of the intestines. Making your own stock is also an important first step toward cooking for a low-FODMAP diet, since most commercial broths have garlic and onion in them. My recipes can be found on pages 140–142. You can also buy collagen peptides and add them to your soups, morning tea (such as Golden Glow Latte, page 157), or smoothies. I've also included a low-histamine broth (page 142).

Cabbage. Certain families of vegetables are specifically rich in L-glutamine, which is a supreme healer of your intestinal lining's tight junctions. Cabbage is one of the most abundant in this amino acid. It is low FODMAP in servings under ¾ cup, but if you're sensitive to the fiber, adding small amounts to your juices, smoothies, or soups is an easy way to pack it in without as much pressure on the gut (Kitchen Sink Crucifer Soup, page 235, is a great option). Once you begin adding fermented foods back into your diet, kraut is an especially beneficial choice. You can also sometimes find kraut juice, which is the brine from making sauerkraut. This is a wonderful drinkable supplement to keep in the fridge and take swigs of throughout the week or to use instead of vinegar in salad dressings.

Turmeric. One class of medications that puts you at a higher risk for intestinal permeability is NSAIDs, such as Advil. Luckily, turmeric, one of the substances that can help heal your gut, also packs enough anti-inflammatory punch to help with pain management. As you know, color is a great indicator of anti-inflammatory properties. And few foods are more vibrant and medicinally powerful than turmeric. The color can be rather obtrusive, but I added it whenever possible to up the nutrition of the recipes in this book. For leaky gut specifically, curcumin, the main compound in turmeric, encourages glands on the surface of your intestines to regenerate. Try Turmeric-Dill Catfish (page 274) or Pumpkin-Chive Risotto (page 202) for some golden goodness.

REMOVING THE INSULT

Gluten. Non-celiac gluten sensitivity has risen to epic proportions in the last decade, spurring numerous theories as to why people are reacting to a protein that has been our civilization's culinary lifeline for centuries. One potential reason: Wheat has been hybridized over the years to withstand increased levels of pesticides, most notably glyphosate, the main ingredient in Roundup. In addition to being as disruptive to beneficial flora in our gut as it is to pests in nature, a meta-analysis also calculated that exposure to glyphosate increases cancer risk by 41 percent.

Bread is made very differently than it was a century ago, with the starkest change being the rise time. A higher percentage of gluten allows factories to develop the elasticity in bread much faster—from twenty-four hours to a mere twenty minutes—through a creepy stabilizing ingredient called vital wheat gluten, which is now added to the majority of processed baked goods. Gluten itself has posed a risk in the autoimmune era because of molecular mimicry, a phenomenon when a foreign player is so structurally similar to your body's own tissues that when your immune system creates antibodies to attack the invader, it mistakenly attacks your own body in the process. Gluten is structurally similar to a number of your body's tissues, particularly the thyroid gland, making it both a contributing factor for autoimmune thyroid diseases and an ingredient that fans the flames of those already struggling with high thyroid antibody counts. Gluten intolerance is also commonly associated with yeast overgrowths (SIFO) because of this cross-reactivity issue.

Dairy. The majority of the world's population stops producing lactase, the enzyme that breaks down lactose in dairy, once they've finished breastfeeding. If you have SIBO, reducing the quantity of lactose in your diet is another way of reducing your bacteria's favorite food sources, which is why a low-FODMAP diet only allows aged cheeses and highly fermented twenty-four-hour yogurt, which has very little lactose. However, I've excluded most dairy products from these recipes, with the exception of ghee and fermented yogurt, due to the potential for cross-reactivity. Similar to gluten, many people experience dairy sensitivities because they do not tolerate casein or whey (two proteins found in milk). Conventional dairy also tends to be full of hormones and antibiotics, both of which can promote imbalances in gut flora.

Corn and soy. Corn and soy are two of the most commonly genetically engineered foods, with about 90 percent of their crops being GMO. There are many people who argue that these modifications pose no issue for the human body. But once you consider what they were engineered to accomplish, it's clear that our gut gets caught in the crosshairs. Many GMO crops were designed to produce their own insecticide, called Bt-toxin, which kills insects by destroying the lining of their digestive tract. Studies have shown that this action is effective on human cells, damaging the intestines and causing leaky gut. The only soy product in this book is gluten-free tamari, which you can buy organic or omit entirely in favor of paleo and SCD-friendly coconut aminos.

Sugar. I explained earlier how volatile blood sugar levels can have a downwind effect on your whole digestive system, making your liver less capable of regulating hormones and flushing out toxins. More significantly, several studies illustrate how high-glucose and -fructose diets can fundamentally change the balance of bacteria in your microbiome, limiting diversity and increasing intestinal permeability. In addition to the effects that sugar alcohols have on overgrowth (just refer back to that handy high-FODMAP chart, page 83), recent evidence suggests that artificial sweeteners are actually even more likely to induce glucose intolerance than consumption of pure sugar, even the refined stuff. During your healing period, it might be worth breaking up with the idea of dessert at every meal, avoiding overly sweet cuisines, such as barbecue, pan-Asian, and southern food when eating out, and relying instead on natural options, such as pure maple syrup and clover honey, in modest amounts to add a balance of flavor to your recipes. Plus, a square of good-quality dark chocolate at the end of the meal, if you need it!

Coffee. Coffee is a polarizing ingredient in the wellness world, seen as a drug by some and a superfood by others. Your tolerance really comes down to how well you metabolize it, which varies from person to person and can be affected by a number of variables (hormonal birth control being a biggie). Coffee competes for precious enzyme resources that are also needed to process estrogen during the detoxification process. This is one reason that women taking hormone replacement drugs metabolize caffeine more slowly and can feel its effects longer. When estrogen levels are elevated, as can happen when your liver isn't efficiently sorting the excess and eliminating properly, it creates a chain reaction through other parts of the body, especially the thyroid. We talk about the impact of estrogen dominance on the gut on page 33. Especially for women, morning pick-me-ups such as organic green tea or matcha are better options.

Alcohol. Before you start hating me for taking away all the fun, let me just point out that you've probably experienced the argument for not drinking on many hazy mornings. In addition to the raging headache, you might have seen what happens to your digestion after overimbibing. The issue really involves quantity: consecutive vodka tonics in one evening can overwhelm your liver. Order a sugary, caffeinated rum and Coke, and you've got triple the trouble. While I'd assume most of you can probably dial it back on the quantity during a healing period, there's also the lesser discussed issue of frequency. Having a glass of wine every night with dinner is sometimes worse than having several on a Saturday night, as your liver then never fully gets time to catch up. To do your gut the biggest favor, try to at least exclude alcohol from your diet while on antimicrobials, so as to not undo their efficacy. But moreover, make sure you're giving yourself a few consecutive days of detox a week in addition to moderating your overall consumption. Even though most alcohol (with the exception of rum) is low FODMAP, we don't want to interfere with all the other good work we're doing.

Cheap oils. One of my healthy hedonism saving graces during SIBO treatment was that French fries (from a dedicated gluten-free fryer) were technically allowed on a low-FODMAP diet. I ate them sparingly as a treat, while also keeping in mind that cheap oils used in restaurants for everyday cooking, and more notably in the deep fryer—such as soy, corn, peanut, and canola oil—are often a source of digestive woes. Too many saturated fatty acids in your diet has been shown to decrease microbial diversity and trigger a host of metabolic diseases. If you eat out at a restaurant and wonder why you feel crappy afterward, it might not be an ingredient on your plate, but the oils being used to cook them.

INGREDIENT TROUBLESHOOTING

Hero foods can also hurt, depending on the person. If you're reacting to something in these recipes, it might be for one of the following reasons. Be your own gut detective and use these suggestions for tweaking dishes when necessary.

Coconut. For various reasons, coconut is an underappreciated allergen these days, and one that can make many "healthy" spins on comfort foods difficult. That said, coconut milk is one of my favorite ways to add both creaminess and thickness to recipes that usually have heavy cream. If you find that you're sensitive to coconut milk, it could be due to some of the gums and additives in many canned varieties. My favorite brand is Native Forest, as its "Simple" formula doesn't use any guar gum. If you are certain your reaction is to the coconut itself, you can sub any other nondairy milk— almond, flax, hemp, oat—or use other means of thickening like adding ½ cup of mashed potatoes to a soup, stew, or curry. It should be noted that bottled and boxed nut milks also tend to have additives and sweeteners, so it's best to make your own using one of the recipes on page 156.

Fiber. Although the low-FODMAP diet removes many forms of resistant starch and insoluble fiber, there will still be plenty of plant roughage in your meals. If your gut is seriously inflamed, things in the fiber department that might be difficult to process include whole nuts, seeds, and tough vegetable skins. Before ruling out an ingredient entirely, consider the fiber content. If a vegetable, try first seeding it and removing the skin before adding it to a recipe. Many of the nuts and seeds in these recipes are used as garnish, so feel free to omit them if you know they will be problematic.

Healthy fats & animal protein. Fat malabsorption is common with SIBO, even though healthy fats, such as coconut oil, ghee, and olive oil, are so essential for long-term gut healing and feeling satiated on a restrictive diet. If you're worried about the amount of oil or ghee in a recipe, I urge you to step out of the '90s fat-free dogma that you may have been indoctrinated in and give these ingredients a chance as part of your SIBO diet. On the other hand, if you find that there's greasy discharge in the toilet bowl after you go to the bathroom, that could be a sign that you're not processing fats well. In this case, pay extra attention to increasing your stomach acid and try a digestive enzyme or an ox bile supplement (page 55). You may also find that leaner protein (chicken, turkey, pork tenderloin) is easier to handle until your gut is in better shape.

Nightshades. Ingredients like eggplant, tomatoes, sweet and hot peppers, and potatoes can be problematic for some people with autoimmune issues, due to their lectin, saponin, and/or capsaicin content. These items are removed on an autoimmune paleo (AIP) diet, but are often increased on a SIBO diet, since they are low FODMAP. If you notice an issue with nightshades, it might be worth experimenting with an elimination to gauge your sensitivity. Seeding and removing the skins sometimes helps as well.

Spicy foods. Hot peppers can pose issues for sensitive gut folks for several reasons: The nightshade factor, as just noted; also, the histamine factor, as explained on page 96. And more vaguely, hot foods can fan the flames of gut inflammation. Unfortunately, on a low-FODMAP diet, we often resort to some heat to make our plates more interesting without the use of alliums. If you know spicy foods upset your stomach, make sure to omit the jalapeño, cayenne, chili powder, and red pepper flakes in any recipes that call for it. Black pepper doesn't tend to fall in this category, so see how you tolerate it.

Raw foods. Similar to the earlier tip about fiber, there are many cases where a reaction might not be caused by the ingredient itself but, rather, by how it's prepared. For more information on why cooked foods are easier to process than raw foods, see page 103. If you're in a fragile state, stick with the cooked recipes, like those in the soups and stews section (page 215), and avoid big raw salads.

Eggs. Eggs are used minimally in these recipes, despite their yolks' being one of the best natural sources of choline, an essential nutrient for women during childbearing years. If you can tolerate eggs, they are a fantastic addition to your SIBO pantry. However, since they are a histamine-liberating food, those with histamine issues might notice an increase in symptoms as they become more reliant on eggs as a source of protein. Many autoimmune sufferers also find that they can be sensitive to eggs due to the ability of lysozyme (found in egg whites) to penetrate the gut barrier, which can exacerbate systemic inflammation if they are eaten in larger quantities without other foods, as some people do in the morning with scrambled egg whites. If enjoying eggs, eat the whole egg.

Broth-heavy soups and slow-cooked stews. Although the collagen in bone broth is generally a boon to gut health, if you're experiencing histamine dysregulation, you might notice that soups and stews that rely on slow-cooked broths can cause symptoms. Refer to page 95 on histamine intolerance for how to do a short-term diet to reset. To make any of the soup and stew recipes in this book, simply use the recipe for Low-Histamine Stock (page 142) or water. You may also want to choose quicker-cooking dishes and avoid putting animal protein for extended periods of time in a slow cooker.

Low-FODMAP Cooking 101

As you'll quickly learn from scanning ingredient labels at the supermarket, eliminating garlic, onion, and added sugar from your diet will mean you can no longer rely on many quick-fix packaged foods. Luckily, this gives you an opportunity to do some DIY-ing at home and begin building your "living pantry." This is a concept I learned from chef David Bouley, who has spent the last decade developing nutrition-forward building blocks for his restaurant that further good gut health. The low-FODMAP diet forces you to do this by necessity, but the added benefit is far more nutritious options always at your fingertips for adding flavor to your meals. Here are a few more ways to build your low-FODMAP cooking arsenal.

Infuse your oil with alliums (garlic, shallot, and onion). So often, I get messages or comments about recipes of mine that have garlic in the ingredient list. People get their panties in a low-FODMAP twist without reading the whole recipe to see how they are used. FODMAPs are not fat-soluble, so the simplest way to keep the flavor of garlic, shallot, or onion in your meals is to infuse them into your cooking oil. I have recipes for how to make bulk batches of garlic and shallot oil on page 143. Since olive oil isn't great for high-heat cooking, I'd recommend using these to finish a dish and add a top note of garlic rather than using these premade oils to brown your meat. In some recipes in this book, I call for infusing garlic or shallot into your cooking oil as the first step, so don't be alarmed if you see either on the ingredient list! You can always substitute a premade oil if you have some.

Keep medium-FODMAP "pantry vegetables" on hand. One of the most annoying aspects of the low-FODMAP diet are the medium-FODMAP vegetables that have to adhere to a certain portion size. These aren't always logical, like, say, ⅛ fennel bulb. Although generally I prefer to write recipes that use a vegetable from start to finish, to adhere to the low-FODMAP diet and still keep as many vegetables as possible on your plate, the ingredient list will often call for less than the quantity you would traditionally buy. This works well for some vegetables and not as well for others. The more useful types are those that keep for longer periods of time in the crisper drawer. I call them "pantry vegetables." Broccoli, cabbage, celery, fennel, sweet potato, and winter squash can last for weeks on end, allowing you to slowly work through them. You can find a visual guide to these portions on page 130. Another useful tactic is to buy frozen vegetables, such as broccoli florets, green beans, and sweet peas, so you can siphon off smaller quantities without waste.

Make your own stock. Once you have a hardy stock, you can pretty much make any dish have a sense of depth. Take a whole chicken carcass and add peppercorns, lots of herbs, fresh ginger, carrots, and any other FODMAP-friendly vegetable scraps you have lying around. For set recipes, including a vegetarian option, see page 142.

Use pure maple syrup as your sweetener. Although table sugar is techni-cally considered low-FODMAP, I've focused on natural, less-refined sweet-eners in the occasional recipe where a little sugar is needed. Pure maple syrup for wet measurements and coconut sugar for dry measurements are my preferred substitutions. But those following the SIBO-specific food guide, bi-phasic diet, or SCD can sub in clover honey.

Make your own salad dressing. On a low-FODMAP diet, you can have most acids—vinegar, lemon or lime juice—and emulsifiers, such as mayo and mustard, as long as there's no garlic or onion. Really the no-nos are sweeteners, like high-fructose corn syrup and honey that are in many store-bought dressings and condiments. Luckily, making your own salad dressing is one of the easiest things to do at home. And having flavorful homemade condiments around at all times makes throwing together a not-sad desk lunch or dinner that much easier. See the "Foundational Dishes" section (page 139) for some of my favorites.

Sub almond, flax, hemp, or coconut milk for dairy. Milk and cream are to be avoided on a low-FODMAP diet, but many nut and seed milks are okay in moderation. Coconut milk poses some issues in quantities greater than ¼-cup servings. Many recipes in this book call for 1 cup total in the recipe, which usually means half of a standard-size can. Save the other half for another use. If the recipe at hand is one that would benefit from extra creaminess, try to use the top half of the can, which is where the cream usually rests. Alternatively, you can often find coconut cream in 5.4-ounce cans, which would be a perfect substitute for a 1-cup measure with a couple extra splashes of water.

Let spices be your friend. Building out your spice rack is one of the best places you can put your money in terms of creating flavorful meals out of humble ingredients. A bold curry doesn't need a whole lot of other aromat-ics to make the main ingredients taste wonderful. Spices are also a great way to jazz up plain roasted vegetables, such as carrots or potatoes (see Moroccan Carrot Salad, page 211; Smoky Fingerling Steak Fries, page 195). You can slowly build your collection, but many will lose their punch and medicinal efficacy after a year or two.

Add some heat! For those who can tolerate peppers, jalapeño and hot sauce can add a much-needed punch to everyday cooking. Just make sure to read labels to avoid onion, shallot, garlic, and added sugar in store-bought options, such as sriracha. My favorite brand is Cholula, which has just peppers, water, salt, and vinegar on the ingredient list.

Make your own sausage. All meat, seafood, and poultry is fair game on a low-FODMAP diet, with the exception of processed meats, which could contain flavorings like onion and garlic. The solution is to simply make your own sausage—and it's easy! All you need is ground meat and the herbs and spices of your choice. For sweet Italian, see page 155. To make your own cho-rizo, just add cumin and coriander. Sausage is a fun canvas to get creative.

Brown your meat and deglaze the pan. Understanding basic cooking techniques for layering flavor will be a huge asset in cooking without onion, garlic, and shallots. First and foremost, you want to cook your meat, seafood, and poultry as simply and perfectly as possible. This means giving it a good sear on the stovetop. Get your pan (preferably cast-iron) nice and hot, using an appropriate oil with a high burning point (refined coconut, avocado). Dry the protein with paper towels and season it generously with salt and pepper. Add it to the pan, making sure you're not packing it to the gills with food (crowding diffuses the heat). Then, DON'T TOUCH IT. Your meat needs to hang out on the surface area of the pan undisturbed to develop that beautiful sear. Once you notice the bottom of the meat forming a brown crust, it's time to flip it. If the meat clings to the pan when you try to move it, that's an indication that it's not ready. When it's finished cooking, transfer the protein to a plate and allow it to rest there for at least half of the time it spent in the pan. While it rests, make use of all those brown bits on the bottom to create a pan sauce.

Bacon makes everything better, even a low-FODMAP diet. Okay, it isn't the healthiest or most gut-friendly. But when in doubt, or in extreme diet depression, a little crispy bacon goes a long way. Make sure to check the ingredient labels for added flavors and sugar. Buy organic and nitrate-free. Then, sprinkle it on salads or eggs, or enjoy a slice or two just because.

Have five back-pocket recipes. This book makes the question of what's for dinner a little easier. But it's still most helpful to have a few recipes top of mind that are your go-tos, especially for those of you who have a very restrictive diet. Here are some of mine!

---

5 BACK-POCKET LOW-FODMAP, ONE-PAN DINNERS

1. Chili-Lime Sheet Pan Chicken with Delicata Squash and Kale (page 243)
2. Sesame Sheet Pan Salmon with Radishes (page 276)
3. West African Yam and Peanut Stew (page 225)
4. Beef Negimaki Stir-Fry with Green Beans and Watercress (page 259)
5. Summer Squash Moqueca (page 229)

10 BACK-POCKET LOW-FODMAP, LOW-SUGAR BREAKFASTS

1. BLT Frittata (page 270)
2. Sausage and Sweet Pepper Hash (page 269)
3. Very Berry Smoothie (page 162)
4. Hormone-Balancing Energy Balls (page 153)
5. Scrambled eggs with sautéed spinach
6. Two coconut oil–fried eggs with homemade Sausage Patties (page 155)
7. Overnight oats with mixed berries
8. 24-Hour Yogurt (page 163) with kiwi and pineapple
9. Gluten-free toast with peanut butter and sliced banana
10. Leftovers—any recipe in this book will work!!

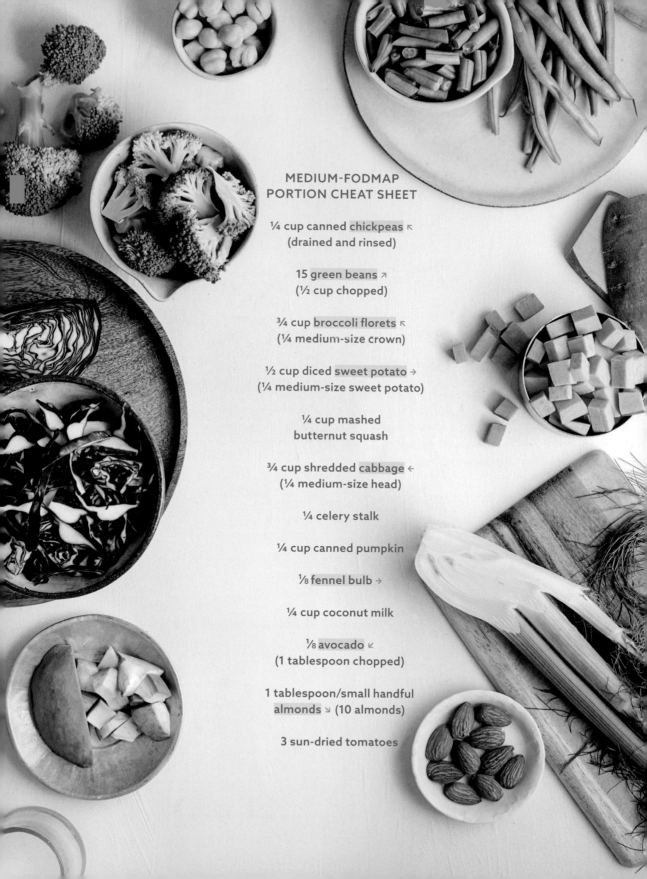

MEDIUM-FODMAP PORTION CHEAT SHEET

¼ cup canned chickpeas ↖
(drained and rinsed)

15 green beans ↗
(½ cup chopped)

¾ cup broccoli florets ↖
(¼ medium-size crown)

½ cup diced sweet potato →
(¼ medium-size sweet potato)

¼ cup mashed
butternut squash

¾ cup shredded cabbage ←
(¼ medium-size head)

¼ celery stalk

¼ cup canned pumpkin

⅛ fennel bulb →

¼ cup coconut milk

⅛ avocado ↙
(1 tablespoon chopped)

1 tablespoon/small handful
almonds ↘ (10 almonds)

3 sun-dried tomatoes

MEDIUM-FODMAP PORTION CHEAT SHEET

Since a low-FODMAP diet is portion-specific, you need to be careful when exceeding the recommended serving size of these recipes in one sitting. For example, ¼ cup of coconut milk is low-FODMAP, but ½ cup of coconut milk is high-FODMAP. If you enjoy more than one portion of the Orange Remedy Soup (page 217), you'll be exceeding the coconut milk quantity. Of course, if you end up eating half of the soup pot and not feeling any worse for it, don't stress. Coconut milk might not be a trigger for you.

The point is: I've done all the hard math for you in this book. For a quick reference guide on some of the most-used medium-FODMAP ingredients in Chapter 5, I've created the list on page 130 based on the Monash University guidelines.

Meal Prep Like a Pro

Everyone has their own method to the madness of preparing their meals for the week in one or two cooking sessions. The way I recommend tackling "batch cooking" is to block off **four hours over the weekend** to get intimate with your kitchen. You'll allocate one hour for each activity: shopping, prepping, cooking, and cleanup. Compared to the time you would spend to do all of these things every night, four hours doesn't seem like such a big commitment. And having something delicious and nutritious already made in your fridge will make you much less likely to order in or dine out. Not that those quick fixes are even a possibility on a SIBO diet...

Besides saving time, one of the big benefits of preparing your meals in advance is that it makes you less wasteful, which in turn will have a positive impact on your budget. Planning ahead forces you to buy fewer veggies and use them start to finish. The key is to choose a menu of four or five dishes while keeping the following tips in mind. I've also put together some sample menus on page 285 that fit the bill.

Make sure it's make-ahead. A dressed salad will be soggy within hours, whereas a simple yellow rice pilaf (page 197) will last for days. In general, hearty grains and anything that's slow cooked (e.g., soups or stews) will keep well, whereas raw foods with lots of added acid will spoil more easily. For chopped salads, such as my Garden Salad (page 181), just store each element separately and assemble to order.

Don't bite off more than you can chew. The menu should be easy enough to fit within a one- to two-hour cooking window. Look for recipes that have limited ingredient lists (fewer than ten items) and don't require a lot of active work at the stove so you can be working on several things at once. Most of the recipes in this book are fairly streamlined and meant to be either quick at the stovetop or hands-off in the oven.

Mix one-pot meals with simple sides. Choose a few dishes, such as those in the "Main Event" section (page 239) that hit all the food groups and can be made from start to finish (think: stir-fries, casseroles, sheet pan meals), and then round out those mains with simple building blocks, such as roasted vegetables and premade grains, or some of the recipes from the "Salads & Veggie Sides" and "Careful Carbs" sections (pages 169 and 191).

Keep your "night of" cooking to ten minutes or less. There are certain things that won't keep well if premade, such as panfried fish or those dressed salads. Often, though, they'll also be the quickest things to fire off or assemble right before you eat.

Use a variety of techniques. If you choose four dishes that all require sautéing, you're going to get overwhelmed. Instead, look for a mix of roasting, stewing, and raw, and try not to have more than two things on the stovetop at once.

Stick with complementary flavor profiles. Since you're going to be mixing and matching your premade meals, you want to make sure that all the flavors go together. Stick with Italian, Thai, Mediterranean, or Indian, instead of a menu that includes all of the above. This will also make your time and budget more efficient by allowing you to use the same herbs and condiments across all dishes.

Use your pantry to fill out the fresh ingredients. This will make your shopping trips less stressful, and keep you on task with your budget. Generally, pantry grains are items that keep just as well precooked for the week ahead as they do on the shelf. If you are eating very limited grains, having one batch in the fridge for the week will allow you to slowly work through them, adding ½-cup portions to your plate at each meal. Another tactic? Freeze them! Cooling grains and potatoes increases their bioavailability and ups the amount of resistant starch, which is beneficial for the bacteria in your large intestine.

Avoid obscure odds and ends. If a recipe calls for three types of herb garnishes or a specialty ingredient you're never going to use again, consider omitting those items, or choosing a dish that's simpler to begin with. If it's something you already have in your pantry, like raw nuts or seeds, then great! But don't be shy about skipping what doesn't seem necessary. Same goes for the recipes in this book!

Add acid and herbs last. If you're reading through a recipe that's finished with freshly squeezed lemon juice, vinegar, or herbs, save those elements for right before you're ready to eat. Lemon can cause the color of your food to go off over time, and herbs have the tendency to spoil unless they are blended or fully incorporated. Plus, a fresh garnish before eating can make your leftovers feel that much more new and exciting.

Freeze extra portions. If you have histamine issues, you might think that meal prep is off-limits. However, it's still possible to make your meals in advance if you use your freezer. You can avoid further waste or cut down your meal prep in future weeks if you siphon off some portions of your meals and freeze them for down the road.

SIBO-FRIENDLY LAST-MINUTE ACCENTS

Here are some of my favorite things to keep on hand to supplement my premade meals. Often these are items that are best left to the last minute anyway, but are also easy enough to prepare in under ten minutes.

Eggs. Maybe you only have a small portion of Spinach-Ghee Mashed Potatoes (page 201) at the end of the week and it doesn't really feel like a meal without a protein. Solution: put a fried egg on it.

Rotisserie chicken. If you're someone who needs a little extra meat to feel full, you might want to pick up a rotisserie chicken to pull apart and add to some of your meals. You can use the carcass to make homemade low-FODMAP stock for the month! If you can't find a plain or herb-roasted chicken, simply try to scrape off the skin to avoid garlic seasoning. Otherwise, you can always make your own by following the recipe for Lemon-Rosemary Roast Chicken (page 241).

Salad greens. The easiest way to stretch your meals and balance your plate in the process is to fill half of it with a simple green salad. I find that baby arugula keeps the best out of all the bagged greens, but you can also buy a head of romaine or other lettuce and prep the leaves yourself during your batch cooking session. You can't go wrong with freshly squeezed lemon juice, sea salt, and olive oil, but there are also plenty of dressing options in the "Foundational Dishes" section (page 139). If raw greens are not in the cards for you, a batch of wilted spinach can serve the same purpose—it takes two minutes to sauté or steam.

Tomatoes. As long as you're not sensitive to nightshades or histamines, take advantage of gorgeous summer tomatoes. There's no simpler side around than a plate of sliced tomatoes with sea salt and olive oil.

Fish fillets. Wild, sustainable fish (such as those discussed on page 120) are a great option to keep on hand in your freezer. They thaw in warm water fairly quickly and usually cook up in less than ten minutes. For recipes like my Blackened Salmon Burrito Bowls (page 281), you can make all the elements in advance and broil the fish right before eating.

Eating Out on a SIBO Diet

Eating well during SIBO recovery is not an issue (just see Chapter 5). Eating well at a restaurant while on a SIBO diet, on the other hand, is a taller order. It's much easier to have restrictive food rules within the four walls of your home, but life is much more enjoyable if you venture outside of them! Learn the things on a menu that you can be flexible around and the things you can't. If eating out is causing you stress, make sure to read the mindset tips and takeaways for staying sane around food on page 99. You may also want to explore some of the ongoing anxiety and stress management tools on page 65.

Not all cuisines are created equal. When you're avoiding major allergens and low-FODMAP ingredients, some restaurants will be easier to navigate than others. Chinese cuisine is a land mine for gluten (soy sauce), cornstarch, added sugar, and cheap oils. This may not be true for certain authentic, regional Chinese cuisines, but soy sauce is fairly ubiquitous. Japanese is slightly easier for low-FODMAP eating, since you can reduce your dishes to their core elements: fish, rice. If avoiding gluten, bring your own gluten-free tamari sauce or coconut aminos, or check whether the restaurant has some—many do these days. If prone to food poisoning, consider sticking with cooked sushi rolls, such as shrimp or salmon skin. French and Italian cuisine are harder due to the amount of garlic used in most marinades, but usually a restaurant will be able to provide a plain piece of protein and a side salad. The best cuisines for SIBO diets are Mediterranean, Middle Eastern, Moroccan, Greek, Brazilian, Indian, South American, Spanish (watch out for stale bread in sauces), Thai, and Vietnamese (unlike Chinese food, Southeast Asian cuisines use very little soy sauce).

Call ahead during nonbusy hours. Usually midday if the restaurant is open for lunch, or around 5:00 p.m. if it's a dinner-only establishment, are the best times to commandeer a few minutes of the kitchen's attention. Ask whether the chef is able to offer you any alternatives on the menu. A plain piece of chicken or fish done simply with olive oil, salt, and pepper is usually a possibility if the staff knows in advance. When you get to the restaurant, just let your server know that you called ahead, especially if it's a place that doesn't like substitutions. If you can tolerate it, a side salad with olive oil and freshly squeezed lemon juice is pretty much always on offer.

Watch out for red-flag terms. The hardest ingredient to spot on a menu is gluten. It comes in so many forms, and is used in a variety of different culinary techniques. Big hidden sources of gluten are soy sauce, creamy condiments and dressings (sadly not every restaurant makes its own in-house), beer, roux or béchamel sauces used to thicken soups and stews, deli meats, and imitation crab (as well as licorice, sour candies, and chewing gum). Red-flag words and dishes include chowders and bisques, stews, chili, breaded, mole sauce, soy glaze, ponzu, miso, dashi, gochujang, romesco (often includes stale bread), crispy vegetables, panfried, hash browns, barbecue sauce, and malt. Many of these condiments and sauces will also be red flags for added sugar.

Have a snack or bite beforehand. If I know I'm going to feel disappointed in my meal or possibly not have enough options to feel satiated, I always try to eat a light meal at home, just in case. Think of it as your new pregame routine. Sometimes in work situations or when a friend is hosting, you don't have full control over your circumstances. Do your best to prepare, or per the next tip, just let yourself go.

Remember healthy hedonism. Are you going to be more miserable being a little bloated after your meal or feeling hungry and deprived? Social and emotional wellness are often more important than a little physical discomfort. Being low-FODMAP doesn't mean every night has to be a FODMAP-free night. And if you stray from your diet a few times, it will not impact your SIBO recovery, even if you experience some consequences on the toilet the next day.

Don't let the food be the enemy of the company. Always let hosts know your needs far in advance and offer to contribute to the meal. But more important, don't turn down an invitation just because you're worried about your diet. It's already so easy to feel isolated and lonely while dealing with a chronic illness. Being around your loved ones is the best medicine. If you're not someone who usually cooks for others or hosts, use this as an excuse to put on your entertaining cap. I threw dozens of dinner parties while dealing with SIBO and recipe testing for this book, and no one had any idea there was no garlic or onion in my food.

The SIBO Amigo Digest: 10 Cooking Rules of Thumb

1
Adapt, tweak, and get creative; cooking is not an exact science.

2
Add, don't just take away; your healing relies on both.

3
Make your kitchen a place where you truly want to spend time.

4
Don't bite off more than you can chew; start small and build your skills from there.

5
Build your "living pantry" with from-scratch condiments, allium oils, sauces, and stocks.

6
Keep medium-FODMAP pantry vegetables on hand to slowly work through.

7
Practice meal prep. It can make cooking a source of joy rather than a chore you can never fully keep up with.

8
Batch cook on weekends and make your freezer your new BFF.

9
Read ingredient labels and restaurant menus for red-flag words.

10
Put on your hosting hat and bring the party to you.

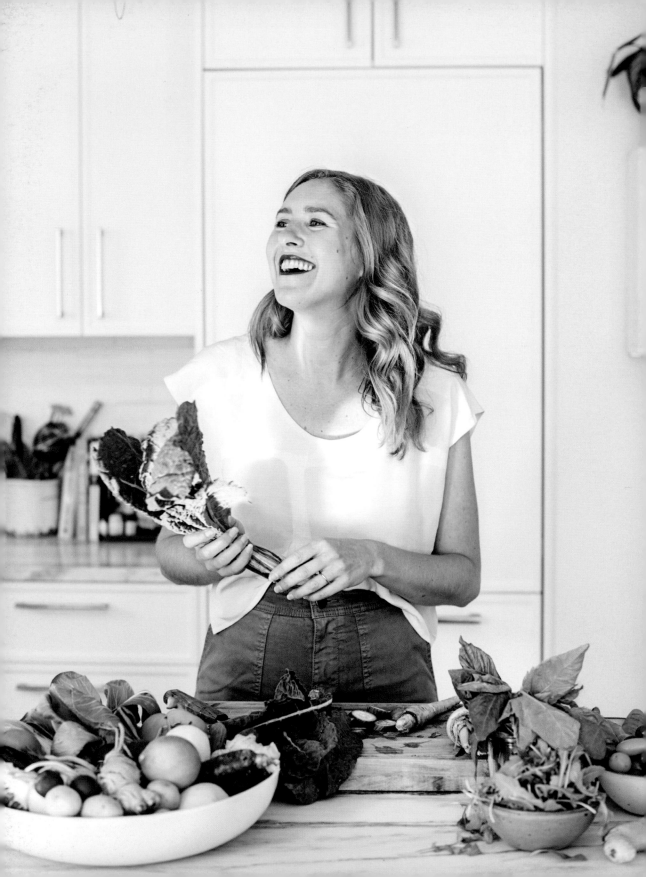

Chapter Five

THE RECIPES

*Really Delicious Dishes for
Every Stage of Your SIBO Journey*

―――――――――

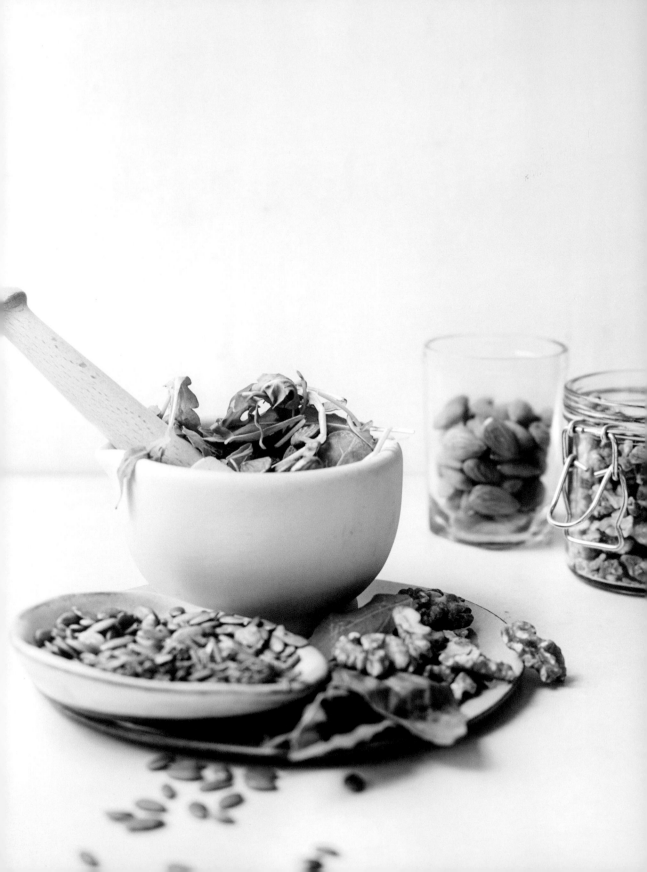

FOUNDATIONAL DISHES

Sauces, Snacks, Drinks & Condiments

Gut-Building Broth, Four Ways

Bone broth is literally so hot right now, and for good reason. As animal bones simmer for hours, they release amino acids, collagen, and nutrients that help your body rebuild tissue. This is especially important for repairing the tight junctions of your intestines. Since most store-bought versions use garlic and onion, I've included recipes for making several varieties of broth (the artist formerly known as stock). While these recipes are starting points, homemade broth and stock are also a fantastic way to compost kitchen scraps and be a little greener at home. Especially the veggie version, which allows you to "recycle" whatever wayward herb stems, carrot peelings, and other random hunks of this and that you have lying around. I keep a resealable plastic bag in the freezer and add to it throughout the week as I do my meal prep, then make a big batch of broth or stock over the weekend. Try to avoid citrus rinds, starchy vegetables, bitter greens, and sulfurous veggies in the brassica family.

Low-FODMAP Basic Chicken Bone Broth

MAKES ABOUT 3 QUARTS BROTH OR STOCK

- 1 chicken carcass, or 2 pounds uncooked chicken wings
- 2 carrots, halved widthwise
- 4 thyme sprigs, or 2 rosemary sprigs or ½ teaspoon dried
- 2 bay leaves
- 1 tablespoon black peppercorns
- 1 tablespoon sea salt
- 4 quarts filtered water

1 Place the chicken carcass, carrots, thyme, bay leaves, peppercorns, and salt in a 6- to 8-quart stockpot or slow cooker. Cover the ingredients with 4 quarts of filtered water, or enough to submerge them while leaving an inch of room at the top. Cook over low heat for at least 4 hours, or up to 12 if using a slow cooker. Skim any foam off the top with a ladle.

2 Over a large bowl or liquid measuring cup, strain the stock through a fine-mesh sieve, discarding the solids once or twice if there's too much pileup. Taste for seasoning and add more salt as necessary.

3 Transfer the chicken broth to three 1-quart mason jars or airtight containers and store in the fridge to sip throughout the week. Alternatively, you can freeze the containers for future cooking.

Onward Add 1 **celery** stalk, ½ **onion**, and 2 **garlic** cloves.

recipe continues →

LF	SCD	SSFG	BPD1R	BPD1	BPD2	P	SF

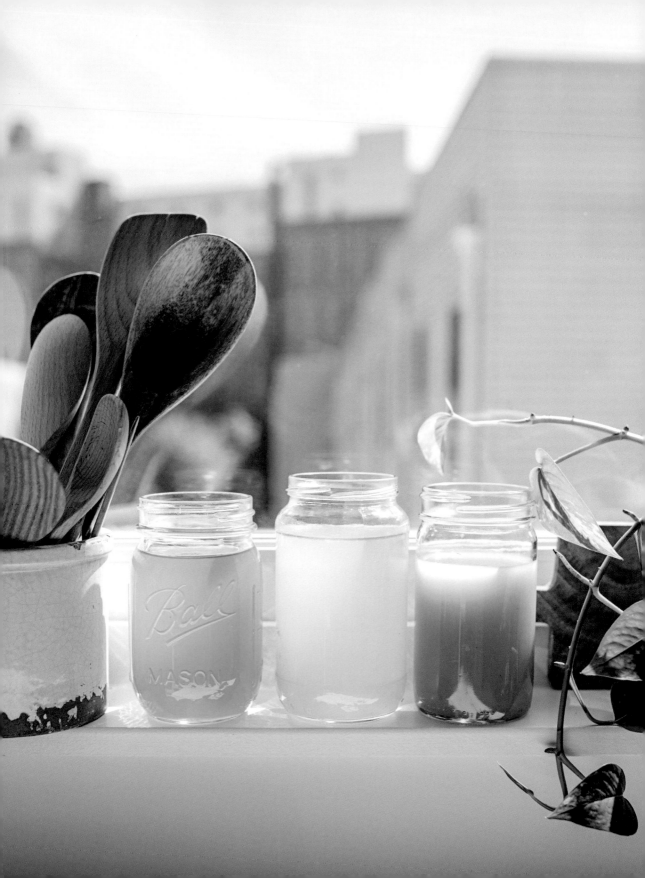

Low-FODMAP Beef Bone Broth

Substitute **4 pounds of beef bones** (ask your butcher for knuckle bones, oxtails, or marrow bones cut 2 inches thick) for the chicken carcass. To prepare them for an extra-flavorful broth, roast the bones on a rimmed baking sheet in a 450°F oven, flipping every 10 minutes, until the bones are deeply browned and fragrant, about 30 minutes total. Transfer the whole contents of the pan (bones, juices, etc.) to a 6- to 8-quart stockpot or slow cooker, and proceed with the main recipe.

Low-FODMAP Vegetable Stock

Omit the chicken bones, double the carrots, and add **1 cup of roughly chopped fresh flat-leaf parsley** (stems and leaves), **½ roughly chopped bell pepper**, and **2 tablespoons of tomato paste.** For even more flavor, roughly chop the carrot and sauté over medium-high heat in 2 tablespoons of Garlic-Infused Oil (page 143) before adding the pepper and tomato paste and cooking for 1 minute more. Add the remaining ingredients and the water. Proceed with the main recipe.

Low-Histamine Stock

You can make any of the preceding broths or stock low-histamine by simmering for a maximum of 2 hours over medium heat on the stovetop. Even better, use a pressure cooker!

Low-FODMAP Vegetable Stock ↓		Low-Histamine Stock ↓	
V		HI	YC

Garlic-Infused Oil

Since FODMAPs are not fat-soluble, the secret weapon to cooking on a SIBO diet is to infuse your oil with alliums, which are so often the building blocks of sauces and condiments. You can use the garlic-infused oil (and shallot-infused oil; recipe follows) anywhere that olive oil is called for in this book. I prefer to use these oils either raw or stirred in toward the end of the cooking process, rather than for sautéing over high heat. Use your judgment and think of them as a condiment for whenever your dishes feel like they could use the scent of garlic or shallot. Finally, infusing oil works for many flavors. Get creative and add fresh rosemary, thyme, or oregano to your garlic or shallot oil. Red pepper flakes also are fantastic for making a spicy oil.

MAKES 2 CUPS OIL

2 cups extra-virgin olive oil

6 garlic cloves, crushed with the back of a knife

1 In a small saucepan or pot, gently heat the olive oil and garlic over very low heat until warm to the touch. Remove from the heat and allow the oil to sit for at least 2 hours, or until you've reached your desired potency.

2 Strain the garlic oil through cheesecloth to remove the cloves or fish them out with tongs. Transfer the garlic oil to an airtight glass jar or bottle and store in the refrigerator for up to 1 week. You can also transfer to silicone ice cube trays to freeze individual portions for future uses. The cubes will keep for at least 2 months, potentially longer.

Shallot-Infused Oil

Replace the garlic with 1 medium-size shallot, quartered.

LF	SCD	SSFG	BPD1R	BPD1	BPD2	P	SF	HS	V	HI	YC

Basic Lemon-Dijon Vinaigrette

This is the only technique you need to make a vinaigrette by hand. Every combination starts with an acid, an oil, and an emulsifier. You can get creative from there, swapping out the lemon juice for red wine vinegar if you want an even more traditional bistro option, or using mayonnaise instead of Dijon for a creamier base. This would also be a fantastic opportunity to swap out regular olive oil for one of the infused oils on page 143!

MAKES ABOUT ⅓ CUP DRESSING

- 1 tablespoon Dijon mustard
- 2 tablespoons freshly squeezed lemon juice (from ½ lemon)
- ¼ teaspoon sea salt
- ¼ cup extra-virgin olive oil

❶ In a small bowl or food processor, whisk or pulse together the mustard, lemon juice, and salt until combined.

❷ Working slowly, add 1 teaspoon of the olive oil in a thin drizzle and whisk or pulse until incorporated. Repeat with 3 additional teaspoons of the oil, 1 teaspoon at a time. Once the oil is taking, slowly drizzle in the remaining olive oil, whisking or pulsing throughout.

❸ Taste for seasoning and add more salt or oil as necessary. The best way to test it is by dipping whatever leaf of lettuce you'll be eating into the dressing.

Onward Add 1 minced **garlic** clove to the dressing.

LF	SCD	SSFG	BPD1R	BPD1	BPD2	P	SF	V

Creamy Cilantro-Jalapeño Ranch

This mayo-based dressing is a lightened-up version of my favorite gloppy Hidden Valley condiment. The flavor profile is slightly spicy and southwestern, but you can get creative and make it an Asian-inspired dressing by substituting 1 inch of peeled fresh ginger for the jalapeño. This swap is also a great option for those who don't tolerate heat.

MAKES ABOUT 1 CUP DRESSING

⅓ cup mayonnaise

3 tablespoons rice vinegar or apple cider vinegar

½ cup fresh cilantro leaves and stems

1 jalapeño pepper, ribs and seeds removed

½ teaspoon sea salt

⅓ cup extra-virgin olive oil

In a small food processor, puree the mayonnaise, vinegar, cilantro, jalapeño, and salt. Slowly add the olive oil, pulsing to incorporate, until completely combined. Taste for seasoning and add more olive oil or salt as necessary.

Onward Sub ¼ cup of plain Greek **yogurt** or **kefir** for the mayonnaise.

					Use apple cider vinegar ↓			
LF	P	SF	V	SCD	SSFG	BPD1R	BPD1	BPD2

Aioli, Three Ways

Making homemade aioli (or mayonnaise) is much easier than people think, especially if you have a small food processor or immersion blender to help the oil emulsify quickly. And doing so gives you full agency over the quality of eggs, oil, and vinegar used. It's also a perfect opportunity to use garlic- or shallot-infused oil. To make your life even easier, or if raw egg freaks you out, feel free to skip the yolks and oil, and start with ½ cup of store-bought mayonnaise (just make sure you buy one without added sugar). These mix-in options will jazz up even the most mediocre jarred variety.

MAKES ⅔ CUP AIOLI

- 2 large egg yolks
- 1 teaspoon Dijon mustard
- 1 tablespoon freshly squeezed lemon juice (from ½ lemon)
- ¼ cup Garlic-Infused Oil (page 143) or extra-virgin olive oil
- ¼ cup melted refined (triple-filtered) coconut oil, organic canola oil, or other neutral oil
- ½ teaspoon sea salt
- 2 tablespoons finely chopped fresh basil, tarragon, chives, parsley, or dill

Lemon-Herb Aioli

In a small bowl or food processor, whisk or pulse the egg yolks, mustard, and lemon juice until smooth. Working slowly, add 1 teaspoon of the infused oil and whisk or pulse until incorporated. Repeat with 3 additional teaspoons of the oil, 1 teaspoon at a time. Once the oil is emulsifying easily, slowly drizzle in the remaining infused oil and the coconut oil, whisking or pulsing throughout. Once the mixture is thick, season with the salt and fold in the herbs. The aioli will keep for up to a week.

Spicy Lime Aioli

Substitute freshly squeezed **lime juice** for the lemon juice. Swap out the herbs for **2 teaspoons of sambal oelek** or any other low-FODMAP hot sauce.

Antipasti Bar Aioli

Replace the herbs with 1 tablespoon of minced **green olives** and 1 tablespoon of minced **capers**; reduce the salt to ¼ teaspoon. Optional: Add 1 tablespoon of finely chopped fresh parsley or chives.

Onward Use 1 small, minced **garlic** clove and sub regular olive oil for garlic-infused oil.

LF	SCD	SSFG	BPD1R	BPD1	BPD2	P	SF	V

Pesto, Three Ways

If the SIBO treatment options in this book have taught you anything, it should be that *herbs are powerful*. Pesto is a fantastic way to pack plenty of them into your diet, or simply work your way through the slowly wilting bunches in your fridge. These are three of my favorite combinations of greens and nuts or seeds. Pine nuts are used in traditional basil pesto, but since they tend to be expensive, I've gone with the poor man's version using walnuts. Chive pesto is a magical condiment, especially for adding that onion flavor to low-FODMAP recipes. And finally, arugula pesto is delicious as a dressing for nonleafy salads and boiled baby potatoes.

MAKES ABOUT ¾ CUP PESTO (SAFE SERVING: ¼ CUP)

- 2 cups tightly packed fresh basil leaves
- ¼ cup toasted walnuts
- 1 tablespoon freshly squeezed lemon juice
- ½ cup extra-virgin olive oil or Garlic-Infused Oil (page 143)
- ¼ teaspoon sea salt
- ⅛ teaspoon red pepper flakes (optional)

Poor Man's Basil Pesto

Combine the basil, walnuts, lemon juice, olive oil, salt, and red pepper flakes (if using) in a food processor or blender and puree until smooth, adding more olive oil as necessary.

Pumpkin Seed–Chive Pesto

Substitute ¼ **cup of pumpkin seeds** for the walnuts and ½ cup of roughly chopped **fresh chives** plus ½ **cup of tightly packed fresh parsley leaves** for the basil.

Arugula-Almond Pesto

Substitute ¼ **cup of almonds** for the walnuts and **2 cups of tightly packed baby arugula** for the basil. Up the **lemon juice to 2 tablespoons**.

Onward Add 1 small **garlic** clove.

										Use lime juice instead of lemon, unless tolerated ↓
LF	SCD	SSFG	BPD1R	BPD1	BPD2	P	SF	V	YC	HI

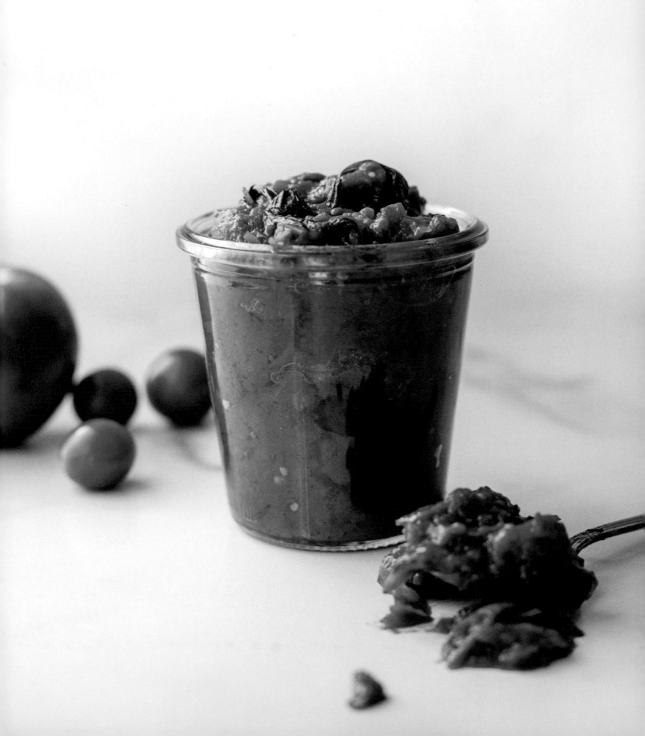

Low-FODMAP Pasta Sauce

This tomato-basil sauce is inspired by Marcella Hazan's famous recipe that uses just three ingredients: whole tomatoes, onion, and a very generous amount of butter. The longer simmer time is the best possible way of coaxing tons of flavor out of just a few simple ingredients. In this version, you make shallot- and garlic-infused oil using a mixture of olive oil and ghee. Alternatively, you can substitute 2 tablespoons of Shallot-Infused Oil (page 143) and 1 tablespoon of Garlic-Infused Oil (page 143), or whatever combination you like, and skip Step 1 if you happen to have either premade on hand. If you prefer a creamier sauce, you can transfer the end result to a blender. For a spicy arrabbiata version, add ½ teaspoon of red pepper flakes. You can also make a dairy-free faux vodka sauce by adding 1 cup of full-fat coconut milk.

MAKES 2 CUPS (16 OUNCES) SAUCE (SAFE SERVING: 1 CUP)

- 3 tablespoons extra-virgin olive oil
- 2 tablespoons grass-fed ghee
- 2 garlic cloves, crushed
- 1 shallot, halved
- 1 (28-ounce) can whole peeled San Marzano tomatoes
- 1 teaspoon sea salt
- 10 fresh basil leaves

1 In a large saucepan, heat the oil, ghee, garlic, and shallot over medium-low heat. Allow the oil to infuse and the alliums to gently sizzle, rotating occasionally, until just beginning to turn golden brown, about 5 minutes. Remove the garlic and shallot and discard.

2 Carefully pour in the tomatoes and their juices and season with the salt. Add ½ cup of water to the tomato can and swirl it around to catch any extra juices. Transfer the tomato liquid to the pan. Using the back of your spoon, roughly puncture the tomatoes so more of their juices are released. Arrange the basil leaves on top of the sauce. Increase the heat to medium and bring to a simmer. Cook, uncovered, over medium-low heat for about 45 minutes, stirring every 10 minutes or so, and breaking up any large pieces of tomato with a spoon. If the tomatoes are on the harder side, you can use a potato masher.

3 Taste for seasoning and add more salt as needed. Transfer the sauce to a quart-size glass jar or airtight container. It will keep for up to 2 weeks in the refrigerator and can be used for 12 ounces of gluten-free pasta.

Onward Thinly slice the **shallot** and don't remove from the sauce.

LF	P	SF	V	HS	YC	Skip garlic and shallot oil ↓ HS	Use 2 pounds of chopped fresh Roma tomatoes or a boxed variety ↓			
							SCD	SSFG	BPD1R	BPD1	BPD2

Roasted Carrot Hummus

Although canned chickpeas are allowed on a low-FODMAP diet in quantities of ¼ cup per serving, to make a whole batch of hummus, it helps to have something else to add volume to the dip. Roasted carrots provide a subtle sweetness to the hummus. You can use the remainder of your can of chickpeas in the Lamb & Sweet Potato Chili (page 236) or Green Falafel with Magic Tahini Sauce (page 198). For a more traditional hummus, omit the carrots and use the whole can; just make sure to limit your intake to ¼ cup total per sitting.

MAKES ABOUT 2 CUPS HUMMUS (SAFE SERVING: ½ CUP)

1 pound carrots (about 8 medium), unpeeled and cut into 1-inch pieces

2 tablespoons extra-virgin olive oil

1 teaspoon sea salt

1 teaspoon ground cumin

1 cup canned chickpeas, drained and rinsed

¼ cup tahini

3 tablespoons freshly squeezed lemon juice (from 1 lemon)

Garlic-Infused Oil (page 143), for garnish (optional)

❶ Preheat the oven to 425°F. Line a baking sheet with parchment paper.

❷ On the prepared baking sheet, toss the carrots with the olive oil, ½ teaspoon of the salt, and ½ teaspoon of the cumin and arrange in an even layer. Roast in the oven until the carrots are tender and caramelized, about 30 minutes.

❸ Remove the pan from the oven, and transfer the carrots to a high-powered blender or food processor, along with the chickpeas, tahini, lemon juice, the remaining ½ teaspoon of salt, remaining ½ teaspoon of cumin, and ¼ cup of water. Puree until smooth, adding more water as needed to reach your desired consistency. Taste for seasoning and add more salt as necessary. Garnish with a drizzle of olive oil or garlic-infused oil.

❹ Serve the hummus alongside crudités or low-FODMAP, gluten-free crackers.

Onward Add 1 small **garlic** clove.

			Sub lime juice for lemon, unless tolerated ↓
LF	SF	V	HI

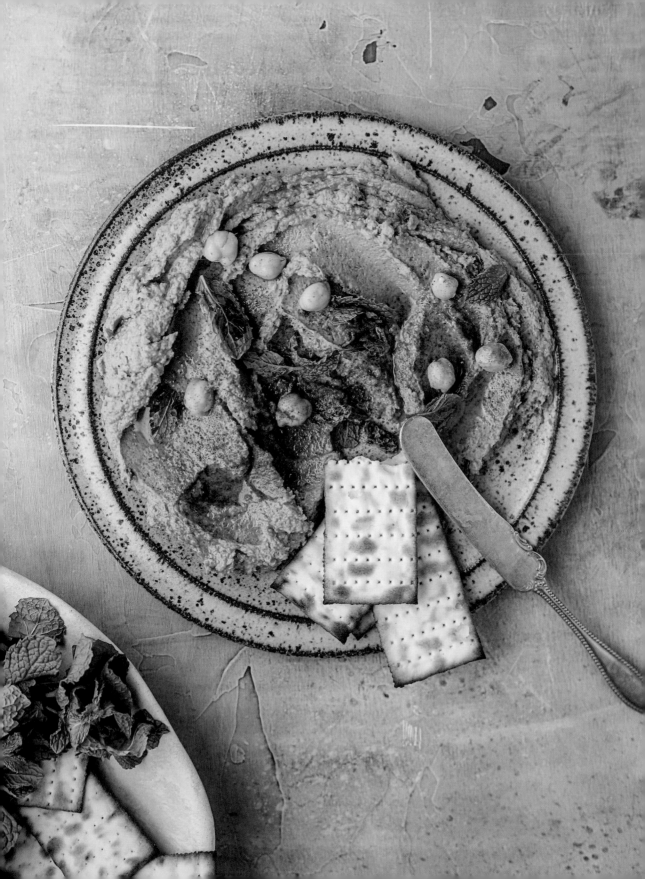

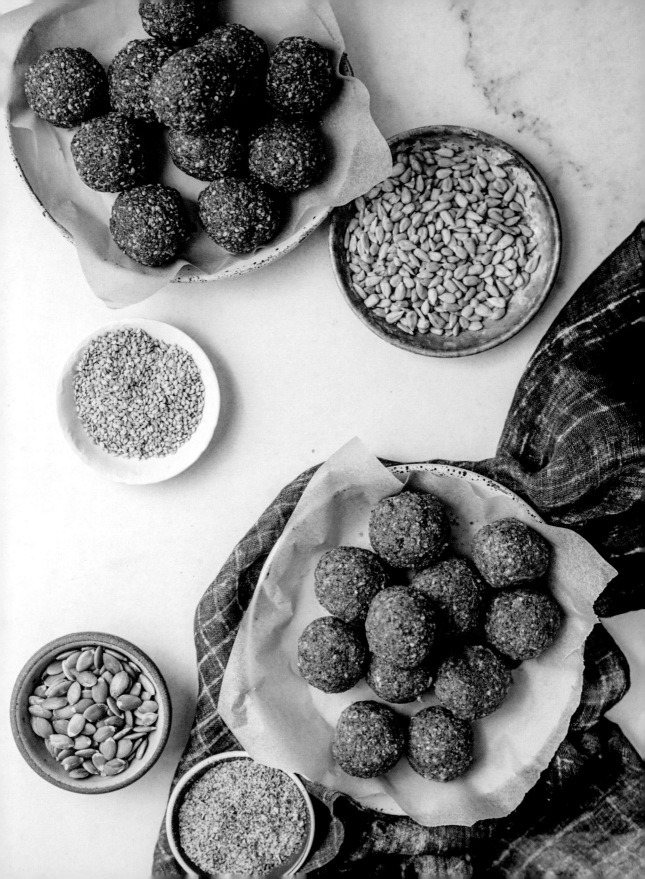

Hormone-Balancing Energy Balls, Two Ways

These grain-free energy bites are packed with healthy fats and are the perfect snack to both stabilize your blood sugar and satisfy your sweet tooth (at least a little bit). The seed pairings are based on a concept for hormone balancing that uses the power of certain seeds to support estrogen production and metabolism during a woman's cycle. Toward the beginning, from menstruation until ovulation (around Day 14), the best seeds to eat are ground flaxseeds and raw pumpkin seeds, whereas during the second half of your cycle, your hormones are best supported by raw sunflower and sesame seeds. If you've been struggling with period problems, seed cycling is an easy enough concept to follow, and these balls make the application even more delicious!

**MAKES ABOUT 20 BALLS
(SAFE SERVING: 4 BALLS)**

- ½ cup finely shredded unsweetened coconut
- ½ cup walnuts
- ½ cup flaxseed meal
- ½ cup pumpkin seeds
- 2 teaspoons ground turmeric
- ½ teaspoon ground cinnamon
- ¼ teaspoon ground ginger
- ¼ teaspoon sea salt
- 2 tablespoons pure maple syrup or clover honey
- ½ cup melted unrefined virgin coconut oil
- ¼ cup almond butter
- ¼ cup nondairy milk (almond, hemp, or flax)
- ¼ cup grass-fed collagen (optional)

Flax & Pumpkin Golden Milk Balls

❶ Line a baking sheet or plate with parchment paper and set aside. In a large food processor, pulse together the coconut, walnuts, flaxseed meal, pumpkin seeds, turmeric, cinnamon, ginger, and salt until ground into a fine meal. Add the maple syrup, coconut oil, almond butter, dairy-free milk, and collagen (if using). Puree until smooth and forming into a batter.

❷ Using 2 teaspoons or a melon baller, gather the batter into balls and roll in your hands until compact (it will be quite greasy). Place on the prepared baking sheet or plate with a little room between the balls and chill in the fridge for 10 minutes, or until solid and easy to peel off the paper. Transfer to an airtight container and store in the fridge or freezer for up to a month.

Sunflower & Sesame Mexican Chocolate Balls

Substitute ½ **cup of sesame seeds** for the flaxseed meal and ½ **cup of sunflower seeds** for the pumpkin seeds. Omit the ground ginger and turmeric. Add ¼ **cup of unsweetened cocoa powder**.

Onward Swap in 2 Medjool **dates** for the maple syrup or honey.

Use maple syrup ↓	Use honey ↓						Omit collagen ↓	
LF	SCD	SSFG	BPD1R	BPD1	BPD2	P	V	HI

Low-FODMAP Restaurant-Style Salsa

If done right, Mexican food is one of the most fun and rewarding cuisines to adapt to a SIBO diet. The base seasonings—lime juice, ground cumin, and loads of leafy cilantro—are all excellent detox ingredients. The key is to make sure the rest of the dish stands up to those same standards. This fresh version of a typical cantina salsa is perfect as a topping for organic grilled meats or to use as a dipping sauce for a low-FODMAP-friendly crisp or chip.

MAKES 2 CUPS SALSA

- 2 large vine tomatoes (1 pound), stems removed and cored
- 1 jalapeño pepper, ribs and seeds removed
- 2 tablespoons finely chopped fresh cilantro leaves
- 1 tablespoon freshly squeezed lime juice
- ½ teaspoon ground cumin
- ½ teaspoon sea salt

1 Finely chop the tomatoes and jalapeño. Transfer half to a food processor or blender. Pulse until the ingredients are pureed. Alternatively, you can skip the food processor, chop by hand, and keep it chunkier. Transfer the pureed tomatoes and the remaining chopped tomatoes and jalapeño to a medium-size bowl. Stir in the cilantro along with the lime juice, cumin, and salt.

2 Serve the salsa alongside crudités or low-FODMAP tortilla chips, or store in an airtight container for up to a week in the refrigerator.

Onward Add 1 tablespoon of finely chopped **onion**.

										Omit cilantro ↓
LF	SCD	SSFG	BPD1R	BPD1	BPD2	P	SF	V	YC	HS

Sausage Patties, Three Ways

Making homemade sausage is one of the easiest ways to get creative in the kitchen. And since most fresh butcher station options have garlic or onion, you will need to. You can use any type of ground meat as your base. I love keeping several varieties in my freezer for weekends, or using it immediately in Sausage and Sweet Pepper Hash (page 269).

MAKES 1 DOZEN SMALL PATTIES

1 pound ground pork

1 teaspoon fennel seeds

1 teaspoon paprika

½ teaspoon smoked paprika

¼ to ½ teaspoon red pepper flakes, depending on your tolerance

½ teaspoon sea salt

Oil, for frying

Hot Italian Sausage

❶ In a medium-size bowl, combine the pork, fennel seeds, paprika, smoked paprika, red pepper flakes, and salt. Mix until the spices are fully incorporated.

❷ Roll a heaping tablespoon of the meat mixture into a small ball, then flatten between your palms to form a ¼-inch-thick patty. Place on a plate and repeat with the remaining meat. You should get twelve small patties.

❸ Transfer the sausage directly to the freezer to save for another time, then transfer to a bag or lidded storage container once solid. To cook immediately, panfry the patties in a very thin layer of oil in a skillet over medium-high heat until golden brown and cooked through on both sides, about 4 minutes per side. Alternatively, bake them on a baking sheet in a 425°F oven for 20 minutes, or until browned.

Sweet Italian Sausage

Omit the smoked paprika and red pepper flakes. Add **¼ teaspoon of dried thyme**, **¼ teaspoon of dried oregano**, and **1 teaspoon of coconut sugar**.

Lamb Merguez Sausage

Omit the fennel seeds, paprika, and red pepper flakes. Substitute **1 pound of ground lamb** for the pork. Add **1 teaspoon of ground cumin**, **½ teaspoon of ground coriander**, **¼ teaspoon of ground ginger**, and **⅛ teaspoon of cayenne pepper**.

Onward Add 1 small, minced **garlic** clove.

LF	SCD	SSFG	BPD1R	BPD1	BPD2	P	Use ground chicken instead of pork or lamb ↓		Omit sugar in Sweet Italian Sausage recipe ↓	
							HS	HI	YC	SF

Plant-Based Milk, Two Ways

Nondairy "milks" are a dime a dozen these days at the grocery store. Well, more like sixty dollars a dozen. Saving money is just one of the many reasons to try making your own nut- or seed-based milks at home. You'll also avoid the many additives on the ingredient label. Plus, these homemade versions just taste better. If you want a little sweetness, you can add a smidge of pure maple syrup or clover honey to taste and a splash of pure vanilla extract. Store the milk in an airtight container in the refrigerator for up to five days. Shake well before drinking, as it will separate without stabilizers.

MAKES 1 QUART MILK

1 cup raw almonds (soaked overnight in room-temperature water or for 1 to 2 hours in boiling water)

4 cups filtered water

Pinch of sea salt

Almond Milk

❶ Drain the almonds of their soaking water and rinse thoroughly.

❷ Add the almonds, 4 cups filtered water, and the salt to a high-powered blender. Puree on the highest setting for 1 to 2 minutes, until all the nuts are broken down and the liquid is creamy.

❸ Pour the almond mixture into a nut milk bag or strainer layered with cheesecloth set over a large bowl. If using a nut milk bag, squeeze immediately until all liquid is extracted from the nut solids. For the strainer method, allow gravity to do most of the work, then gather the corners of your cheesecloth and gently squeeze before discarding. Transfer to a 1-quart mason jar or bottle.

Hemp Milk

Swap out the almonds for 1 cup of raw hemp seeds (unsoaked): combine with the water and salt in the blender and puree on the highest setting for 1 to 2 minutes. You don't need to soak or strain this one! The yield will be 5 cups of milk.

Onward Puree 1 Medjool **date** with the nuts, for sweetness.

LF	SCD	SSFG	BPD1R	BPD1	BPD2	P	HI	YC	SF	Hemp version only ↓
										HS

Golden Glow Latte

If you're feeling achy and inflamed, add a little medicine from your spice rack with this golden milk latte. Turmeric is basically Ayurvedic Advil, making this caffeine-free beverage the perfect anti-inflammatory way to start your day. When using spices in cooking, you always want to add a little heat to turn them "on." In this case, the hot water brings out the full golden hue of the turmeric. If you don't have a high-powered blender to help add more heat, alternatively you can simmer the ingredients over low heat in a saucepan. Just wait until the end to whisk in the collagen. And if you're sensitive to histamine, omit it entirely.

MAKES 1 DRINK

1 tablespoon coconut butter

1 teaspoon pure maple syrup or clover honey

2 tablespoons grass-fed collagen powder

¾ teaspoon ground turmeric

¼ teaspoon ground ginger

⅛ teaspoon ground cinnamon

1 cup nondairy milk (almond, hemp, oat, or flax)

❶ Bring a kettle of water to a boil.

❷ In a blender, combine the coconut butter, maple syrup, collagen powder, turmeric, ginger, and cinnamon.

❸ Cover the spice mixture with ½ cup of boiling water, followed by the nondairy milk.

❹ Puree the golden milk until frothy and transfer to a mug. Enjoy immediately.

Use maple syrup ↓	Use honey ↓							Omit collagen ↓			Omit sweetener ↓	
LF	SCD	SSFG	BPD1R	BPD1	BPD2	P	V	HS	YC	HI	YC	SF

Happy Tummy Digestive Tea

This peppermint-ginger tea is minty, spicy, and slightly woody, thanks to the whole cumin seeds, which are commonly used in Ayurvedic medicine to treat digestive discomfort. If you're feeling lazy, you can skip the peppermint leaves and cumin entirely and just submerge sliced fresh ginger in hot water. This recipe calls for an infuser or cheesecloth, but if you don't have one, place the spice and herb mixture in a teapot or heatproof bowl, then strain through a mesh sieve after ten minutes.

MAKES 1 CUP TEA

- 1 teaspoon dried peppermint leaves
- 1 teaspoon cumin seeds
- 1 heaping teaspoon minced fresh ginger (from 1 inch of peeled ginger)
- 8 ounces boiling water

❶ Combine the peppermint leaves, cumin seeds, and minced ginger in an infuser or cheesecloth sachet, and place it in a heatproof mug.

❷ Pour the boiling water over the tea blend. Steep for 10 minutes, remove the infuser or sachet, and enjoy.

Onward Add 1 teaspoon of **chamomile** flowers and/or **fennel seeds**.

LF	SCD	SSFG	BPD1R	BPD1	BPD2	P	V	HS	HI	YC	SF

Hibiscus Arnold Palmers

The hibiscus flower has been touted for many medicinal uses: lowering blood pressure, balancing blood sugar levels, and supporting liver function. It's also used as a digestive aid, especially for those prone to constipation. This drink is a healthy spin on an Arnold Palmer using homemade hibiscus tea. If you can't find hibiscus petals, simple look for a bagged hibiscus tea that doesn't include other ingredients or additives. You can adjust the sweetness level, but with your critters in mind, I kept it purposefully on the tart side. I love making a big batch of this tea, especially in the summer months, and keeping it in the fridge for occasional sipping. Fresh lemon juice is a wonderful addition in the morning, and combined with the hibiscus, it can give your liver a much-needed boost.

MAKES FOUR 16-OUNCE DRINKS

- 8 cups filtered water
- ¼ cup dried hibiscus petals
- 2 tablespoons pure maple syrup or honey
- ½ cup freshly squeezed lemon juice (from 2 to 3 lemons)

❶ Bring 4 cups of the water to a boil. Place the hibiscus and maple syrup in a 2-quart carafe or heatproof bowl, and pour the hot water over it. Steep the hibiscus for 15 minutes.

❷ Strain the tea mixture through a fine-mesh sieve into a 3-quart (or larger) container. Add the remaining 4 cups of water and the lemon juice. Chill until ready to serve, or pour the Arnold Palmers immediately over ice.

Use maple syrup ↓	Use honey ↓					Omit sweetener ↓					Sub lime juice for lemon, unless tolerated ↓
LF	SCD	SSFG	BPD1R	BPD1	BPD2	YC	SF	P	HS	V	HI

Green Immunity Smoothie

This drink is closer to a juice than a smoothie, and not for the vegetable lover faint of heart. If you want to get your green on in the morning without any blood sugar spikes or added sweetness, this is basically a salad in a glass. The cucumber and spinach are on the sweeter side, while the kale, ginger, and lime juice give it a slight bitter, spicy punch. For best results, I'd recommend using a high-powered blender that can make short work of the seeds and fiber. If you really don't love that pulpy consistency, you can strain the liquid through a fine-mesh sieve to make it more juice-like.

MAKES ONE 16-OUNCE DRINK

- 1 cup loosely packed baby spinach
- 1 kale leaf, stemmed
- 2 medium-size cucumbers, peeled and roughly chopped
- 1 (1-inch) piece fresh ginger, peeled
- 2 tablespoons freshly squeezed lime juice (from 1 lime)
- Pinch of sea salt

1 In a high-powered blender, combine the spinach, kale, cucumber, ginger, lime juice, and salt. Puree until the mixture is frothy and smooth. You want the consistency to be somewhere between a juice and a smoothie.

2 Pour the drink into a pint-size mason jar or glass and enjoy.

Onward Add 1 **celery** stalk or ¼ **green apple**.

LF	SCD	SSFG	BPD1R	BPD1	BPD2	P	SF	V	YC	Omit spinach ↓
										HI

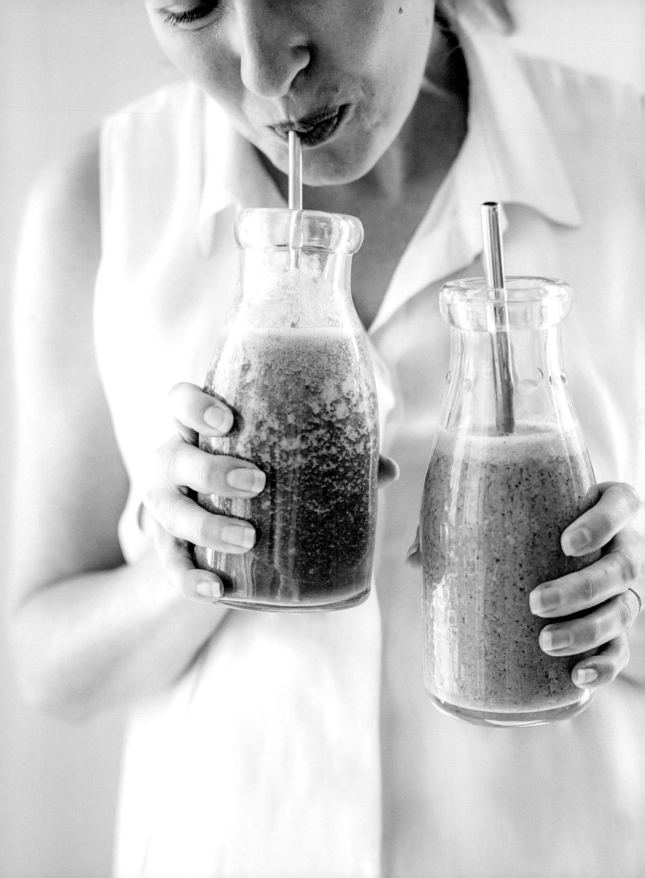

Very Berry Smoothie

I find that forming a smoothie habit is much easier when starting with frozen produce. I usually get a market haul at the beginning of the week, prep the fruit and veg, and freeze the pieces for future use as part of my batch-cooking routine. You can, of course, use fresh produce instead. Since SIBO Amigos benefit from warmer foods, I'd recommend leaving your fruit to thaw for a few minutes if using frozen. This berry smoothie was designed with your blood sugar in mind and is on the tarter side. If you need extra sweetness, you can add a splash of pure maple syrup or honey. Half of a banana also works, as specified in the "Onward" section. Finally, smoothies are some of my favorite ways of packing in gut-promoting powders. Depending on where you are in your treatment, add collagen powder, prebiotic powders (e.g., partially hydrolyzed guar gum), or your favorite adaptogens (maca, in particular, is great for thyroid health).

MAKES ONE 16-OUNCE DRINK

- 1 cup frozen strawberries (about 10)
- ¼ cup frozen blueberries
- ¼ cup frozen kale or spinach
- 1 tablespoon peanut or almond butter
- 1 cup nondairy milk (almond, flax, or hemp)

❶ In a high-powered blender, combine the strawberries, blueberries, kale, peanut butter, and nondairy milk. Puree until smooth, adding more nondairy milk if necessary to reach your desired consistency.

❷ Pour the drink into a pint-size mason jar or glass and enjoy.

Onward Add ½ **banana**.

LF	SCD	SSFG	BPD1	BPD2	P	SF	V	YC	Omit greens and almond butter ↓	Use kale ↓
									HS	HI

24-Hour Yogurt, Two Ways

The longer yogurt ferments, the less lactose it has. This is why homemade 24-hour yogurt is low-FODMAP, whereas most generic store-bought yogurts are not. Luckily, it's very simple to make using one of two methods: an Instant Pot with a yogurt function, or a stovetop. All you need is a store-bought starter or a little leftover yogurt to get your fermentation going. The following recipes make perfectly creamy yogurt, but if you would like a thicker consistency that's closer to Greek yogurt, you can place the finished yogurt in a strainer lined with cheesecloth or a clean, thin dish towel. Set it over a large bowl and allow the whey to strain from the yogurt for three to five hours, depending on your desired thickness. Both varieties will keep for at least two weeks in the fridge. Since this is the only recipe in this book that uses cow's milk, remember to buy organic to avoid unwanted hormones!

MAKES 2 QUARTS YOGURT (6 CUPS IF STRAINED)

2 quarts organic whole milk

Yogurt starter culture (use the amount specified on the package instructions), or 2 tablespoons plain organic yogurt with live active cultures

▷ Special equipment

Instant Pot with yogurt setting

Instant Pot Homemade 24-Hour Yogurt

❶ Pour the milk into the basin of your Instant Pot. Press the **YOGURT** button and adjust to the **BOIL** mode. Let the milk heat until the Instant Pot beeps to indicate the cycle is finished.

❷ Allow the milk to cool to between 95° and 110°F, about 30 minutes. If you don't have a thermometer, a good rule of thumb is that when it's the right temperature, you should be able to hold your (clean!) finger in the milk for 10 seconds. If it's too hot to handle for that amount of time, it's still too hot. You can speed up the process by placing the basin of the Instant Pot in an ice bath and stirring the milk for a few minutes until cool.

❸ When the milk has come down to temperature, ladle ½ cup into a small bowl, add the yogurt starter or plain yogurt, and whisk until smooth. Transfer the starter mixture back to the basin of milk, whisking well to combine.

❹ Turn the Instant Pot **YOGURT** function back on, close the lid, and adjust the time to 8 hours. Begin checking the yogurt at 4 hours by carefully removing the lid (there will be condensation, and you want to avoid it dripping into the yogurt) and gently tilting the basin. When the yogurt is ready, it will have set into a soft gelatin-like texture that jiggles when the basin is jostled. It may also come away from the sides of the basin. If your yogurt is not set after 4 hours, continue checking every hour until it has the texture described (it could take up to 8 hours).

recipe continues →

5 Once the yogurt is set, remove the Instant Pot basin and place your yogurt in the refrigerator, being careful not to disturb it. Allow the yogurt to cool for at least 2 hours, then scoop into an airtight container and enjoy for up to 1 week.

Stovetop 24-Hour Yogurt

1 Pour the milk into a large (4-quart or more), heavy lidded pot or Dutch oven. Heat over medium-low heat, whisking constantly until the milk reaches 185°F or is quite frothy.

2 Remove from the heat and allow the milk to cool down to 116°F, about 30 minutes. (See Step 2 of the Instant Pot directions for how to hack this without a thermometer.)

3 When the milk has come down to temperature, ladle ½ cup into a small bowl, add the yogurt starter or yogurt, and whisk until smooth. Transfer the starter mixture back to the pot of milk, whisking well to combine.

4 Cover the pot with a lid. If you are using a Dutch oven or other very heavy-sided pot, transfer it immediately into your oven with the pilot light on. If you are using a standard thin stockpot, wrap the pot completely in a towel or a large blanket before moving it to the oven. You are aiming to keep the pot as insulated as possible as the yogurt incubates. Set a timer for 6 hours and be careful not to turn your oven on at all during the incubation process!

5 Begin checking the yogurt at 6 hours by carefully removing the lid and following the specifications in Step 4 of the Instant Pot recipe. Follow the remaining instructions in Step 5 of that recipe.

LF	SCD	SSFG	BPD2	P	V	SF

Sauerkraut

Making sauerkraut could not be easier. It takes only fifteen minutes to an hour to prepare your jar for fermentation. Then, the process is fairly hands-off: simply start tasting your kraut on Day 3 and move it to the refrigerator when you're satisfied (leave a week to ten days total, depending on the temperature in your home). Besides the following ingredients, you'll also need the special equipment listed below. One of the only things that can go wrong is for mold to form on the top of the kraut if there isn't enough brine to submerge it. If the cabbage isn't submerged after twenty-four hours, dissolve 1 teaspoon of salt in 1 cup of water and add enough to cover the vegetables. This technique works for all sorts of vegetables; try it with cucumbers and radishes!

MAKES 1 PINT KRAUT (SAFE SERVING: 1 TABLESPOON)

- 1 small green cabbage (about 1 pound)
- 2 teaspoons fine sea salt

▷ Special equipment

- 1 quart-size sterilized mason jar
- 1 small (8-ounce) jelly-size jar
- 1 square of cheesecloth

  Rubber band

① Remove the thick outer layers of the cabbage until you reach the smooth, light green interior. Cut the head into quarters lengthwise. Remove the core at the center and thinly slice. You should have about 6 cups of shredded cabbage.

② In a large bowl, toss the cabbage with the salt. With clean hands, massage the shredded cabbage for 2 to 5 minutes, or until it begins to release some of its liquid and soften. You may want to rush this step, but don't—it's really important for making sure you have enough liquid later on to submerge the cabbage.

③ Transfer the cabbage to a quart-size sterilized mason jar along with any liquid. Using a wooden spoon, push the cabbage down until it compacts into the bottom half of the jar, releasing more juices in the process. Allow to sit for an hour, then tamp down the cabbage again with your wooden spoon—muddling the cabbage like this will continue to release more liquid.

④ Place the smaller jar inside the larger jar. You can weight it down with a rock, but just the jar is usually heavy enough to make sure the shredded cabbage stays beneath the brine (see note). Cover the top of the jar with the cheesecloth and secure with a rubber band so no flies or bugs can get in.

⑤ Set the jar in a shaded area of your countertop and allow to ferment for 3 to 10 days. For the first 24 hours, tamp it down every couple hours by placing some pressure on the smaller interior jar. Start tasting it after the first few days, and when the cabbage tastes sufficiently fermented, cover and store in the refrigerator. The kraut will keep for a month.

LF	SCD	SSFG	BPD1R	BPD1	BPD2	P	SF	V

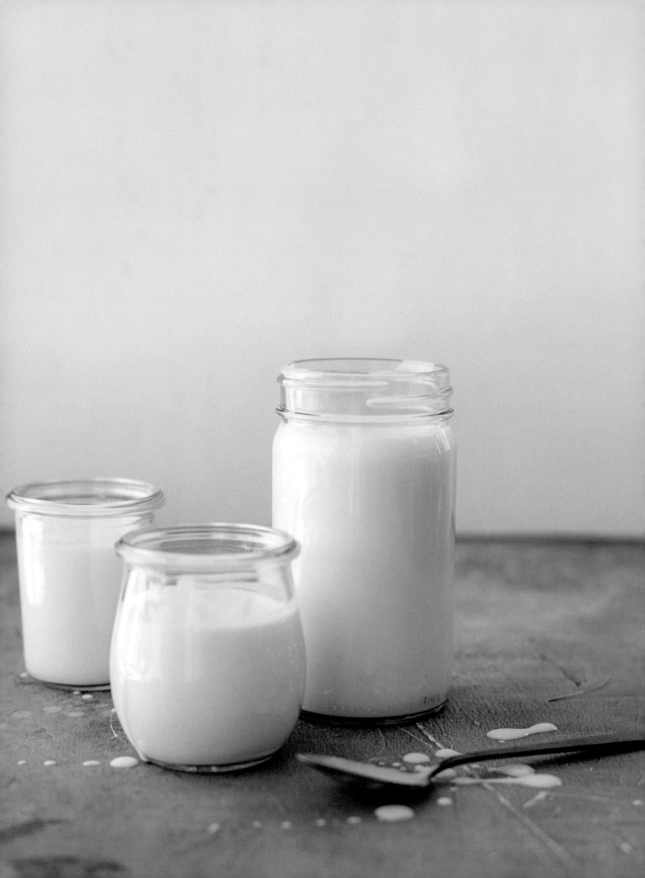

Coconut Kefir

You can buy prepared kefir, a fermented drink with a pleasantly sour taste, a lot of places these days—but it is also easy to make. Although homemade kefir does take much longer than most recipes in this book (one to two days), the process is completely hands-off once you have the right ingredients. I adapted this recipe from Dana Shultz at Minimalist Baker, and if you have any issues or fears, I'd highly recommend checking out the troubleshooting section on her site. The following brands are her recommendations. Whichever probiotic you use, make sure it's a capsule, so you can easily open and empty it into the coconut milk. Lastly, the kefir plain is a bit tangy. If you don't mind a little added sugar, feel free to sweeten modestly with pure maple syrup or clover honey. It's lovely drizzled over granola or in savory sauces and dressings. There's some controversy over the place of fermented foods in a SIBO diet (more about this on page 121), but the rule of thumb is easy to remember: if you tolerate it, eat it!

MAKES 2 CUPS KEFIR (SAFE SERVING: ¼ CUP)

1 (14-ounce) can organic full-fat coconut milk (Whole Foods 365 brand)

2 capsules high-quality probiotic (Renew Life Ultra Flora 50 Billion)

▷ Special equipment

1 quart-size sterilized mason jar

1 square of cheesecloth

Rubber band

❶ Sterilize a 1-quart mason jar by rinsing with boiling water and letting it dry completely. Let cool to room temperature.

❷ Shake your can of coconut milk well, and pour the contents into the sterilized, cooled jar. Whisk the coconut milk until smooth.

❸ Empty your probiotic capsules into the coconut milk and use a wooden or plastic spoon to stir, making sure there are no clumps. (Note: Metal utensils can react negatively with probiotics.)

❹ Cover the mixture with a double layer of cheesecloth and secure with a rubber band.

❺ Let the coconut milk sit for at least 24 hours in a warm area (75°F is ideal) and up to 48 hours, until thick and tangy. (For coconut yogurt, simply allow the milk to thicken and sit for longer.) The longer the kefir sits, the thicker and tangier the end result will be. If your home is too cold, store the jar in the oven (unheated) with the light on to create a warm environment.

❻ Cover with an airtight lid and refrigerate until ready to eat. The kefir will thicken more in the fridge, but will keep for up to a week.

LF	SCD	SSFG	BPD2	P	SF	HS	V

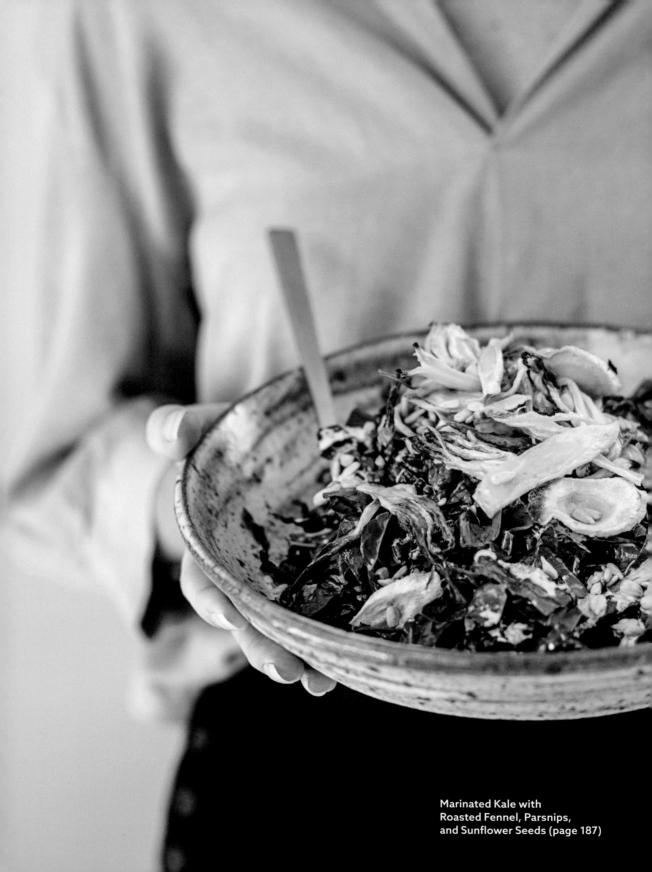

Marinated Kale with
Roasted Fennel, Parsnips,
and Sunflower Seeds (page 187)

SALADS & VEGGIE SIDES

French Bean and Carrot Salad with Green Harissa Sauce

This is the consummate crowd-pleasing side dish. The green harissa is both delicious and perfect for detoxing, as it's packed with cilantro, spinach, and gut-aiding spices. The only dietary note is to roughly monitor the quantity of green beans: if you are sensitive, aim for about fifteen to remain low-FODMAP.

MAKES 6 SIDE SERVINGS (SAFE SERVING: 15 GREEN BEANS)

- 1 pound carrots (about 8 medium), preferably assorted colors
- Extra-virgin olive oil
- Sea salt
- 1 pound French green beans, ends trimmed
- 1½ cups coarsely chopped fresh cilantro leaves and stems
- 1½ cups tightly packed baby spinach leaves
- 1 jalapeño pepper, ribs and seeds removed, coarsely chopped
- 2 tablespoons freshly squeezed lime juice (from 1 lime)
- ½ teaspoon ground cumin
- ½ teaspoon ground coriander

1 Preheat the oven to 425°F. Line a baking sheet with parchment paper.

2 Trim the carrots and cut them lengthwise in half (or quarters, if on the thicker side). On the prepared baking sheet, toss the carrots with 2 tablespoons of olive oil and ½ teaspoon of salt until coated. Arrange in an even layer, cut side down, and roast in the oven for about 30 minutes, or until the carrots are tender and caramelized.

3 Meanwhile, bring a large pot of salted water to a boil.

4 Add the beans to the boiling water and cook for 4 minutes, until vibrant and al dente. Drain the beans in a colander and run under cold water to stop the cooking. Shake out all the excess water.

5 Meanwhile, combine the cilantro, spinach, jalapeño, lime juice, cumin, coriander, ¼ cup of olive oil and ¾ teaspoon of salt in a blender or food processor and puree until smooth; then add water, 1 tablespoon at a time, until the harissa is slightly thinner than pesto (2 tablespoons of water should do it). Taste for seasoning and add more salt as necessary.

6 Arrange the carrots and green beans on a platter and drizzle with half of the sauce. Add more, if necessary, or save the remaining as a marinade for grilled meats or salad dressing.

Onward Garnish the salad with 2 tablespoons of roughly chopped, toasted **pistachios**.

										Omit jalapeño; replace spinach with arugula ↓
LF	SCD	SSFG	BPD1R	BPD1	BPD2	YC	P	V	SF	HI

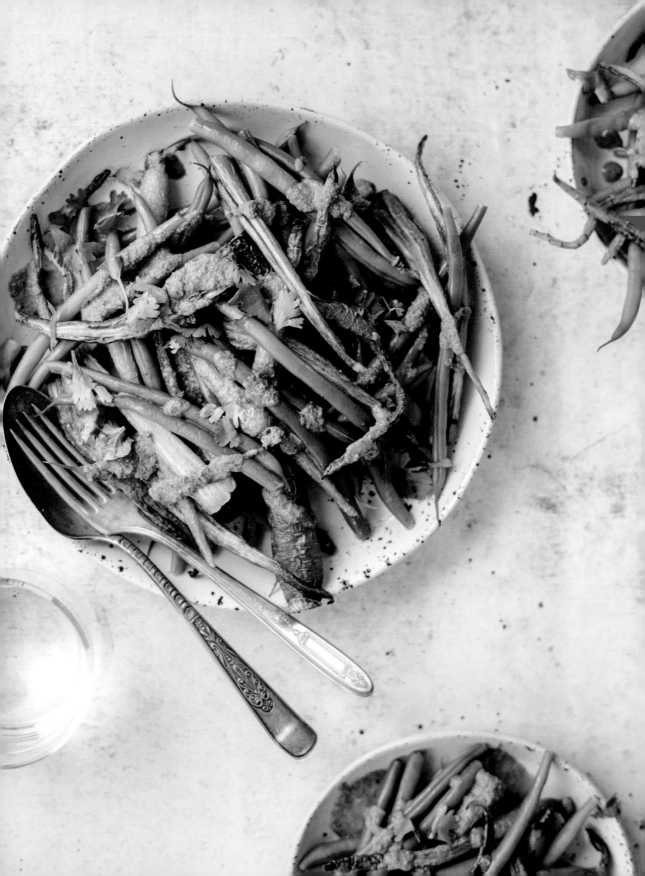

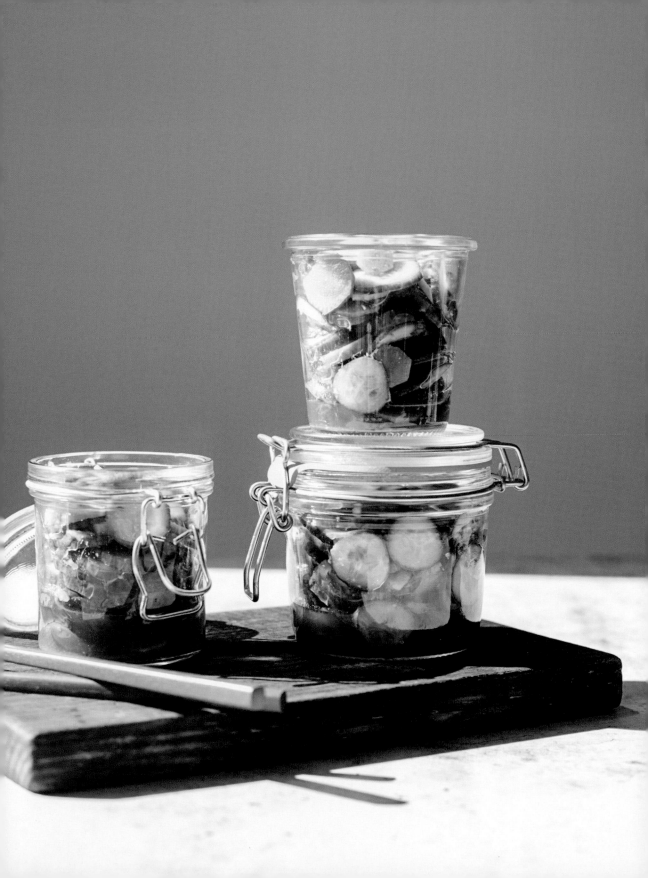

Heat-Free Cucumber Kimchi

This cucumber salad is more of a quick pickle than a long-fermented kimchi. Instead of loading it up with Korean chili flakes that might upset your gut, I rely on the natural heat from raw ginger to add a kick. Ordinarily, you'll notice that gluten-free tamari and coconut aminos are interchangeable in these recipes. But I opted for the fermented coconut in this case, since it brings with it some sweetness, which allows you to skip the sugar that's normally found in a quick pickle. This is a great side for so many dishes in this book, but I particularly enjoy serving it with the Larb Lettuce Wraps (page 265), Thai Green Curry Chicken (page 246) or Vietnamese Roasted Eggplant Salad (page 174).

MAKES 4 CUPS KIMCHI

- 1 pound Persian cucumbers (the small, seedless ones), unpeeled, thinly sliced
- 1 medium-size carrot, peeled and thinly sliced
- 1½ teaspoons sea salt
- 1 (1-inch) piece fresh ginger, peeled
- 2 scallions, green parts only
- 2 tablespoons rice vinegar or apple cider vinegar
- 2 tablespoons freshly squeezed lime juice (from 1 lime)
- 1 tablespoon Asian fish sauce (I like Red Boat brand)
- 1 tablespoon coconut aminos

❶ In a medium-size bowl, sprinkle the cucumbers and carrots with the salt. Toss a few times until coated and set aside to soften while you make the dressing.

❷ In a small food processor, combine the ginger, scallions, vinegar, lime juice, fish sauce, and coconut aminos. Puree until everything is well minced. Alternatively, you can finely chop by hand.

❸ Pour the sauce over the cucumbers and toss to combine. Serve as a condiment or side salad.

Onward Add 1 small **shallot** and/or 1 small **garlic** clove to the paste.

Use pure maple syrup ↓	Use honey and apple cider vinegar ↓				Omit fish sauce ↓	Omit scallions ↓	
LF	SCD	SSFG	BPD1	BPD2	V	HS	P

Vietnamese Roasted Eggplant Salad

Vietnamese cuisine essentially treats fresh herbs how Applebee's treats shredded iceberg. It's always piled onto plates as a miscellaneous garnish, and eaten in larger quantities (often in one mouthful) than most Americans allot to their total daily vegetables. This is one of the reasons that the region makes for such great healthy hedonist inspiration. Even when the centerpiece (in this case, roasted eggplant) is crisped or charred, the herbs transform it into something light and summery. Since the marinade renders plenty of sauce, you can serve the eggplant as a main course over rice or as a grain-free filling for Bibb lettuce cups. In warmer weather (and when my gut is on the stronger side), I like tossing the whole thing together with a 5-ounce bag of watercress or baby arugula, since there's a built-in dressing. Although the roasting process is fairly hands-off, an alternative is to grill the eggplant in slabs, then roughly chop and toss with the sauce.

MAKES 4 SIDE SERVINGS

- 2 medium-size eggplant (about 1½ pounds), cut into ½-inch cubes
- 2 tablespoons extra-virgin olive oil
- ½ teaspoon sea salt
- ¼ cup gluten-free tamari or coconut aminos
- ¼ cup freshly squeezed lime juice (from 2 limes)
- ¼ teaspoon cayenne pepper (optional)
- 1 tablespoon minced fresh ginger
- ¼ cup roughly chopped fresh cilantro leaves
- ¼ cup roughly chopped fresh mint leaves

❶ Preheat the oven to 425°F. Line two baking sheets with parchment paper.

❷ In a large bowl, toss the eggplant with the olive oil and salt. Divide between the two prepared baking sheets and arrange in an even layer on each pan. Transfer to the oven and bake until soft and beginning to brown, about 30 minutes, swapping the pans halfway through for even color.

❸ While the eggplant is roasting, whisk together the tamari, lime juice, cayenne, and ginger in the same large bowl, then set aside.

❹ Add the cooked eggplant to the bowl along with the cilantro and mint. Toss to combine and taste for seasoning.

❺ Serve the eggplant salad immediately warm, or later at room temperature.

Onward Thinly slice 1 **leek** and roast with the eggplant.

				Use coconut aminos ↓				Omit cilantro ↓
V	SF	LF	SCD	SSFG	BPD1	BPD2	P	HS

Zucchini Carpaccio with Pine Nuts and Crispy Prosciutto

When summer vegetables are at their peak, I try not to cook them to death or gild the lily with too many fussy garnishes. But since SIBO folks with inflamed guts benefit from their food being warm or partially broken down, I like using fresh lemon juice as a marinade to help soften fresh vegetables. In this case, the zucchini and summer squash coins "cook" in the acid, similar to a ceviche. You can substitute toasted walnuts for the more expensive pine nuts (but in this recipe, which has so few ingredients, they really shine and are worth the investment).

MAKES 4 SIDE SERVINGS

3 ounces prosciutto di Parma (about 6 slices)

¼ cup pine nuts

8 ounces zucchini (1 medium)

8 ounces summer squash (1 medium)

Sea salt

¼ cup freshly squeezed lemon juice (from 1 to 2 lemons)

¼ cup extra-virgin olive oil

5 ounces baby arugula (about 5 cups, tightly packed)

❶ Preheat the oven to 375°F. Line a baking sheet with parchment paper.

❷ Arrange the prosciutto on the prepared baking sheet. Transfer to the oven and cook until dark and crispy, about 10 minutes. Allow to cool on the pan and break apart with your fingers into large pieces.

❸ While the prosciutto cooks, toast the pine nuts: arrange the nuts in a small skillet and cook over medium-low heat until golden brown and fragrant, about 5 minutes.

❹ **Prep the zucchini and squash:** with a sharp knife, slice as thinly as you can into rounds (¹/₁₆ inch thick with a mandoline). Arrange the zucchini and squash on a large platter, fanning out the rounds as much as possible and alternating sections of color. Season lightly with salt.

❺ In a small bowl or a jar with a lid, combine the lemon juice, olive oil, and ½ teaspoon of salt. Stir or shake until well mixed. Pour half of the dressing evenly over the zucchini and squash.

❻ In a large bowl, toss the arugula with the remaining dressing and pile on top of the squash coins. Garnish with the pine nuts and flecks of crispy prosciutto.

Onward Thinly slice 2 **celery** stalks and toss with the arugula.

LF	SF	SSFG	BPD1R	BPD1	BPD2	P	SF	Omit prosciutto; sub lime juice for lemon, unless tolerated ↓	Omit prosciutto ↓
								YC	HI	V

Southwestern Wedge Salad with Sweet & Smoky Pepita Brittle

BREAKING NEWS: I just welcomed your grandma's wedge salad into this century, and boy, is it happy to be here for the fiesta! This is one of the most glamorous recipes in the book, and yet also one of the easiest to make. It might seem like a lot of elements, but they are all quick to throw together and last all week long. If raw foods are a little much for your digestive system, you can give the wedges a quick sear on the grill or stovetop.

MAKES 6 SIDE SERVINGS

▷ Brittle

½ cup pepitas (pumpkin seeds)

1 tablespoon extra-virgin olive oil

2 teaspoons clover honey or pure maple syrup

¼ teaspoon smoked paprika

¼ teaspoon ground cumin

¼ teaspoon sea salt

▷ Salad

1 bunch radishes, thinly sliced

2 tablespoons apple cider vinegar

½ teaspoon sea salt

3 hearts romaine lettuce, halved lengthwise

1 cup Creamy Cilantro-Jalapeño Ranch (page 145)

1 Make the brittle: Preheat the oven to 350°F, and position a rack in the center of the oven. Line a baking sheet with parchment paper.

2 In a large bowl, combine the pumpkin seeds, olive oil, honey, smoked paprika, cumin, and salt. Arrange the mixture in an even layer on the prepared baking sheet, doing your best to separate any clumps. Bake for about 15 minutes, or until browned and crunchy.

3 Remove from the oven and allow the pepitas to cool completely on the pan. Break up any remaining clusters with with your hands and store in an airtight container until ready to use. The seeds will keep for up to a week on the counter.

4 Make the salad: In a medium-size bowl, toss the radishes with the vinegar and salt. Allow to sit for 5 to 10 minutes, or until light pink and pliable.

5 To serve, arrange the romaine wedges on a platter and drizzle with the cilantro-jalapeño ranch. Top with the sliced radishes and pepita brittle.

Onward Top the salad with 1 thinly sliced **avocado** or ¼ cup of crumbled **cotija cheese**.

Use pure maple syrup ↓		Use honey ↓					Omit radishes; sub oil and vinegar for dressing ↓
LF	V	SCD	SSFG	BPD1	BPD2	P	HS

SIBO Made Simple

176

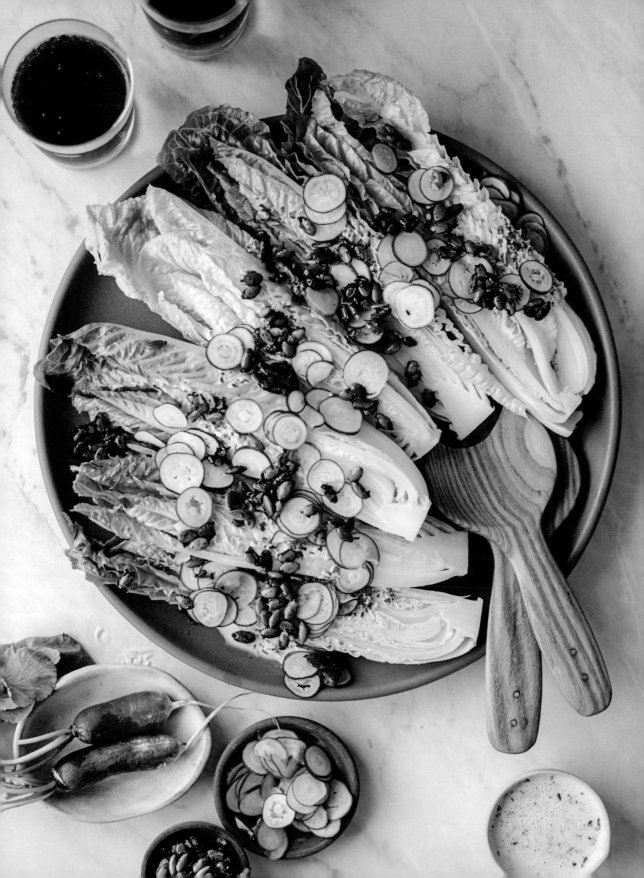

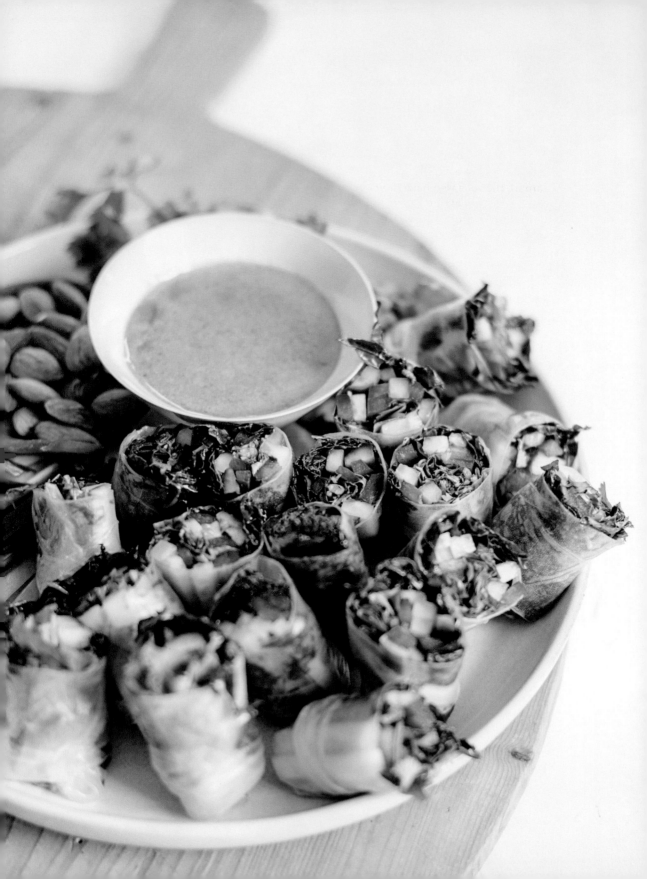

Zesty Kale Summer Rolls with Almond-Tamari Dipping Sauce

Kale ribbons replace the usual vermicelli noodles in these summer rolls, adding extra bulk without the needless carbs. Since the greens are dressed with lime juice and tamari, the rolls also have their own internal sauce so you won't be *as* tempted to double dip (my almond-tamari mixture is so addictive, who could blame you!). If you don't feel like going the extra mile to prepare the kale, you can also just use plain undressed Bibb lettuce or mounds of mint and basil leaves as your greens. Same goes if you don't like cilantro. The beauty of summer rolls is that you can individualize them. Lastly, if following a carb-free diet, you might enjoy a deconstructed version of this dish—just toss all the veggies together as a salad and use the dipping sauce as your dressing.

MAKES 12 ROLLS OR 4 APPETIZER SERVINGS

▷ **Sauce**

½ cup almond butter

¼ cup freshly squeezed lime juice (from 2 limes)

¼ cup gluten-free tamari or coconut aminos

2 teaspoons clover honey or pure maple syrup

1 teaspoon sea salt

½ teaspoon ground ginger

▷ **Rolls**

1 medium-size bunch lacinato kale, thick stems removed, thinly sliced (4 cups, packed)

1 tablespoon freshly squeezed lime juice (from ½ lime)

1 tablespoon gluten-free tamari or coconut aminos

1 tablespoon extra-virgin olive oil

Sea salt

2 small Persian or Kirby cucumbers, or 1 seedless regular cucumber, julienned

1 red bell pepper, julienned

1 bunch cilantro, coarse stems removed (the bottom third)

12 (8-inch) rice paper spring roll wrappers

❶ **Make the sauce:** In a medium-size bowl, combine the almond butter, lime juice, tamari, honey, salt, and ginger. Whisk until smooth, adding 1 tablespoon of water at a time until it reaches the consistency of ranch dressing.

❷ **Make the rolls:** In a large bowl, combine the kale, lime juice, tamari, and olive oil. Massage with your hands until the kale is fully coated in the dressing and has begun to wilt. Season to taste with salt.

recipe continues →

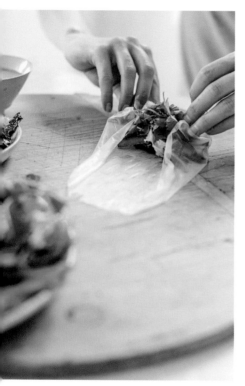

❸ Heat 4 cups of water in a kettle until just shy of boiling. Pour the water into a baking dish so it comes up the sides by at least ½ inch. Keep the remaining hot water handy, in case the water in the dish begins to cool.

❹ Arrange the cucumber, red pepper, and cilantro in neat piles on a plate or shallow bowl.

❺ When cool enough to touch, dip one spring roll wrapper in the baking dish of hot water to coat on both sides, shaking off any excess. Immediately place on a large cutting board or clean work surface. Wait about 15 seconds for the skins to soften. Add a small handful of kale to the bottom half of the wrapper closest to you. Then, top with three to four cucumber spears, three to four red pepper slices, and a few cilantro sprigs, arranging the veggies parallel to the edge of your cutting board. Fold in the sides of the wrapper lengthwise—you should have about an inch on either end to play with. Fold over the long flap closest to you and pull it tight around the vegetable pile so it seals with the paper on the other side. Then, roll the whole thing up like a burrito. It's easiest to do this in one motion, holding the veggies in with your fingers as you roll so you have a tight package.

❻ Repeat with the remaining skins. If your roll tears, have no fear. You can double wrap. Simply repeat with a second skin. Cut each roll in half and serve alongside the almond-tamari sauce.

Onward Add a few spears of julienned **mango** to each roll.

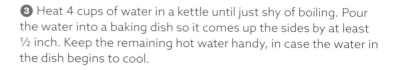

Use honey and coconut aminos ↓	Use honey and coconut aminos; omit rice paper (see headnote) ↓		Use maple syrup ↓	Omit sweetener ↓	
BPD2	SSFG	BPD1	P	LF	SF	V

Garden Salad with Carrot-Ginger Dressing

This dressing is modeled after the slightly alarming bright orange version you see at many sushi restaurants. Once I started making my own at home, I couldn't get over how sweet the one at my local joint tasted. Especially when using carrots from a farmers' market (or your garden) at the peak of their season, you hardly need any added sugar. In fact, I like adding even more acid and probiotic goodness by mixing in some fermented cabbage. If you are sensitive to fermented foods, just omit it. This salad might seem a little simple, but consider it a blank canvas for your reintroductions. A handful of snap peas, corn, or avocado are my favorites during the summer months.

MAKES 4 SERVINGS

▷ Dressing

2 medium-size carrots (about 4 ounces), peeled and roughly chopped

1 (2-inch) piece fresh ginger, peeled

¼ cup sauerkraut or fermented cabbage (see headnote)

2 tablespoons apple cider vinegar

½ teaspoon clover honey or pure maple syrup

2 tablespoons mayonnaise

½ teaspoon sea salt

¼ cup extra-virgin olive, grapeseed, or avocado oil

▷ Salad

2 heads romaine lettuce, thinly sliced

1 cup thinly sliced red or green cabbage

1 seedless cucumber, finely diced

1 cup cherry tomatoes, halved, or 2 vine tomatoes, chopped

Sea salt

2 tablespoons black sesame seeds, for garnish

❶ Make the dressing: Combine the carrots, ginger, kraut, vinegar, honey, mayonnaise, and salt in a food processor or blender and puree until smooth. Add the oil and whiz a few more times to incorporate. Add water, 1 tablespoon at a time, until the mixture is the consistency of ranch dressing (about 2 tablespoons total). Set aside or store until ready to eat (the dressing can be made up to a week in advance).

❷ Assemble the salad: On a large platter, scatter the romaine and cabbage. Drizzle lightly with dressing, then arrange the cucumbers and tomatoes on top. Season the veggies lightly with salt and the sesame seeds. Serve immediately with the remaining dressing on the side.

Onward Add ½ cup of finely sliced **sugar snap peas**, ½ cup of **sweet corn**, and/or 1 sliced **avocado**.

Use honey ↓				Omit sweetener ↓		Use maple syrup ↓			Omit mayo, kraut, and cabbage ↓
SCD	SSFG	BPD1	BPD2	BPD1R	SF	LF	P	V	HS

Chicory Salad with Jammy Eggs and Bagna Cauda Dressing

A lot of SIBO survivors complain that their diet has become completely made up of chicken and salad while reducing their carbs and FODMAPs. But even if you stick to those two basic dishes, there's a whole spectrum of leafy green options that are vibrant and full of flavor. Chicories are bitter lettuces that are often the unsung heroes of the salad world. Radicchio and Treviso add a gorgeous pop of color to your plate; curly escarole and frisée offer plenty of nooks and crannies for your dressing to cling to. This dressing is based on the Italian anchovy dip *bagna càuda*, and is a trifecta of healthy fats. You'll love the salty bite it adds to the rich, oozy eggs and bitter lettuces.

MAKES 4 MAIN COURSE SERVINGS; 6 TO 8 SIDE SERVINGS

- 4 large eggs
- 1 (2-ounce) can anchovy fillets in oil
- 2 tablespoons drained capers
- Zest of 1 lemon
- ¼ cup freshly squeezed lemon juice (from 1 to 2 lemons)
- 1 tablespoon red wine vinegar
- ¼ cup grass-fed ghee, melted
- ¼ cup extra-virgin olive oil
- ¼ teaspoon fine sea salt
- 10 cups assorted chicories (such as Belgian endive, Treviso, escarole, frisée, and/or radicchio), roughly chopped or torn into bite-size pieces
- Coarse sea salt (such as Malden)

❶ Bring a large saucepan of water to a boil over medium-high heat. Using a slotted spoon, carefully lower the eggs into the water, one at a time. Cook for 6½ minutes, adjusting the heat to maintain a gentle boil. Transfer the eggs to a bowl of ice water and chill until just slightly warm, about 2 minutes. Peel and set aside.

❷ Meanwhile, make the dressing: In a small food processor, pulse the anchovies with the capers, lemon zest, lemon juice, and vinegar until finely chopped. With the machine on, drizzle in the melted ghee and olive oil and puree until smooth. Season the dressing with ¼ teaspoon of fine sea salt.

❸ Arrange the chicories on a platter and drizzle with the dressing. Arrange the eggs around the perimeter and garnish them with coarse sea salt.

Onward Top the salad with 1 cup of canned **white beans**, drained and rinsed.

								Omit eggs; sub regular lettuce ↓
LF	SCD	SSFG	BPD1R	BPD1	BPD2	P	SF	HS

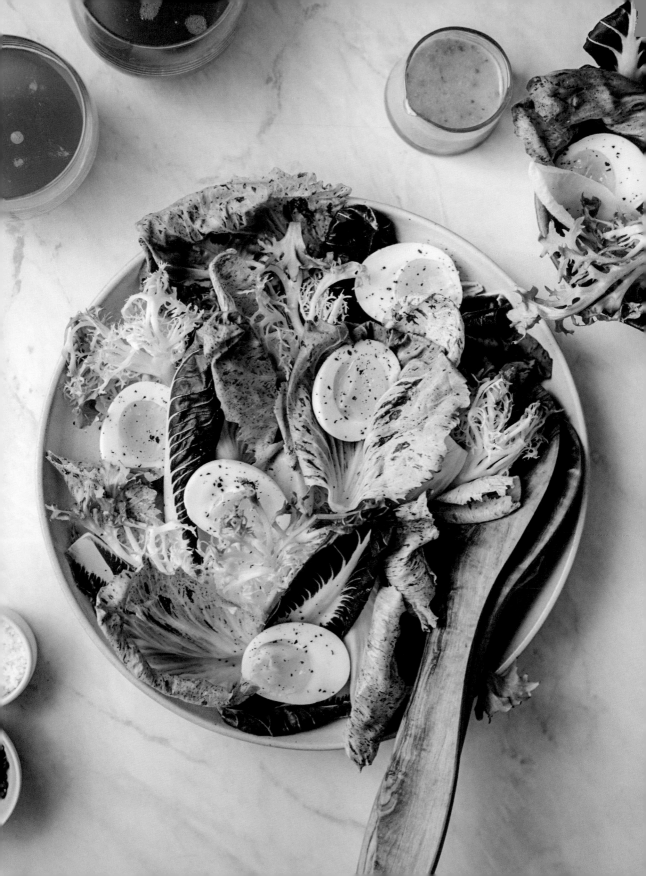

Nutty Steamed Greens

Gomaae is another one of my favorite Japanese salads that I've taken to making at home to be able to enjoy a gluten-free version with minimal sugar. It's made from blanched whole-leaf spinach and is served chilled mixed with a nutty paste of sesame seeds or peanut butter. I opted for the latter, but you can easily use tahini if you're allergic. I've made this recipe with both frozen and fresh spinach. If using fresh, heat 4 cups of water in Step 1 to blanch the leaves in. This is a fantastic accompaniment for some of the Japanese-inspired dishes in the book, such as the Teriyaki Pork Tenderloin (page 266) or Sesame Sheet Pan Salmon with Radishes (page 276).

MAKES 4 SIDE SERVINGS

1 pound frozen whole-leaf spinach (if using fresh spinach, see headnote)

1 tablespoon gluten-free tamari or coconut aminos

1 tablespoon creamy peanut butter

1 tablespoon mirin or rice vinegar

1 teaspoon clover honey or maple syrup

1 teaspoon toasted sesame oil

2 tablespoons white sesame seeds

❶ In a medium-size saucepan, bring 1 cup of water to a boil. Add the frozen spinach. Simmer, covered, over medium heat until fully defrosted, about 3 minutes. Remove from the heat and carefully pour out as much water as you can without losing the spinach down the drain.

❷ Transfer the spinach to a baking sheet lined with a clean dish towel. Gather the spinach up and squeeze as much water as you can into the sink. Transfer the dry spinach to a medium-size bowl, and put it into the fridge to cool.

❸ Meanwhile, make the sauce: In a small bowl, whisk together the tamari, peanut butter, mirin, honey or maple syrup, and sesame oil.

❹ In a small, dry skillet, toast the sesame seeds over medium-low heat until golden and nutty.

❺ Once the spinach is cool, add the sauce and toasted sesame seeds and stir to combine. Taste for seasoning and serve.

Onward Add 1 small **garlic** clove, minced, to the dressing.

Use maple syrup ↓		Use honey and coconut aminos; sub white vinegar ↓				
LF	V	SCD	SSFG	BPD1	BPD2	P

Turmeric-Ginger Stewed Eggplant

I like to think of *baingan bharta* as the baba ghanoush of Indian cuisine. But instead of getting eaten cold with a side of pita, the spiced eggplant is served over rice as a warming, tomatoey stew. This vegetarian entrée only gets better the longer it sits in the fridge, where the garam masala, ginger, and turmeric have a chance to grow in intensity. It also makes a great accompaniment to the Mild and Creamy Butterless Butter Chicken (page 255). Traditionally, this dish uses serrano peppers to give it some heat. If you can tolerate the extra kick, feel free to roast one along with the eggplant or add a dash of cayenne.

MAKES 4 SERVINGS

2 pounds eggplant (about 2 large)

3 large vine or Roma tomatoes (1 pound), halved

Extra-virgin olive oil

2 tablespoons refined virgin coconut oil or grass-fed ghee

1 tablespoon minced fresh ginger

2 teaspoons garam masala

1 teaspoon ground turmeric

1½ teaspoons sea salt

2 tablespoons freshly squeezed lime juice (from 1 lime)

2 tablespoons golden raisins

½ cup roughly chopped fresh cilantro

❶ Preheat the oven to 500°F. Line a rimmed baking sheet with parchment paper.

❷ Pierce the eggplant all over with a knife, and place it on the prepared baking sheet. Arrange the tomatoes, cut side down, around the eggplant. Drizzle the vegetables lightly with olive oil. Bake, turning the eggplant a couple of times during cooking, until it is soft to the touch and the tomatoes are well charred with the skin puckered, about 30 minutes. Remove from the oven and set aside.

❸ When cool enough to handle, peel and discard the stem and skin of the eggplant and tomatoes. Roughly chop the vegetables and transfer to a medium bowl.

❹ In a large skillet, heat the coconut oil over medium heat. Add the ginger, garam masala, and turmeric. Cook for 2 minutes, or until very fragrant. Stir in the eggplant mixture and season with the salt. Cook, stirring occasionally and breaking up any larger pieces of eggplant, until the vegetables are well combined and completely softened, about 10 minutes. Fold in the lime juice and golden raisins. Garnish with the cilantro and serve alongside rice or gluten-free naan.

Onward Sauté ½ small **onion** along with the spice mixture until soft.

LF	SCD	SSFG	P	V	Omit raisins ↓					Omit raisins and cilantro ↓
					BPD1R	BPD1	BPD2	YC	SF	HS

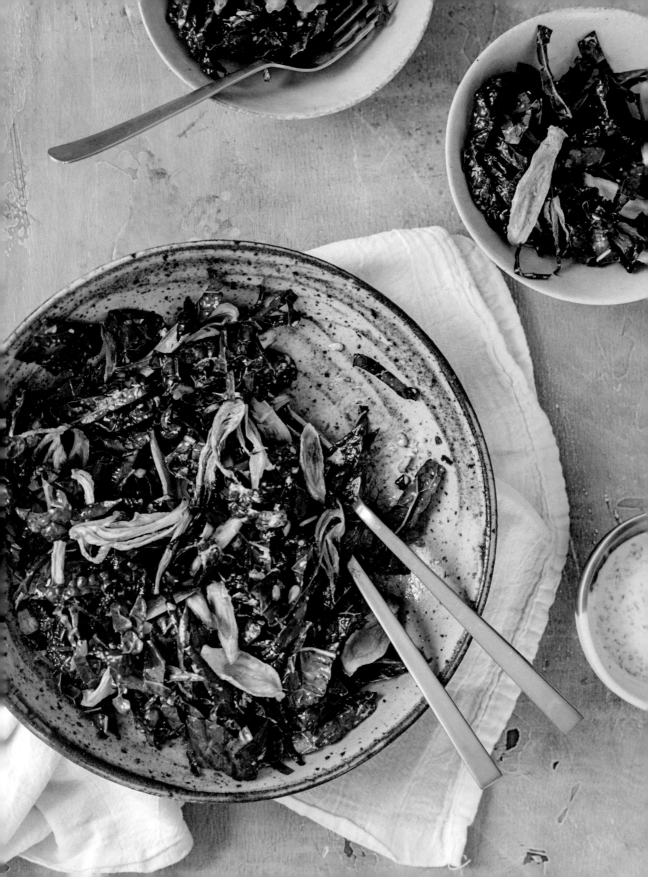

Marinated Kale with Roasted Fennel, Parsnips, and Sunflower Seeds

Kale is a terrific ingredient for meal prep because, unlike regular lettuce, it can be dressed in advance without becoming soggy. You may in fact find the opposite: that the leaves dry out as the week goes on and you need to add additional olive oil. Luckily, in this recipe, you also have a delicious tahini dressing to add even more flavor. Using half of a fennel bulb might seem strange, but it's to stay within the low-FODMAP limits. If you find you can tolerate more, feel free to use the whole bulb. Or use the remaining fennel in the Greek Chicken Zoodle Soup (page 221) or Baked Halibut with Green Olive and Fennel Tapenade (page 273). To make this a main course salad, add some protein, such as roasted chicken or a fillet of wild salmon.

MAKES 4 SIDE SERVINGS

½ medium-size fennel bulb, cut in half lengthwise through the heart, then thinly sliced into wedges

2 medium-size parsnips (about 5 ounces), peeled and thinly sliced on a diagonal

Extra-virgin olive oil

Fine sea salt

1 large bunch lacinato kale

3 tablespoons freshly squeezed lemon juice (from 1 lemon)

2 tablespoons tahini

2 tablespoons finely chopped fresh flat-leaf parsley leaves

2 tablespoons sunflower seeds

❶ Preheat the oven to 425°F. Line a baking sheet with parchment.

❷ On the prepared baking sheet, toss the fennel and parsnips with 2 tablespoons of olive oil and ½ teaspoon of salt. Arrange the veggies in an even layer and roast in the oven until tender and caramelized, about 30 minutes.

❸ **Meanwhile, prepare the kale:** Remove the thick stem by carefully tearing away the bottom part of the leaves, then grabbing hold of the stem and yanking upward. The leaf should come away intact, missing the center stem. Stack the leaves with the largest at the bottom, smallest at the top, and roll into a cigar. Thinly slice into ribbons and place in a large bowl. You should have 4 cups, packed.

❹ Add 1 tablespoon of the lemon juice, 1 tablespoon of olive oil, and ¼ teaspoon of salt. Toss the kale with clean hands until it's very well coated with the mixture—don't be afraid to manhandle it!

❺ **Make the tahini sauce:** In a medium-size bowl, whisk together (a fork is fine) the tahini, remaining 2 tablespoons of lemon juice, and ¼ teaspoon of salt. A thick paste will form—culinary magic! Whisk in water, 1 tablespoon at a time, until the dressing is pourable (around 2 tablespoons of water total). Taste for seasoning and add more salt or lemon juice as necessary. Fold in the parsley.

recipe continues ↓

6 **Assemble the salad:** top the kale with the crispy fennel and parsnips. Drizzle with the tahini sauce and garnish with sunflower seeds.

Onward **Add** ½ cup of diced roasted **beets** to the salad.

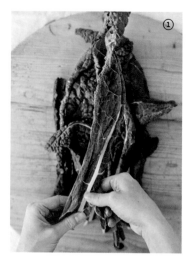

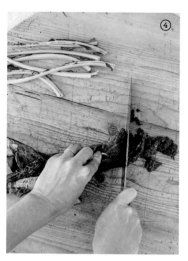

Prepare the kale:
① Remove the thick stem by carefully tearing away the bottom part of the leaves, **②** then grabbing hold of the stem and yanking upward. **③** Stack the leaves with the largest at the bottom, smallest at the top, and roll into a cigar. **④** Thinly slice into ribbons.

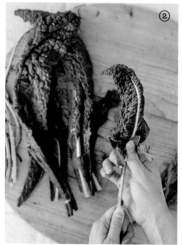

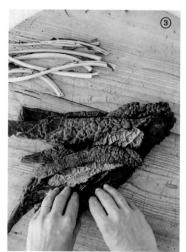

LF	SCD	SSFG	BPD1	BPD2	P	V	SF	YC	Sub lime juice for lemon, unless tolerated ↓	Omit parsnips ↓
									HI	BPD1R

Balsamic Roasted Radicchio and Endive

If your digestive system is really in need of a break, it's always best to give tough greens some gentle heat. For this reason, I absolutely adore radicchio, which can be cut into wedges and roasted in the oven until tender and slightly crisped on top. This bitter powerhouse lettuce is incredible for helping your liver cleanse itself, and therefore, getting your digestive system back on track. The sweet balsamic helps offset some of the bitterness, which is a trick I learned from my mother who is the queen of cooking her lettuces. If you're new to bitter greens and require more sweetness, you can add a little pure maple syrup or clover honey to the vinegar. This would also be fabulous with generous flakes of a low-FODMAP cheese, such as Parmesan or pecorino, if you tolerate dairy.

MAKES 4 SIDE SERVINGS

2 heads radicchio

2 heads endive

¼ cup extra-virgin olive oil

   Sea salt and freshly ground black pepper

3 tablespoons balsamic vinegar

❶ Preheat the oven to 450°F. Line a baking sheet with parchment paper.

❷ Cut each radicchio head in half lengthwise, then cut each half into thirds, making sure to cut on an angle through the core so each wedge holds together. Cut the endive heads into quarters lengthwise.

❸ Arrange the radicchio and endive in an even layer on the prepared baking sheet. Drizzle with the oil and season with salt and pepper to taste. Toss gently to coat, then position each wedge so a cut side faces the pan. Transfer to the oven and roast until the radicchio leaves are wilted and slightly charred, 12 to 15 minutes.

❹ Remove from the oven and drizzle with the vinegar. Serve warm or at room temperature.

Onward Serve over half a thinly sliced Granny Smith or Pink Lady **apple** or garnish with 2 tablespoons of chopped **pistachios**.

					Replace balsamic with lime juice ↓					
LF	P	V	SCD	SF	SSFG	BPD1R	BPD1	BPD2	HI	YC

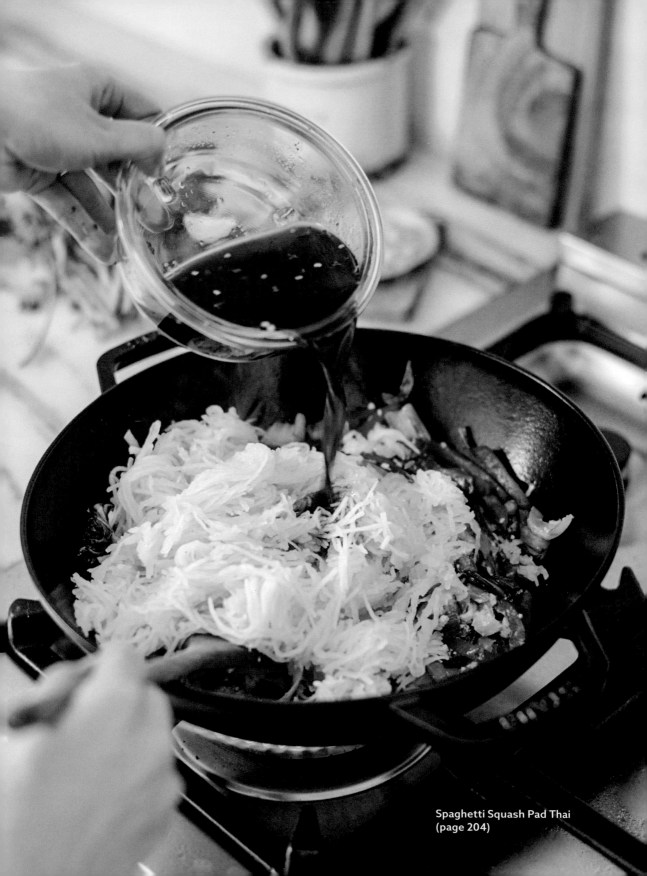

Spaghetti Squash Pad Thai
(page 204)

...

CAREFUL CARBS

Brown Rice Kitchari

Similar to congee in Chinese medicine, *kitchari* is a staple of healing Ayurvedic cuisine. Rice and lentils are cooked until they turn into an easily digestible porridge. The base is also layered with supportive digestive ingredients such as ginger and fennel seeds. This version omits the lentils, keeping it low-FODMAP. Although many people may find that reintegrating legumes is not in the cards, lentils are generally one of the easiest to tolerate, especially when cooked until quite soft. This recipe is a great one to use during your reintroduction.

MAKES 6 SERVINGS

- 3 tablespoons grass-fed ghee or virgin coconut oil
- 2 tablespoons minced fresh ginger
- 2 teaspoons ground cumin
- 1 teaspoon ground coriander
- 1 teaspoon fennel seeds
- 1 teaspoon ground turmeric
- 1½ cups long-grain brown rice
- 5 cups Low-FODMAP Vegetable Stock (page 142)
- 2 teaspoons sea salt
- 2 small zucchini, coarsely grated (about 2 cups)

- 1 small crown broccoli, florets only, finely chopped (about 3 cups)
- 5 ounces baby spinach (about 6 cups, tightly packed)

- ½ cup roughly chopped fresh cilantro stems and leaves
- 1 lemon, cut into wedges, for garnish

❶ In a large, lidded saucepan or 5-quart Dutch oven, heat the ghee over medium heat. Add the ginger, cumin, coriander, fennel seeds, and turmeric. Cook for 30 seconds, or until fragrant. Add the rice and stir to coat in the spices. Cook for 1 minute more, then add the vegetable stock and salt.

❷ Bring to a boil, cover, and lower the heat to medium-low. Simmer for about 40 minutes, stirring occasionally, until the rice is tender but not mushy and most of the liquid has been absorbed. If there seems to be too much liquid, uncover and simmer until you reach this outcome.

❸ Stir in the zucchini and broccoli. Cover and cook for another 5 minutes. Fold in the spinach and cilantro, then remove from the heat and leave to stand for 5 minutes, uncovered. Serve warm alongside the lemon wedges.

Onward Substitute ½ cup of dried **red lentils** for ½ cup of rice.

			Sub kale for spinach; use Low-Histamine Stock (page 142) ↓	Substitute white rice and reduce stock by 1 cup; limit to serving size of ¾ cup ↓		Omit broccoli, spinach, and cilantro ↓
LF	V	SF	HI	YC	BPD1	BPD2	HS

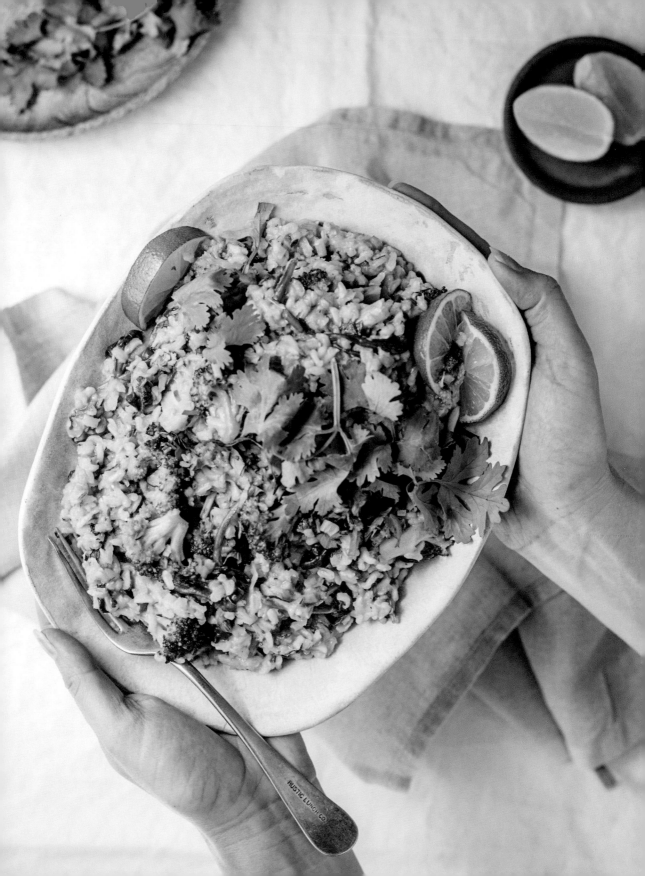

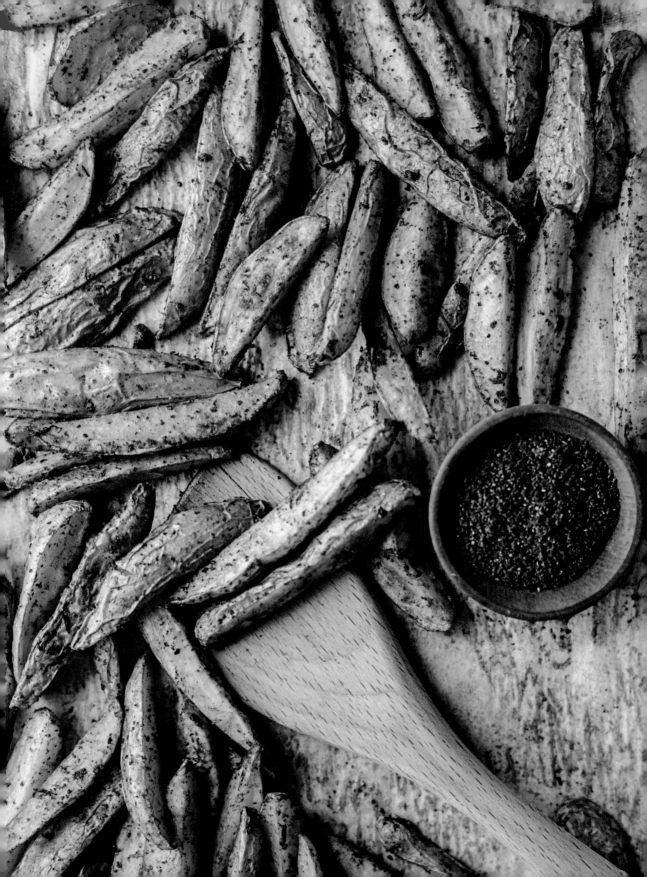

Smoky Fingerling Steak Fries

Like bacon, fries are a rare treat on a SIBO diet, as long as you can find them in a dedicated gluten-free fryer. Keep in mind, though, that most restaurants use cheap oils that can be irritating to an already inflamed system. The best way to enjoy them is to make your own, which allows you to go for a more healthful technique (baking) and get creative with your spice rack. Smoked paprika (also called pimentón de la Vera) is common in Spain and gives these fries a lovely earthiness. Serve them alongside whatever low-FODMAP dipping sauce you like. I'm partial to the Euro way and highly recommend homemade aioli (page 146).

MAKES 4 SIDE SERVINGS

- 2 pounds fingerling potatoes
- 2 tablespoons extra-virgin olive oil
- 1 teaspoon smoked paprika
- ½ teaspoon dried thyme leaves, or 1 teaspoon fresh
- ½ teaspoon sea salt

❶ Preheat the oven to 425°F. Line two baking sheets with parchment paper.

❷ On a clean work surface, halve the potatoes lengthwise and cut into thin wedges. Depending on the thickness of the potato, you might just need to quarter them lengthwise.

❸ In a medium-size bowl, toss the potatoes with the oil, smoked paprika, thyme, and salt. Divide between the two prepared baking sheets and arrange in an even layer, cut side down. Roast in the oven until nicely browned on the bottom and crispy, about 40 minutes, swapping the pans from top to bottom 30 minutes into cooking. Transfer to a serving bowl and enjoy alongside your dipping sauce of choice.

Onward Add ½ teaspoon of **garlic** powder to the spice mixture.

LF	P	V	HI	SF	HS	Limit to serving size of ½ cup ↓	
						YC	BPD2

Gingery Stir-Fried Collards and Quinoa

The trick to cooking collard greens is that you either have go fast (stir-fry) or slow (braise). This recipe uses the former technique for a little Asian-southern fusion that doesn't require three hours and a ham hock, but tastes equally delicious. As always you can omit the jalapeño if sensitive to heat, or double it for extra kick. Like fried rice, this stir-fry tastes best with day-old, dried-out quinoa, so feel free to make it in advance or use leftovers. If you're starting from scratch, combine 1 cup of quinoa with 1¾ cups of water and a sprinkle of salt. Bring to a boil, lower the heat, and cook for 17 minutes until pearly. Allow the moisture to evaporate, uncovered, while you proceed with the rest of the recipe. Add a fried egg to transform this bowl into a main course, or serve it as a side for Larb Lettuce Wraps (page 265) or Thai Green Curry Chicken (page 246).

MAKES 4 SIDE SERVINGS

- 2 tablespoons grass-fed ghee or unrefined coconut oil
- 2 garlic cloves, lightly crushed
- 1 tablespoon minced ginger
- 1 jalapeño pepper, ribs and seeds removed, thinly sliced
- 1 large bunch collard greens, thick stems removed, coarsely chopped
- Sea salt
- 3 cups cooked quinoa (from 1 cup dried; see headnote)

- 2 tablespoons coconut aminos or gluten-free tamari
- 1 tablespoon apple cider vinegar
- 1 teaspoon toasted sesame oil

❶ In a large, nonstick skillet or wok, heat the ghee or oil over medium-low heat. Add the garlic and cook until golden brown on all sides and the oil is infused, 5 minutes. Remove the cloves and discard.

❷ Increase the heat to medium-high and add the ginger and jalapeño; stir-fry until soft, about 2 minutes. Add the collard greens and cook, tossing frequently, until bright green and wilted. Season the greens generously with salt. Fold in the quinoa and cook for 3 minutes more, until toasting slightly. Remove from the heat and season with the coconut aminos, vinegar, and sesame oil, scraping up any quinoa that's stuck to the pan. Taste for seasoning and add more salt as necessary. Transfer the collards and quinoa to a platter. Serve warm.

Onward Add 1 thinly sliced small **shallot** to the ginger and/or whisk 1 tablespoon of white **miso** paste into the vinegar mixture.

			Omit the quinoa and double collard greens; use coconut aminos ↓			Limit to serving size of ¾ cup ↓		Omit vinegar, coconut aminos, and jalapeño ↓	
LF	V	SF	SSFG	SCD	P	BPD1	BPD2	YC	HI

Better-Than-the-Box Yellow Rice Pilaf

When I ask my culinary students what a pilaf is, often their only reference point is Rice-A-Roni, which is one of the reasons I love teaching this dish in my classes. Contrary to popular belief, a pilaf is not ingredient-specific, and has nothing to do with little flecks of dried carrots or peas. Rather, it's a technique that involves sautéing your grains in a mixture of oil and aromatics instead of steaming them with water alone. Although it takes a few more steps than a standard pot of white rice, this yellow rice pilaf has so much flavor thanks to anti-inflammatory turmeric. It looks just like what you get out of the box without much added effort.

MAKES 4 SERVINGS

- 2 tablespoons extra-virgin olive oil
- 2 garlic cloves, peeled and crushed
- 1 cup long-grain white rice
- ½ teaspoon ground turmeric
- ½ teaspoon sea salt
- 1½ cups water or Low-FODMAP Vegetable Stock (page 142)
- 1 tablespoon freshly squeezed lemon juice (optional)
- 2 tablespoons chopped fresh mint (optional)

❶ Heat the oil in a medium-size Dutch oven or lidded saucepan. Add the garlic and brown over low heat until golden all over, about 5 minutes. Discard the cloves.

❷ To the pan, add the rice, turmeric, and salt. Cook over medium heat, stirring occasionally, for 2 minutes, or until the rice is quite yellow and beginning to toast. Carefully pour in the water or stock and bring to a boil. Cover the pot, return the heat to low, and cook until the rice is tender and all the water is absorbed, about 15 minutes. Remove from the heat and allow to sit for 10 minutes, covered, until steamed.

❸ Fluff with a fork and stir in the lemon and mint (if using). Taste for seasoning and add more salt as necessary. Serve alongside any of the main courses in this book.

Onward Sauté 1 thinly sliced **leek** (white and light green parts) with the spices and/or add ¼ cup of frozen **sweet peas** when the rice is done cooking.

				Omit garlic ↓	Limit to serving size of ½ cup ↓		
LF	V	HI	SF	HS	YC	BPD1	BPD2

197

Green Falafel with Magic Tahini Sauce

Since canned chickpeas are only low-FODMAP in ¼-cup servings, these falafel bites get a little extra substance from ground sunflower seeds, spinach, and parsley. I love serving them as part of a gluten-free meze platter or as a vegetarian main course.

**MAKES 4 SERVINGS
(SAFE SERVING: 6 BALLS)**

- ¾ cup (115 g) hulled sunflower seeds
- 1 cup canned chickpeas, drained and rinsed
- ¼ cup loosely packed flat-leaf parsley
- 4 roughly chopped green scallions
- 16 ounces frozen chopped spinach, thawed
- 2 large eggs
- 2 tablespoons grass-fed ghee
- 1 teaspoon ground cumin
- ½ teaspoon ground turmeric
- 1 teaspoon sea salt

▷ Sauce
- ¼ cup tahini
- ¼ cup freshly squeezed lemon juice (from 1 to 2 lemons)
- ½ teaspoon sea salt

❶ Preheat the oven to 375°F. Position a rack in the center of the oven and line a baking sheet with parchment paper.

❷ In a small food processor, pulse the sunflower seeds until ground into a fine flour. Transfer to a large bowl and set aside.

❸ Add the chickpeas, parsley, and scallions to the food processor. Pulse until everything is well broken down but still a little chunky. Transfer to the bowl of sunflower seed flour.

❹ Place the thawed spinach in a clean dish towel and squeeze the water out. Add to the bowl, along with the eggs, ghee, cumin, turmeric, and salt. Mix until fully combined.

❺ Using a 2-inch ice-cream scoop or a heaping tablespoon, portion the falafel batter into balls. Roll each ball in your hands until smooth, and arrange them evenly distanced on the prepared baking sheet. You should have about two dozen in total.

❻ Bake for 15 minutes, or until a light brown crust has formed on the bottom of the balls. Remove the pan, and flip the balls to rest on the opposite side. Return the balls to the oven for another 15 minutes, or until crispy all around and browned on the second side.

❼ **While the falafel bake, make the sauce:** In a medium mixing bowl, whisk the tahini, lemon juice, 2 tablespoons of water, and the salt together until smooth. Add more water if necessary, to reach the consistency of mayonnaise.

❽ Serve the balls warm or room temperature, alongside the sauce.

Onward Blend 1 clove **garlic** with the chickpea mixture.

LF	V	SF	Sub frozen chopped kale for spinach; omit eggs ↓
			HI

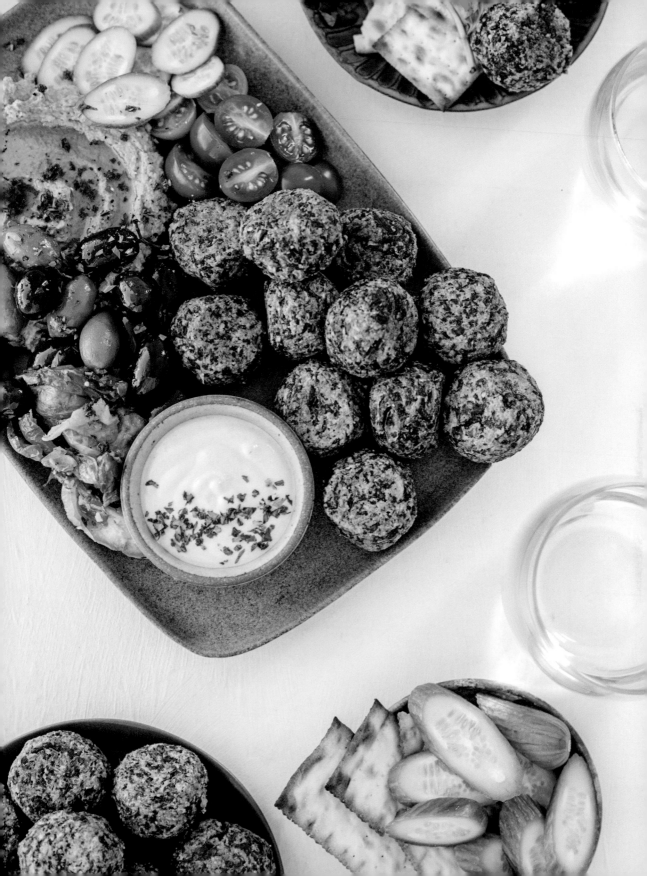

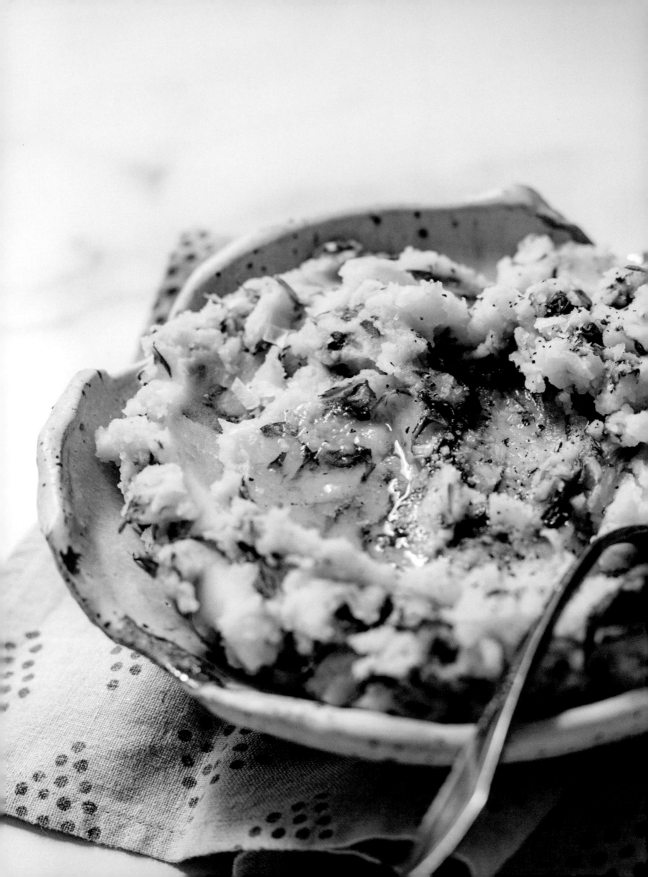

Spinach-Ghee Mashed Potatoes

This dish is a riff on Irish colcannon, which combines mashed potatoes with cooked greens or cabbage. The greens lighten up the spuds and are a sneaky way of getting picky eaters to enjoy more veggies. It's also a wonderful healthy side to add to your Thanksgiving table. Instead of adding cream or butter, I use nutty ghee, a clarified butter that's lactose-free. If you suspect you might be suffering from fat malabsorption, supplements, such as ox bile, taken with meals, might help you get the most out of healthy fats like ghee.

MAKES 4 SERVINGS

2 pounds russet potatoes (about 4 medium), peeled and cut into 2-inch cubes

Sea salt

5 ounces baby spinach (about 6 cups, tightly packed)

2 tablespoons grass-fed ghee

¼ cup Low-FODMAP Vegetable Stock or Basic Chicken Bone Broth (pages 142 and 140)

❶ Place the potatoes in a large pot and cover with cold water by 1 inch. Generously salt the water and bring to a boil. Cook until the potatoes are fork-tender, about 15 minutes. Fold in the spinach and cook for an additional 30 seconds, until wilted. Drain the potato mixture and shake out the excess water.

❷ Return the potatoes to the pot along with the ghee. With a fork or masher, smash the potatoes until semi-smooth. Add the stock if the potatoes seem too thick and dry. Taste for seasoning and add more salt as necessary. Serve immediately.

Onward Sauté 3 cups of chopped **green cabbage** in an additional 2 tablespoons of ghee and add to the cooked potatoes.

				Limit to serving size of ¾ cup ↓	Sub kale for spinach ↓	Omit spinach ↓
LF	P	SF	V	YC	BPD2	HI	HS

Pumpkin-Chive Risotto

Risotto is one of my favorite comfort foods and can be part of a healing diet with the right nutrients added to the mix. In this festive fall version, unsweetened canned pumpkin puree, rosemary, and turmeric make up the base for a rich, aromatic, orange-hued bowl. You can repurpose the remainder of the pumpkin can by whisking it into West African Yam and Peanut Stew (page 225) or Orange Remedy Soup (page 217). A handful of fresh chives at the end will ensure you don't miss that classic Italian onion flavor. You can enjoy this as a vegetarian main course or as a side to accompany Skillet Chicken Cacciatore (page 253). White wine is a staple base of risotto, but if you're avoiding alcohol, you can combine 1 tablespoon of white wine vinegar with ½ cup of water as a replacement.

MAKES 4 SIDE SERVINGS

4 cups Low-FODMAP Basic Chicken Bone Broth or Vegetable Stock (pages 140 and 142)

1⅓ cups pure pumpkin puree

¼ cup extra-virgin olive oil

2 garlic cloves, crushed

½ medium-size fennel bulb, diced

2 teaspoons chopped fresh rosemary, or 1 teaspoon dried

1 teaspoon ground turmeric

1 cup arborio rice

½ teaspoon sea salt

½ cup dry white wine (see note)

¼ cup finely chopped fresh chives

❶ In a medium-size saucepan, whisk together the broth and pumpkin puree. Warm the mixture over low heat.

❷ In a large Dutch oven or saucepan, heat the olive oil. Add the garlic and cook over low heat until very fragrant and lightly toasted, 5 minutes. Discard the garlic. Add the fennel, rosemary, and turmeric; cook over medium heat for about 3 minutes more, until translucent.

❸ Stir in the rice and toast until the edges are opaque and the center pearly white, about 2 minutes. Add the salt and wine to the pan, scraping up any brown bits, and cook until reduced by half, 1 minute.

❹ Add 1 cup of the pumpkin broth to the pan. Bring to a simmer, then lower the heat to medium-low and gently cook until nearly absorbed, about 5 minutes. Repeat this process, adding more pumpkin broth in 1-cup increments and making sure the rice is never sticking to the bottom, until the grains are tender but still hold their shape, about 30 minutes. Taste for seasoning and add more salt as necessary. Stir in half of the chives and garnish with the remaining chives.

Onward Garnish each bowl with a tablespoon of freshly grated Parmesan or **pecorino cheese**.

			Limit to serving size of ½ cup; omit wine ↓		Omit wine; use Low-Histamine Stock (page 142) ↓
LF	V	SF	BPD1	BPD2	HI

Millet Tabbouleh

Millet is an often-overlooked gluten-free grain that can easily moonlight for couscous or bulgur wheat. It understudies for the latter in this Middle Eastern salad and is a perfect make-ahead side for summer picnics or brown bags. Although parsley and mint are the standard flavor base for this salad, it's also a great place to use up any other wayward herbs you have in your crisper drawer (cilantro, dill, chives, basil—anything goes!).

MAKES 6 TO 8 SERVINGS

- 1 cup millet
- ⅔ cup roughly chopped fresh flat-leaf parsley (about 1 bunch)
- ½ cup roughly chopped fresh mint
- 4 thinly sliced green scallions, or ¼ cup chopped fresh chives
- 2 cups cherry tomatoes, quartered
- 2 tablespoons freshly squeezed lemon juice
- 2 teaspoons rice vinegar
- ¼ cup extra-virgin olive oil
- ½ teaspoon sea salt

❶ Bring a large pot of salted water to a boil. Add the millet and cook, uncovered, stirring occasionally, until al dente, about 15 minutes. Drain, then run cool water over the millet to stop the cooking. Shake out all the excess water and transfer to a large bowl.

❷ Toss the grains together with the parsley, mint, scallions, tomatoes, lemon juice, vinegar, olive oil, and salt. Taste for seasoning and add more salt as necessary. Serve at room temperature.

Onward Toss 2 cups of canned quartered **artichoke hearts** (from one 14-ounce can) with 2 tablespoons of olive oil and roast at 425°F for 20 minutes, or until crispy. Sprinkle on top of the millet.

LF	V	SF	Omit tomatoes, vinegar, and lemon juice, unless tolerated ↓	Omit scallion or chives ↓	Omit vinegar; limit to serving size of ¾ cup ↓
			HI	HS	YC

Spaghetti Squash Pad Thai

In addition to SIBO, I suffer from another common affliction: pad thai syndrome. It's a disorder that makes me want to eat pad thai every day of the week. I've been working on a cure for some time, and recently had a breakthrough with this recipe. It tastes just like my favorite noodle dish but without the refined carbs, GMO tofu, and gloppy brown sauce. The spaghetti squash noodles are stretched even further with bok choy and bell peppers, but you can throw in any additional veggies you like. It goes great with Thai Green Curry Chicken (page 246) if you want to mimic my entire takeout order at home. To save on time, you can prep and bake the spaghetti squash up to three days in advance. The stir-fry itself comes together very quickly.

MAKES 4 SERVINGS (SAFE SERVING: 1½ CUPS)

- 1 medium-size spaghetti squash (about 3 pounds)
- Sea salt
- ¼ cup freshly squeezed lime juice (from 2 limes)
- ¼ cup Asian fish sauce (I like Red Boat brand)
- 2 tablespoons gluten-free tamari or coconut aminos

- 2 tablespoons coconut sugar or clover honey
- ¼ teaspoon red pepper flakes (optional)
- 2 tablespoons refined coconut or avocado oil
- 1 red bell pepper, thinly sliced
- 1 baby bok choy, thinly sliced

- 1 bunch scallions, green parts only, cut into 2-inch pieces
- 2 large eggs, beaten
- 2 tablespoons fresh cilantro leaves
- 2 tablespoons roughly chopped peanuts
- 1 lime, cut into wedges, for garnish

1 Preheat the oven to 375°F. Line a rimmed baking sheet with parchment paper.

2 Using the largest chef's knife you have, cut the spaghetti squash in half lengthwise. It's helpful to put a crumpled dish towel on your cutting board to stabilize it, or to remove a little bit from both ends so you can stand the squash upright without its wobbling. Scoop out the seeds and stringy bits from the center cavity. Season the cavity with salt and arrange both cleaned squash halves, cut side down, on the prepared baking sheet. Add ½ cup of water to the pan (this will help steam and soften the squash).

recipe continues →

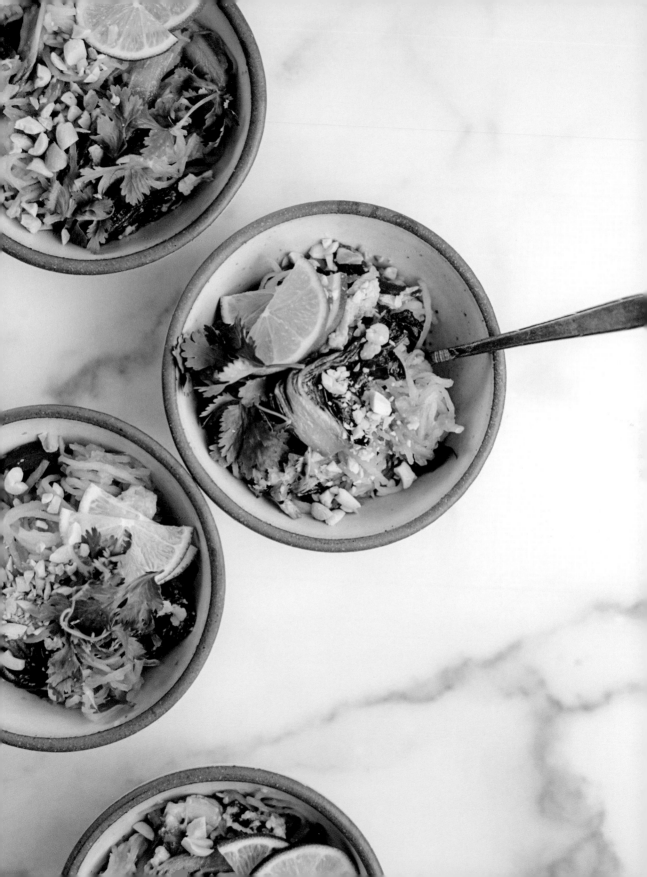

3 Bake until the squash is tender, meaning a fork can easily be inserted from flesh to skin, about 45 minutes. Flip the halves over to allow them to cool. When safe to touch, use a fork to shred the spaghetti strands from the squash: begin along the edges, pulling the strands toward the center, then scoop the bundle into a bowl.

4 **While the squash is cooking, make the sauce:** In a small mixing bowl, combine the lime juice, fish sauce, tamari, coconut sugar, and red pepper flakes (if using). Set aside.

5 In a large wok or nonstick skillet, heat the oil over medium-high heat. Add the red peppers and bok choy; stir-fry until tender and slightly charred, about 3 minutes. Toss in the scallions and cook for 2 minutes more, or until wilted. Push the veggies to the sides of the pan to create a well. Add the eggs to the pan and cook, undisturbed, until set on the bottom, 1 minute. Redistribute with your spatula to cook the other side. Carefully toss with the veggies, making sure not to overly break apart the omelet.

6 When the squash noodles are ready, add to the pan along with the sauce and toss to combine. Stir-fry for a few more minutes, until some of the liquid has evaporated and the squash is fully incorporated into the veggie mixture. Taste for seasoning and add more salt as necessary.

7 To serve, divide the squash among four bowls and garnish with the cilantro, peanuts, and lime wedges.

Onward Add the **scallion** whites.

Limit to serving size of 1½ cups ↓		Use coconut aminos and honey ↓				Omit fish sauce and double tamari or coconut aminos ↓	Omit eggs, fish sauce, and tamari ↓
LF	P	SCD	SSFG	BPD1	BPD2	V	HI

Sweet Potato–Quinoa Burgers with Sprouts and Spicy Lime Aioli

One of the lazy dinners I missed most when my low-FODMAP diet forced me to forgo all my favorite packaged foods was a frozen veggie burger. Especially since eating plant-based is more of a challenge when treating SIBO, I was so excited when I created these southwestern-style Sweet Potato–Quinoa Burgers. Not only are they insanely flavorful, but they also freeze well. Enjoy them on lettuce wraps if you can't find gluten-free buns at the market. You can also make them vegan by omitting the egg—the burger mixture will still hold together nicely. If you haven't salted the quinoa, make sure to taste the burger mix for seasoning before you add the egg.

MAKES 8 SERVINGS

2 medium-size sweet potatoes (about 1¾ pounds), sliced in half lengthwise

Extra-virgin olive oil

2 cups cooked quinoa (from ¾ cup dried; see Step 3)

⅓ cup almond flour

1 large egg, beaten

⅓ cup finely chopped fresh cilantro

1 teaspoon ground cumin

1 teaspoon chili powder

1 teaspoon smoked paprika

1 teaspoon sea salt

Oil, for pan and measuring cup

1 cup Spicy Lime Aioli (page 146; see Step 6)

8 gluten-free burger buns (see headnote), toasted

1 avocado, peeled, pitted, and thinly sliced

2 cups sprouts or microgreens, for serving

❶ Preheat the oven to 425°F. Line a baking sheet with parchment paper.

❷ Lightly brush the cut sides of the sweet potatoes with olive oil and arrange, cut side down, on the prepared baking sheet. Transfer to the oven and cook until quite soft, about 35 minutes. Remove from the oven and set aside to cool, leaving the parchment on the baking sheet.

❸ If making your quinoa from scratch, do so while the sweet potatoes bake.

recipe continues →

4 When the sweet potatoes are cool enough to touch, scoop out the flesh and measure out a total of about 2 cups. Transfer to a medium-size bowl and mash with a fork. Add the cooked quinoa, almond flour, egg, cilantro, cumin, chili powder, smoked paprika, and salt; stir until well incorporated.

5 Lightly oil the parchment paper on the baking sheet. Then oil a 1/3-cup measure and use it to portion the quinoa batter into eight mounds. With your hands, shape the quinoa into balls, then pat into 1-inch-thick smooth disks and arrange an inch or so apart on the prepared baking sheet. Transfer to the oven and bake until the patties have dried out and formed a nice brown crust on the bottom, 30 minutes. Flip the burgers and return to the oven for 10 more minutes, until firm.

6 While the burgers bake, prepare the spicy lime aioli (if you haven't premade it).

7 Top the cut side of each bun with 1 tablespoon of the aioli. Add a quinoa patty to the bottom half and top with 1/8 of the avocado and a small handful of sprouts. Repeat with the remaining burgers and enjoy immediately. Or refrigerate each element separately for later.

Onward Add 1/2 cup of drained and rinsed canned **black beans** to the burger patties in Step 4.

LF	V	SF	Omit egg, avocado, and spicy lime aioli ↓
			HI

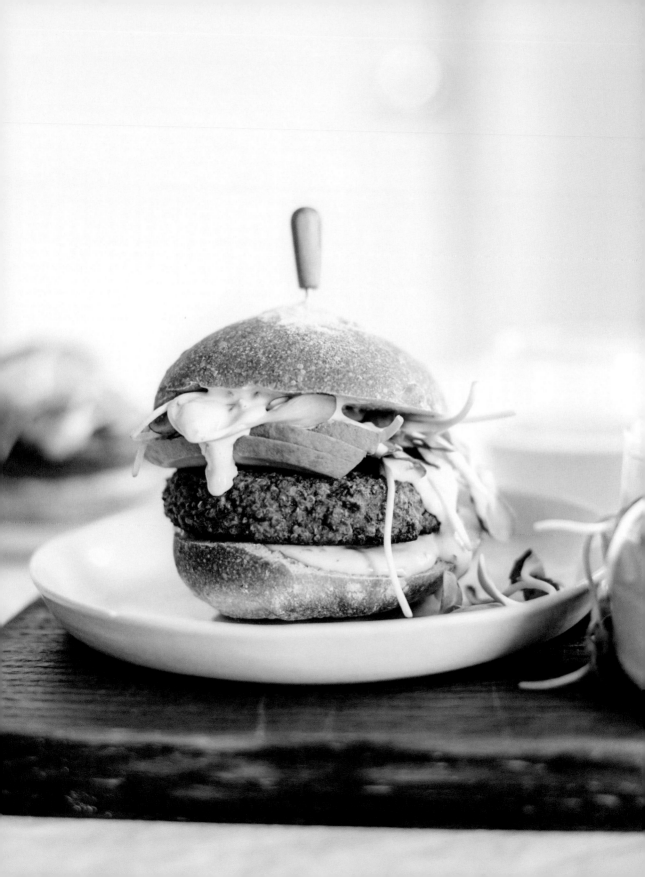

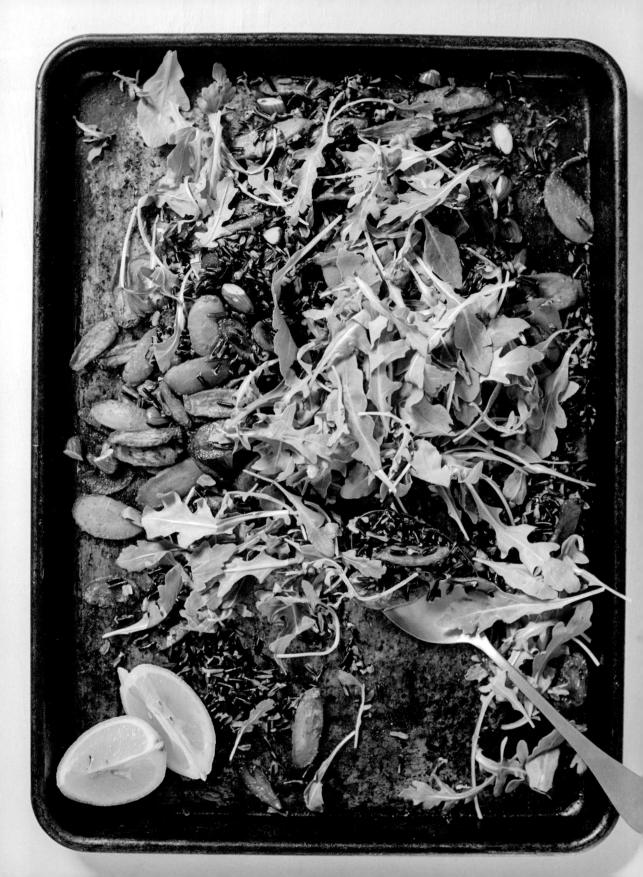

Moroccan Carrot Salad with Wild Rice, Arugula, and Almonds

Many people do just fine eating rice and quinoa during their SIBO treatment. But the trick with any healing diet is making sure that your carb intake isn't also wreaking havoc on your blood sugar, since any sort of hormone dysregulation has negative downwind effects on your digestive system (more about this on page 117). A happy medium on the carb front is wild rice. It's low-FODMAP, yet thanks to its outer husk, it's also high in the kind of insoluble fiber that keeps your blood sugar in check. This salad is a wonderful make-ahead option that's packed with warming Moroccan spices, sweet carrots, and peppery arugula. If making ahead, simply store the greens separately and dress when you're ready to eat.

MAKES 4 SERVINGS

1 cup wild rice, rinsed

Sea salt

1 pound carrots (about 8 medium), cut diagonally into ¼-inch-thick slices

Extra-virgin olive oil

1 teaspoon ground cumin

½ teaspoon ground turmeric

¼ teaspoon ground cinnamon

⅓ cup almonds, roughly chopped

5 ounces baby arugula (about 5 cups, tightly packed)

2 tablespoons freshly squeezed lemon juice (from ½ lemon)

❶ Bring a large pot of salted water to a boil. Add the rinsed wild rice to the pot and cook, uncovered, until al dente, about 45 minutes. Drain the wild rice and return it to the pot. Place a dish towel over the top to catch the steam, and allow it to sit for 10 minutes.

❷ Meanwhile, preheat the oven to 425°F. Line a baking sheet with parchment. On the prepared baking sheet, toss the carrots with 2 tablespoons of olive oil, the cumin, turmeric, and cinnamon, and ½ teaspoon of salt. Arrange in an even layer and bake until tender and caramelized, about 25 minutes. Remove from the oven and add the almonds plus an additional 2 tablespoons of olive oil. Return the pan to the oven for 5 to 10 minutes, or until the nuts are golden brown and toasted.

❸ Add the wild rice to the baking sheet and toss together so it soaks up all the nutty oil. When ready to eat, arrange the arugula on a platter (or just add it to the baking sheet), top with the wild rice mixture, and drizzle with the lemon juice. Serve immediately.

Onward On a second parchment-lined baking sheet, roast 2 cups of thinly sliced **Brussels sprouts** (8 ounces), tossed with olive oil and salt, at the same time as the carrots, until browned.

			Omit lemon juice, unless tolerated ↓	Omit wild rice ↓							Omit arugula and almond ↓
LF	V	SF	HI	SCD	BPD	BPD1R	BPD1	BPD2	P	YC	HS

Caper-Herb Potato Salad

My mother's potato salad recipe is fairly light on the mayo compared to most—and really, compared to all other dishes she makes. To add more bulk, she uses a healthy amount of Dijon mustard and hard-boiled eggs, which make their own sauce. If you don't like the white stuff at all, you can add additional hard-boiled eggs or sub 24-Hour Yogurt (page 163) for those who tolerate fermented dairy. Regardless, don't skimp on the herbs and feel free to use whatever combination you have on hand. Basil and dill also work well.

MAKES 6 SERVINGS

- 6 large eggs
- 2 pounds red or Yukon Gold potatoes, cut into 2-inch pieces

   Sea salt
- ½ cup mayonnaise
- ¼ cup Dijon mustard
- 2 tablespoons capers
- 2 tablespoons finely chopped fresh chives
- 2 tablespoons finely chopped fresh tarragon
- 2 tablespoons finely chopped fresh flat-leaf parsley leaves

❶ Carefully place the eggs in a medium-size saucepan and cover with cold water by 1 inch. Bring to a boil over high heat. Once simmering, remove the pan from the heat and let the eggs stand until cool enough to touch. This is known as the Ina technique for hard-boiling eggs, but use whatever method you prefer if you don't trust the queen.

❷ Meanwhile, place the potatoes in a large saucepan or stockpot and cover with well-salted cold water by 2 inches. Bring to a boil and then simmer until the potatoes are fork-tender, about 15 minutes. Drain well and transfer to a large bowl.

❸ Peel the eggs and add to the potatoes. Using a masher or fork, crush the eggs until the whites and yolks are broken up and the potatoes are still fairly chunky. Stir in the mayonnaise, mustard, capers, chives, tarragon, and parsley. Taste for seasoning and add more salt as necessary.

❹ Transfer to a serving bowl and garnish with additional herbs.

Onward Sub plain Greek **yogurt** for the mayo and/or add 2 thinly sliced **scallions**.

LF	P	SF	Limit to serving size of ½ cup ↓
			BPD2

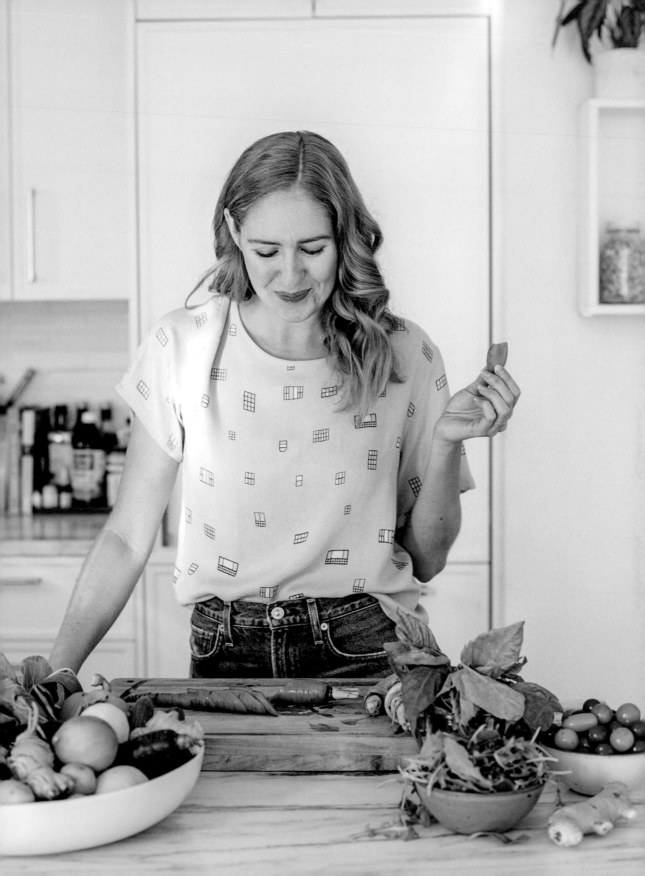

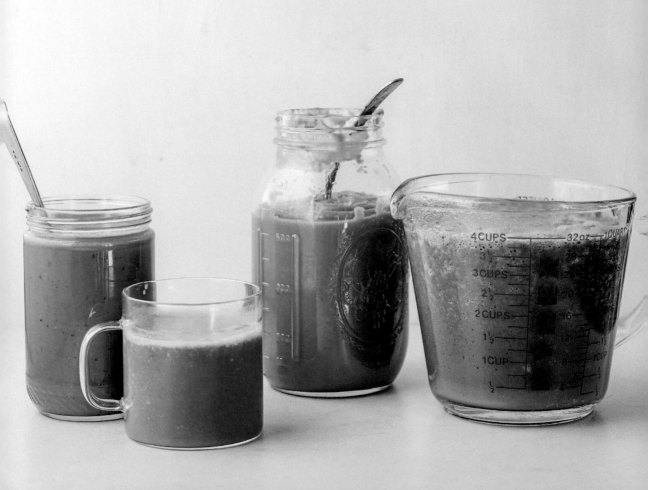

SOUPS
& STEWS

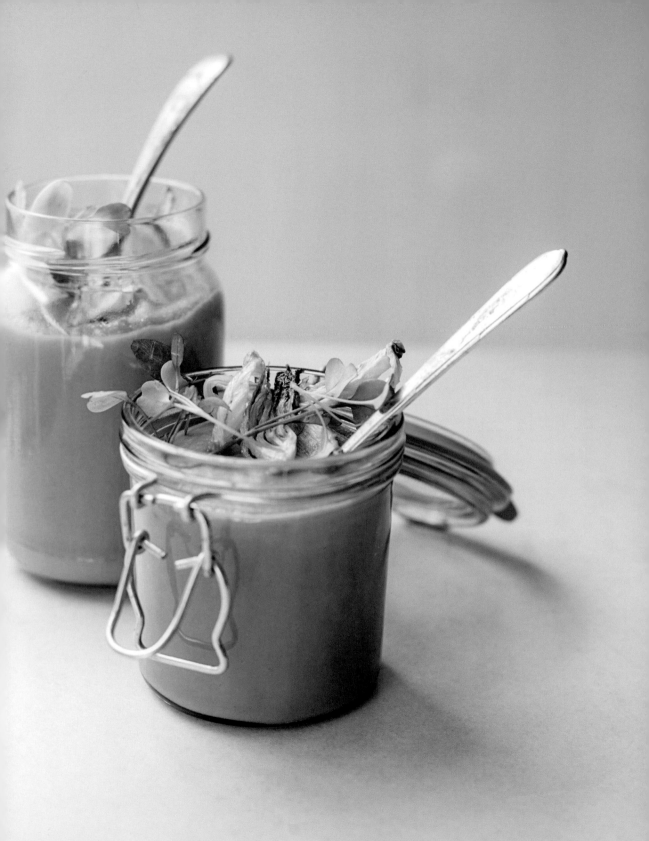

Orange Remedy Soup

Whenever I have a friend who's in need of extra comfort, assistance
I always try to make a homemade delivery. And 90 percent of the time, it's s.
version of this soup. It scores incredibly high on both the health and coziness
spectrum, and is easy to freeze for later. When my friend Rob was battling stomach
cancer, he was craving creamy, non-obtrusive things. So, I found ways to sneak in
more anti-inflammatory properties. Turmeric lights the carrot color on fire. The
parsnips add sweetness. And a little coconut milk gives it a bisque-like texture
without any dairy. It was his absolute favorite soup, and has also been a huge hit
with my postpartum friends and in my own household when I have a gut flare-up that
requires something easy to digest.

**MAKES 6 SERVINGS
(SAFE SERVING: 2 CUPS)**

- 2 pounds carrots (about 16 medium), unpeeled, cut into 1-inch pieces
- 2 tablespoons extra-virgin olive oil
- Sea salt
- 2 tablespoons grass-fed ghee or refined coconut oil
- 2 tablespoons chopped fresh ginger
- 1 teaspoon ground turmeric
- 1 pound parsnips (about 5 medium), peeled and cut into 1-inch pieces
- 1 cup coconut milk
- 4 cups Low-FODMAP Vegetable Stock (page 142)
- 2 tablespoons apple cider vinegar

❶ Preheat the oven to 425°F. Line a baking sheet with parchment.

❷ On the prepared baking sheet, toss the carrots with the olive oil and ½ teaspoon of salt. Arrange in an even layer and roast in the middle of the oven for about 40 minutes, or until caramelized and fork-tender.

❸ Meanwhile, in a large stockpot or saucepan, heat the ghee or coconut oil over medium heat. Add the ginger, turmeric, and parsnips. Sauté for 5 minutes, or until fragrant and beginning to caramelize. Carefully pour in the coconut milk along with the broth and 1 teaspoon of salt. Bring to a boil, then lower the heat to medium-low and simmer until the parsnips are fork-tender, about 10 minutes.

❹ In a high-powered blender, combine the roasted carrots with the parsnip mixture and apple cider vinegar. Puree until smooth, adding more water or stock as necessary to get your desired consistency. Enjoy topped with a drizzle of garlic oil.

Onward Use the full 14-ounce can of **coconut milk** for more creaminess and reduce the quantity of stock to 3 cups. You can also swap in 1 large russet **potato** (peeled and diced) for the parsnips.

								Omit vinegar and use Low-Histamine Stock (page 142) ↓		
LF	SCD	SSFG	BPD1	BPD2	P	V	SF	HS	YC	HI

217

Green Detox Soup

In my first cookbook, there's a story about my mom's famous detox soup and how I used to cringe every time I opened the fridge only to find a few mugs of it sitting there. By Day 3, the color was a sewage-grade green, thanks to the heaps of chard and fresh lemon juice she added. I don't remember how old I was, but I finally got up the nerve to taste it. And—surprise!—after that first taste, I became an official devotee. I make a batch nearly every time I come down with a seasonal illness. The soup requires just a few ingredients—zucchini, chard, cilantro—and is so easy to whip together, it's possible to do so even when you feel like you're on the verge of death. I like to think of it as a hot alternative to green juice, which is a much better choice for a stagnant, SIBO-prone digestive system. If you want the green color to stay as fresh as possible, omit the lemon juice until you're ready to sip it. Contrary to my prior belief, it is not an acquired taste, but something I guarantee you'll love right out of the gate.

MAKES 8 CUPS SOUP (SAFE SERVING: 1½ CUPS)

- 2 tablespoons extra-virgin olive oil
- 2 medium-size zucchini (about 1½ pounds), sliced into 1-inch-thick rounds
- 1 bunch Swiss chard, stems and leaves separated, coarsely chopped (5 cups, packed)
- 4 cups Low-FODMAP Basic Chicken Bone Broth or Vegetable Stock (pages 140 and 142)
- ½ teaspoon sea salt
- 1 bunch cilantro, thick stem ends removed
- 2 tablespoons freshly squeezed lemon juice

1 In a medium-size Dutch oven or stockpot, heat the oil over medium-high heat. Add the zucchini and chard stems. Sauté, stirring occasionally, until the veggies are soft and beginning to brown, 5 to 7 minutes. Add the broth and bring to a boil. Stir in the chard leaves and salt. Simmer until the zucchini is fork-tender, about 5 minutes. Remove from the heat and add the cilantro. Allow to stand for a few minutes, until all the greens are very wilted.

2 Transfer the soup to a food processor or blender and puree until smooth. Add the lemon juice and taste for seasoning.

3 To serve, ladle the soup into bowls or a mug for sipping and drizzle with a little olive oil.

Onward Add 1 peeled and pitted **avocado** to the blender and puree with the rest of the soup.

									Use Low-Histamine Stock (page 142) and omit lemon juice, unless tolerated ↓	
LF	SCD	SSFG	BPD1R	BPD1	BPD2	P	V	SF	YC	HI

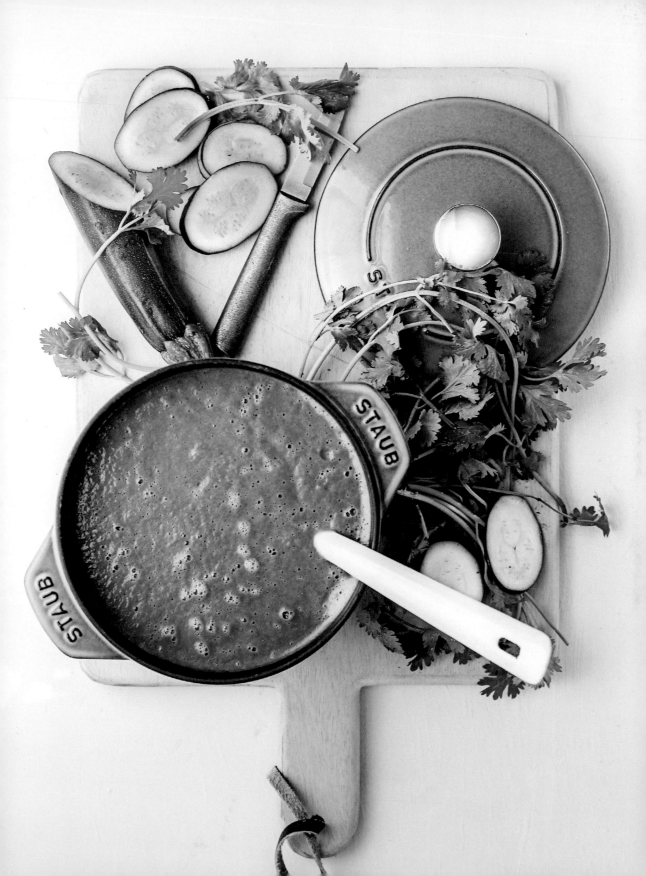

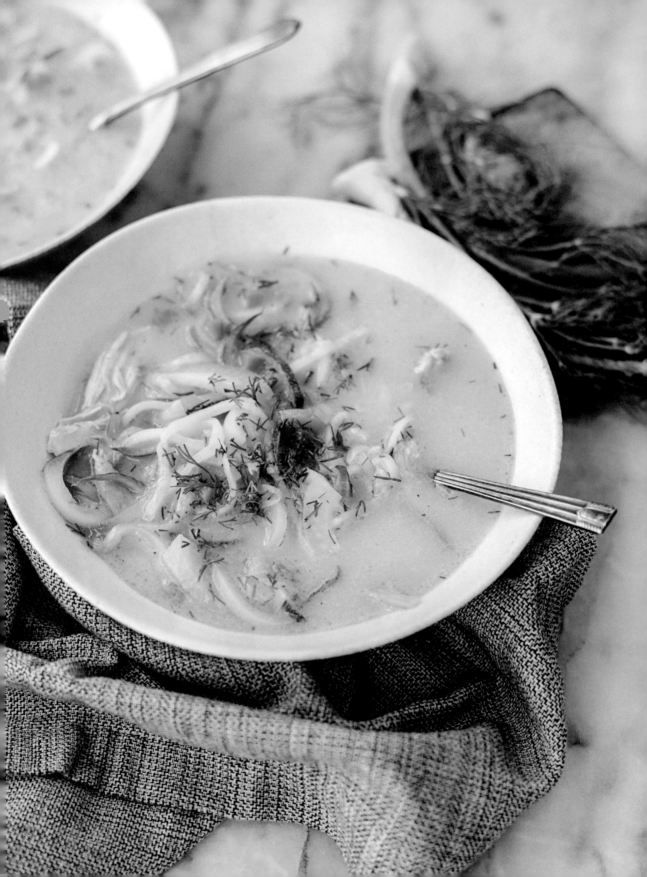

Greek Chicken Zoodle Soup with Dill

This version of avgolemono soup—the classic Greek lemon soup with egg broth—is simmered with fennel, zoodles, and shredded chicken. It's perfect for cold and flu season, but thanks to the zucchini noodles, also works on a chilly summer night. These days you can buy zoodles premade at most grocery stores, but if you're limiting your carbohydrates as part of your SIBO treatment, I'd highly recommend investing in an Inspiralizer, which puts all other spiralizing apparatuses to shame. The machine was created by my friend Ali Maffucci, who has tons of resources for preparing vegetable noodles on her website and in her many cookbooks. Of course, if you want a traditional chicken noodle soup, you can easily swap in your favorite gluten-free pasta. Just simmer it in the broth until al dente.

MAKES 4 SERVINGS

2 tablespoons extra-virgin olive oil

1 pound boneless, skinless chicken thighs

Sea salt and freshly ground black pepper

½ small fennel bulb, core removed, thinly sliced (about 1 cup)

2 medium-size carrots, finely diced

8 cups Low-FODMAP Basic Chicken Bone Broth (page 140)

1 medium-size zucchini (about 8 ounces), spiralized into noodles

⅓ cup freshly squeezed lemon juice (from 2 lemons)

2 tablespoons chopped fresh dill

4 large eggs

1 In a large stockpot or Dutch oven, heat the oil over medium-high heat. Season the chicken generously with salt and pepper. Add to the pot in an even layer and sear until a nice crust has formed on both sides, about 3 minutes per side. Transfer to a plate.

2 Add the fennel and carrots to the pot. Sweat the veggies over medium heat, stirring occasionally and scraping up any brown bits that may have formed from the chicken, until tender, about 5 minutes. Return the chicken to the pot along with the broth and 1 teaspoon of salt. Bring to a boil, lower the heat, and gently simmer until the carrots are soft and the chicken is tender enough to pull apart with a fork, about 15 minutes.

recipe continues →

3 Remove the chicken from the pot again and transfer to a medium-size bowl. Shred with a fork into bite-size pieces.

4 Meanwhile, add the zucchini noodles to the broth and simmer over low heat until tender, about 3 minutes. Remove the pot from the heat and add the lemon juice, shredded chicken, and dill.

5 In a medium-size bowl or 4-cup measuring cup, beat the eggs.

6 Temper the egg by slowly whisking ¼ cup of the hot broth into them, adding a very small amount at a time so as not to scramble the egg. Repeat with another ¾ cup of broth. Once the egg mixture is warm to the touch and the broth is fully incorporated, stir the mixture into the soup. If your egg "breaks" into stringy bits, don't freak out. It will still taste delicious, but will look a little funky—like Chinese egg drop soup. Pretend that's what you were going for and, either way, serve immediately.

Onward Add 6 spears **asparagus**, thinly sliced, with the zoodles.

								Omit eggs and lemon juice, unless tolerated; use Low-Histamine Stock (page 142) ↓	Omit eggs; use Low-Histamine Stock (page 142) ↓
LF	SCD	SSFG	BPD1R	BPD1	BPD2	P	SF	YC	HI	HS

Basque Cod, Pepper & Potato Stew

The key to Basque cooking is an ultra-flavorful base called sofrito, which is essentially peppers, onion, and garlic cooked low and slow in a large amount of olive oil until caramelized. Obviously, we have to forgo two elements of this holy trinity. However, you get the same effect by sweating several types of peppers in garlic oil. This stew is inspired by a traditional *marmitako*, which loosely translates to "tuna pot." I've swapped the albacore for cod to limit the mercury exposure. You could use any sturdy medium-thickness white fish—hake or haddock would also work well.

MAKES 3 TO 4 SERVINGS

¼ cup extra-virgin olive oil

2 garlic cloves, crushed

1 red bell pepper, finely diced

1 poblano pepper, ribs and seeds removed, finely diced

1 teaspoon sea salt

¼ teaspoon red pepper flakes (optional)

1 pound vine or Roma tomatoes, finely diced

1 pound russet potatoes (about 2 medium), peeled and cut into 1-inch cubes

2 cups Low-FODMAP Basic Chicken Bone Broth (page 140) or water

1½ pounds cod or other semi-firm white fish, cut into 2-inch pieces

2 tablespoons finely chopped fresh flat-leaf parsley leaves

❶ Heat the oil in a large, lidded, heavy-bottomed saucepan or Dutch oven. Add the garlic and cook over low heat until golden brown on all sides, about 5 minutes. Remove the garlic and discard.

❷ Carefully add the peppers, salt, and red pepper flakes (if using). Sauté over medium heat until the vegetables are very soft but not browning, about 10 minutes. Stir in the tomatoes and potatoes. Cover with the broth or water and bring to a boil. Lower the heat to medium-low and simmer, stirring occasionally, until the potatoes are tender and the broth has thickened, about 15 minutes. Season the cod with salt, nestle it into the tomato mixture, and cover with a lid. Simmer until the fish is tender but not falling apart, about 7 minutes.

❸ Garnish with the parsley and serve immediately.

Onward Dice and sauté ½ small **onion** along with the peppers.

					Omit potato ↓			
LF	BPD2	P	SF	SCD	SSFG	BPD1R	BPD1	YC

223

Pre–Breath Test Chicken Congee

Congee has long been a secret weapon of Chinese medicine as a salve for the digestive system. This rice porridge is cooked with a much higher ratio of water to grain, and simmered until mush, making it both easy to digest and incredibly nutritious. It's great for hydration, as the starchy mix in the congee can stay in the body longer than other types of food and allow the system to absorb liquid at a slower pace—a fun fact that my acupuncturist, Dr. Heidi Lovie, taught me. And it also just so happens that the base for any congee requires little more than the approved foods for your SIBO breath test prep day: basically, white rice and lean animal protein. Since congee is a fairly hands-off one-pot meal, it makes cooking the day before your breath test that much more painless. This recipe makes enough for three large servings (if that's all you're eating), or four normal-size ones, should you fall so in love with this congee that you want to make it again at other points during your healing journey. In the case of the latter, consider adding some low-FODMAP-friendly toppings, such as chopped fresh ginger, green scallions or chives, dark sesame oil, gluten-free tamari, or coconut aminos. This recipe makes a looser congee, with a ten-to-one ratio of liquid to rice. For a thicker gruel-like congee, go with a ratio of seven to one.

MAKES 4 SERVINGS (8 CUPS CONGEE)

- 1 cup sushi or jasmine rice
- 4 chicken drumsticks
- 2½ quarts (10 cups) filtered water
- 2 teaspoons pink Himalayan salt
- 1 tablespoon virgin coconut oil

1 In a large pot, combine the rice, chicken, water, and salt. Bring to a boil over high heat, then immediately lower the heat to medium-low. Gently simmer, uncovered, stirring every 15 to 20 minutes to prevent sticking, for about an hour, or until the rice is soft and the broth has thickened into a porridge-like consistency.

2 Transfer the chicken to a medium-size bowl and pull the meat from the bones, using two forks. Discard the skin and bones and return the chicken meat to the pot.

3 Gently stir the coconut oil into the congee and taste for seasoning. Serve alongside the garnishes of your choice (see headnote).

Limit to serving size of ½ cup ↓							
YC	BFD1	BFD2	LF	GF	HI	SF	HS

West African Yam and Peanut Stew

Mafe is a Senegalese dish that simmers peanut butter with tomatoes and spices until it becomes a thick, creamy stew. I've been making riffs on this recipe for years, with chicken or shrimp as the base, but I'm particularly fond of this vegetarian version that uses starchy root vegetables to thicken the broth even further. West African peanut stews often incorporate indigenous greens, which the spinach stands in for in this dish. The curry powder isn't traditional, but it helps cut down the ingredient list, which usually includes a few different spices, while retaining some heat and complexity. Like most stews, this dish gets even more flavorful over time, so it's perfect for make-ahead lunches that will last all week.

MAKES 4 SERVINGS

2 tablespoons extra-virgin olive oil

1 green bell pepper, finely diced

1 pound carrots (about 8 medium), cut into ¼-inch rounds

2 tablespoons minced fresh ginger

2 teaspoons Madras curry powder

1 teaspoon ground turmeric

1 teaspoon sea salt

1 (15-ounce) can diced tomatoes, or 2 cups diced fresh tomatoes

1 medium-size sweet potato (about 8 ounces), cut into ½-inch cubes

3 to 4 cups Low-FODMAP Vegetable Stock (page 142)

¼ cup creamy peanut butter

4 cups tightly packed baby spinach (about 3 ounces)

¼ cup roughly chopped fresh cilantro leaves

1 lime, cut into 4 wedges, for serving

Roasted peanuts, for garnish (optional)

❶ Heat the oil in a large Dutch oven or saucepan over medium heat. Add the bell pepper and carrots to the pan, increase the heat to medium-high, and sauté until soft, about 8 minutes. Stir in the ginger, curry powder, turmeric, and salt. Sauté for 2 more minutes, until very fragrant. Carefully pour in the tomatoes and simmer until the liquid has reduced, about 5 minutes.

❷ Stir in the sweet potatoes and cover with stock until submerged (it might be less than 4 cups, depending on the size of your pot). Bring the liquid to a boil, then lower the heat and

recipe continues →

simmer, uncovered, until the sweet potatoes are just tender, about 15 minutes. Stir in the peanut butter and simmer until slightly thickened, about 3 minutes. Fold in the spinach and cook until the greens are wilted, 1 minute more. Taste for seasoning and add more salt or peanut butter as you see fit.

3 To serve, ladle the stew into four bowls and garnish with the cilantro, lime wedges, and peanuts (if using).

Onward Sub 1 cup of cubed **butternut squash** for 1 cup of cubed sweet potato, and/or add ⅓ cup of frozen **sweet peas** along with the spinach.

LF	P	V	SF	HS	HI	SCD	SSFG	BPD1	BPD2
				Omit peanut butter, spinach, and cilantro ↓	Omit tomatoes; sub kale for spinach; use Low-Histamine Stock (page 142) ↓		Sub parsnips for sweet potato; use fresh tomatoes ↓		

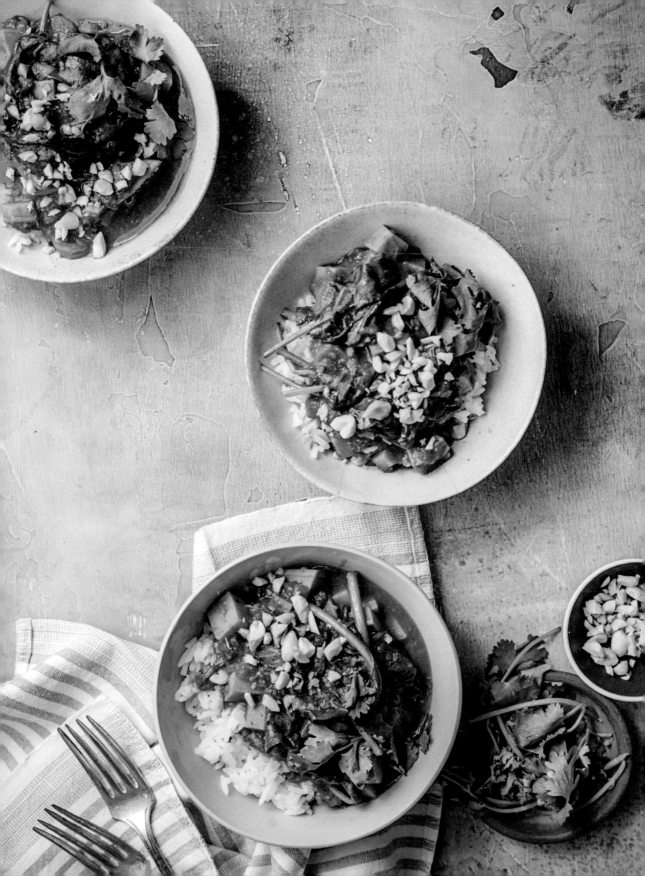

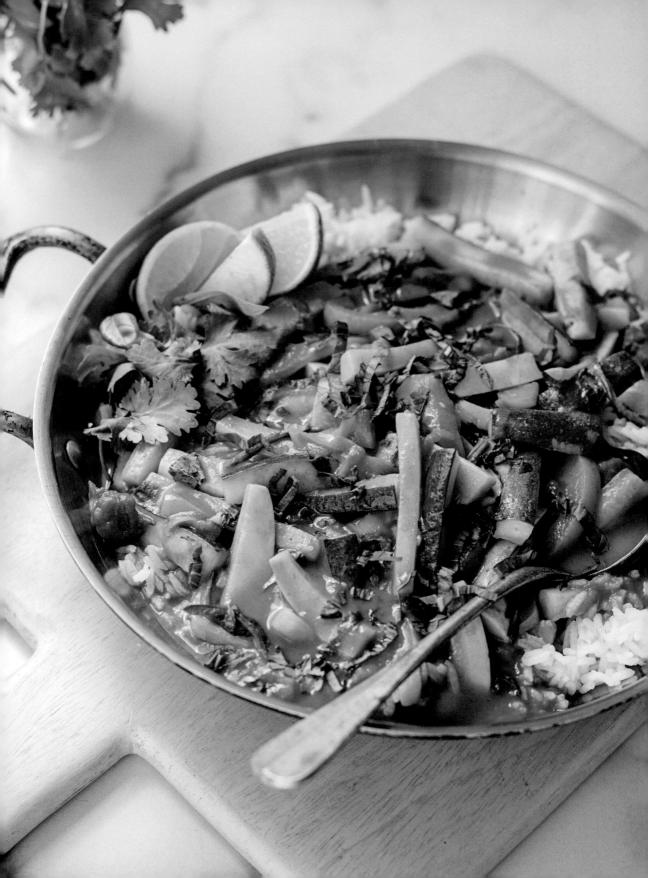

Summer Squash Moqueca

This hardy summer stew is a vegetarian version of the traditional Brazilian fish dish *moqueca*. It's usually made from a rich seafood stock with a creamy, red finish, thanks to coconut milk, tomatoes, and paprika. I've found that even this quick version is just as vibrant and comforting. If you want a more traditional flavor profile, you can add cubed cod, haddock, or shrimp along with the coconut milk. For more veggies, I love adding chopped hearts of palm, which is another Brazilian staple (I couldn't find any information on their FODMAP content, so incorporate at your own risk!).

MAKES 4 SERVINGS (SAFE SERVING: 1½ CUPS)

- 2 tablespoons extra-virgin olive or virgin coconut oil
- 1 medium-size orange bell pepper, thinly sliced
- 1 Fresno or jalapeño pepper, ribs and seeds removed, thinly sliced
- 2 medium-size zucchini (12 ounces), cut into ½-inch-thick matchsticks
- 2 medium-size summer squash (12 ounces), cut into ½-inch-thick matchsticks
- 1 vine tomato, roughly chopped
- 2 tablespoons tomato paste
- 2 teaspoons paprika

- 1 cup full-fat coconut milk
- ½ cup Low-FODMAP Basic Chicken Bone Broth or Vegetable Stock (pages 140 and 142)
- 1 teaspoon sea salt

- 2 tablespoons freshly squeezed lime juice (from 1 lime)
- ¼ cup roughly chopped fresh cilantro
- ¼ cup roughly chopped fresh basil leaves

❶ In a large Dutch oven or saucepan, heat the oil over medium-high heat. Add the peppers. Sauté for about 4 minutes, until soft and starting to brown. Stir in the zucchini, summer squash, tomatoes, tomato paste, and paprika. Cook for 4 minutes more, or until very fragrant and the tomato juices have reduced.

❷ Pour in the coconut milk and broth, scraping up any brown bits that may have formed on the bottom of the pan, and season with the salt. Simmer rapidly over medium-high heat for about 5 minutes, or until the squash is fork-tender but not too mushy. Remove from the heat and stir in the lime juice and half of the cilantro and basil. Serve warm over rice, quinoa, or sautéed greens with the remaining herbs as garnish.

Onward Add 1 can **hearts of palm**, thinly sliced, in Step 2, along with the lime juice.

LF	SCD	SSFG	Omit cilantro; use Low-Histamine Stock (page 142)↓	Omit tomatoes, tomato paste, and jalapeño; use Low-Histamine Stock (page 142)↓	Use Low-Histamine Stock (page 142)↓
BPD1R	BPD1	BPD2			
P	V	SF	HS	HI	YC

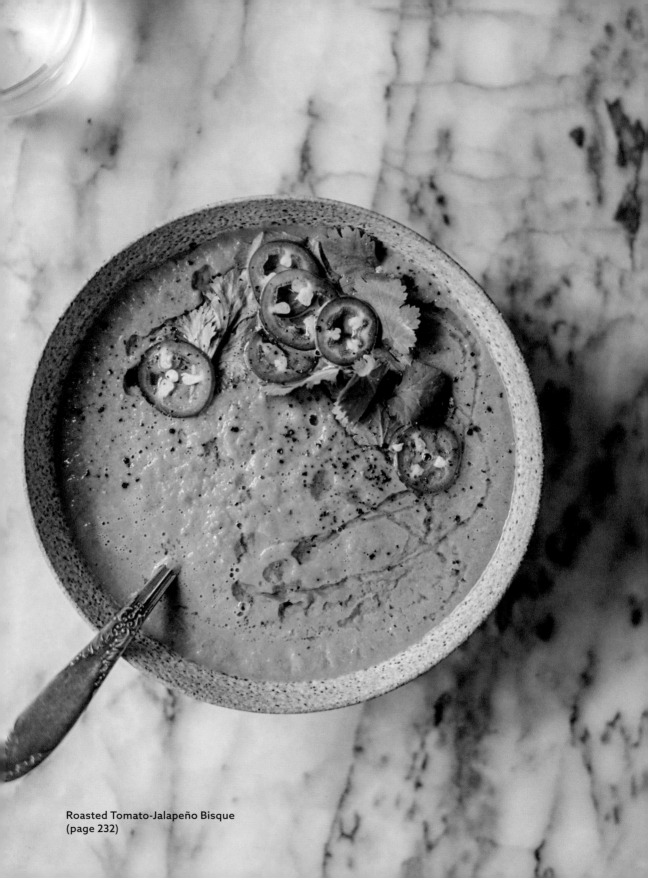

Roasted Tomato-Jalapeño Bisque
(page 232)

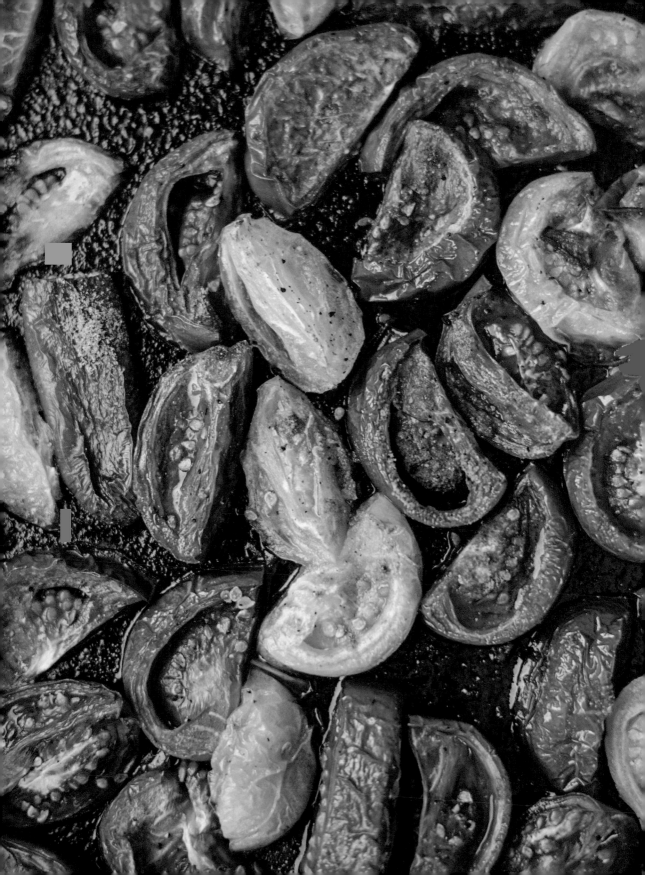

Roasted Tomato-Jalapeño Bisque

Cream of tomato soup gets a little kick in the pantaloons in this recipe. The vine-ripened tomatoes and jalapeño still have a lovely brightness after roasting but also benefit from the oven caramelization. Roasting the tomatoes also lends the broth a handsome orange hue. Since the soup has so few ingredients, it helps to choose really good-quality tomatoes. Just pay attention as you add the coconut milk and stock, as the amount you'll need may vary depending on the water content of your tomatoes. If you want some extra texture and crunch, garnish with the Sweet & Smoky Pepita Brittle on page 176.

MAKES 4 SERVINGS

3½ pounds Roma or plum tomatoes, quartered

1 jalapeño pepper, halved (seeds and ribs removed if you prefer less heat)

½ teaspoon ground cumin

Sea salt

Extra-virgin olive oil

½ cup fresh cilantro leaves and stems

1 cup Low-FODMAP Basic Chicken Bone Broth or Vegetable Stock (pages 140 and 142)

1 cup coconut milk

1 Preheat the oven to 450°F. Line a baking sheet with parchment paper.

2 Arrange the tomatoes and jalapeño in a single layer on the prepared baking sheet and season with the cumin and a sprinkle of salt. Drizzle the vegetables lightly with olive oil and transfer to the oven.

3 Roast until the tomatoes are shriveled and have released their juices, about 45 minutes. Remove the pan from the oven.

4 Transfer the tomatoes and jalapeño to a blender or food processor, along with any juices from the pan, half of the cilantro, and the broth, coconut milk, and ¾ teaspoon of salt. Process the soup until smooth, adding more water or broth if the soup is too thick.

5 Taste for seasoning and divide among four bowls. Garnish with the remaining cilantro.

Onward Substitute ⅓ cup of raw **cashews**, soaked for 10 minutes in 1 cup of boiling water, for the coconut milk.

	LF	SCD	SSFG	BPD1R	BPD1	BPD2	P	V	SF	Use Low-Histamine Stock (page 142) ↓ YC	Sub basil for cilantro; Use Low-Histamine Stock (page 142) ↓ HS

Warming Root Vegetable Chicken Tagine with Chard

As you can probably tell by now, I love borrowing flavor profiles from other cultures to create as much variety as possible on a SIBO diet. This dish is no different. Tagine is named after the terra-cotta pot in which it is traditionally cooked, but it is essentially the Moroccan Arabic word for "stew." Tagines are usually layered with a variety of warming spices and finished with some type of dried fruit. Since most fruit is off-limits for SIBO Amigos, I've instead relied on the sweetness of root vegetables, here parsnip and carrots. Feel free to swap in other starchy vegetables, such as turnips, rutabaga, sweet potato, or baby potatoes, if tolerated.

MAKES 4 SERVINGS

1 pound boneless, skinless chicken thighs

Sea salt and freshly ground black pepper

Extra-virgin olive oil

1 pound carrots (about 8 medium), cut diagonally into 1-inch pieces

1 pound parsnips (about 5 medium), peeled and cut diagonally into 1-inch pieces

1 bunch chard, stems and leaves divided and finely chopped (about 5 cups, packed)

1 tablespoon ground cumin

2 teaspoons ground turmeric

2 teaspoons ground ginger

¼ teaspoon ground cinnamon

¼ teaspoon cayenne pepper

1 (15-ounce) can diced tomatoes, or 2 large vine tomatoes, diced

4 cups Low-FODMAP Basic Chicken Bone Broth (page 140)

2 tablespoons freshly squeezed lemon juice

Fresh parsley or cilantro leaves, for serving

❶ Season the chicken thighs with salt and pepper. In a large pot or Dutch oven, heat a thin layer of olive oil. Sear the chicken in batches over high heat, making sure not to crowd the pot, until golden brown, about 4 minutes per side. Transfer to a bowl.

❷ Add another glug of olive oil along with the carrots, parsnips, and chard stems. Sauté over medium-high heat until soft and beginning to brown, about 7 minutes.

recipe continues →

❸ Stir in the cumin, turmeric, ginger, cinnamon, cayenne, and 2 teaspoons of salt. Cook until the spices are fully incorporated and aromatic, about 2 minutes. Add the tomatoes and cook, scraping up any brown bits that may have formed, until thickened, about 3 minutes. Arrange the chicken on top of the vegetable mixture and cover with the broth.

❹ Bring to a simmer, reduce the heat to low, and cook, uncovered, for at least 30 minutes, until the chicken and carrots are fork-tender, or up to 2 hours, adding more water or broth as necessary.

❺ Add the chard and lemon juice and simmer until wilted, about 3 minutes.

❻ Spoon the tagine into individual bowls and garnish with cilantro or parsley.

Onward Add 1 cup of canned **chickpeas** along with the stock and/or stir in ¼ cup of chopped dried **apricots** in Step 5.

LF	P	SF	SSFG	SCD	BPD1	BPD2	HI	HS	YC
			Use fresh tomatoes ↓				Omit tomatoes and lemon juice, unless tolerated; use Low-Histamine Stock (page 142) ↓	Omit chard and cilantro; use Low-Histamine Stock (page 142) ↓	Use Low-Histamine Stock (page 142) ↓

Kitchen Sink Crucifer Soup

What do broccoli, cabbage, and kale have in common? They are all cruciferous vegetables, or members of the mustard family. Other varieties include cauliflower, bok choy, arugula, Brussels sprouts, collards, watercress, and radishes. Most cruciferous veggies are rich in folate and vitamin K. Without cruciferous vegetables, our liver detox pathways have a harder time running efficiently. And that can get us into big trouble in our hypertoxic environment. This soup is a fantastic way to reap some of these benefits without blowing your FODMAP threshold or battling the woody fiber that might be harder for SIBO sufferers to process when eating these veggies raw. You can use bok choy, watercress, or arugula instead of kale. The cabbage and broccoli add bulk and make the soup feel like a healthy version of some creamy, cheesy concoction you might be served in a bread bowl.

MAKES 4 SERVINGS

¼ cup extra-virgin olive oil

2 cups broccoli florets

2 cups chopped green cabbage

1 medium-size russet potato (8 ounces), peeled and cut into ½-inch cubes

6 cups Low-FODMAP Vegetable Stock (page 142)

1 teaspoon sea salt

1 small bunch kale (any variety works), roughly chopped (3 cups, packed)

6 scallions, green parts only, roughly chopped, or ½ cup chopped fresh chives

2 tablespoons freshly squeezed lemon juice

❶ In a large pot or deep-sided saucepan, heat the olive oil over medium heat. Add the broccoli, cabbage, and potato. Cook, stirring occasionally, until the cabbage is translucent and beginning to brown, about 5 minutes. Pour in the broth and season with salt. Bring to a boil over high heat, then lower the heat to maintain a rapid simmer. Cook the vegetables until the potato is fork-tender, about 8 minutes. Stir in the kale and scallions; cook for 1 minute more, until wilted.

❷ Remove the soup from the heat and transfer to a stand blender (or use an immersion blender) to puree until smooth.

❸ Stir in the lemon juice right before serving and enjoy warm.

Onward Whisk in 2 tablespoons of fermented **white miso** paste along with the lemon juice (Step 3).

									Use Low-Histamine Stock (page 142) ↓	Omit lemon juice, unless tolerated; use Low-Histamine Stock (page 142) ↓
						Omit potato ↓				
LF	P	SF	V	BPD2	SCD	SSFG	BPD1R	BPD1	YC	HI

Lamb & Sweet Potato Chili

You might be wondering how someone pulls off a traditional chili without any beans in the mix. The solution is skirting the traditional components altogether. Since ground lamb pairs so well with Moroccan flavors, I used the spice mix and accoutrements from one of my favorite tagines (more about this on page 233) to form the base. Instead of beans, I use a low-FODMAP-friendly quantity of canned chickpeas. With the addition of sweet potato and kale, this chili covers all the food groups. If you tolerate dairy, you can top it with 24-Hour Yogurt (page 163) as a gut-friendly substitute for the usual sour cream. To make this in a slow cooker, simply transfer to the cooker at Step 2, add the remaining ingredients, and cook on HIGH for four hours.

MAKES 4 SERVINGS

- 2 tablespoons olive oil
- 1 large red bell pepper, finely diced
- 1 pound ground lamb
- 1 tablespoon ground cumin
- 1 teaspoon ground coriander
- 1 teaspoon ground ginger
- ¼ teaspoon cayenne pepper
- 2 teaspoons sea salt
- 1 (28-ounce) can fire-roasted diced or crushed tomatoes
- 1 medium sweet potato peeled and cut into ½-inch cubes (about 2 cups)
- ¾ cup canned chickpeas, drained and rinsed
- 2 cups frozen chopped curly kale, or 4 leaves fresh, stemmed and chopped
- 2 cups Low-FODMAP Beef or Basic Chicken Bone Broth (pages 142 and 140) or water
- Fresh cilantro leaves, for serving
- 24-Hour Yogurt (page 163), for serving (optional)

❶ In a large stockpot or Dutch oven, heat the oil. Sauté the red bell pepper over medium-high heat until soft, about 5 minutes. Push the pepper to the sides of the pan and add the lamb. Brown the meat, breaking it apart with your spatula, until cooked through, 5 minutes. Add the cumin, coriander, ground ginger, cayenne, and salt. Cook for 1 minute, or until the spices are fragrant. Carefully pour in the tomatoes and simmer over medium heat until the liquid has reduced, 10 minutes.

❷ Stir in the sweet potatoes, chickpeas, and kale. Cover with the broth or water. Bring to a boil, lower the heat to low, and simmer, uncovered, for 15 to 20 minutes, or until the sweet potatoes are tender and the chili has thickened.

❸ Serve the chili with cilantro leaves and yogurt (if using) on top.

Onward Use the full 14.5-ounce can of **chickpeas**.

		Omit sweet potato and chickpeas; use 1½ pounds fresh tomatoes; double kale ↓					Omit chickpeas ↓
LF	SF	SCD	SSFG	BPD1R	BPD1	BPD2	P

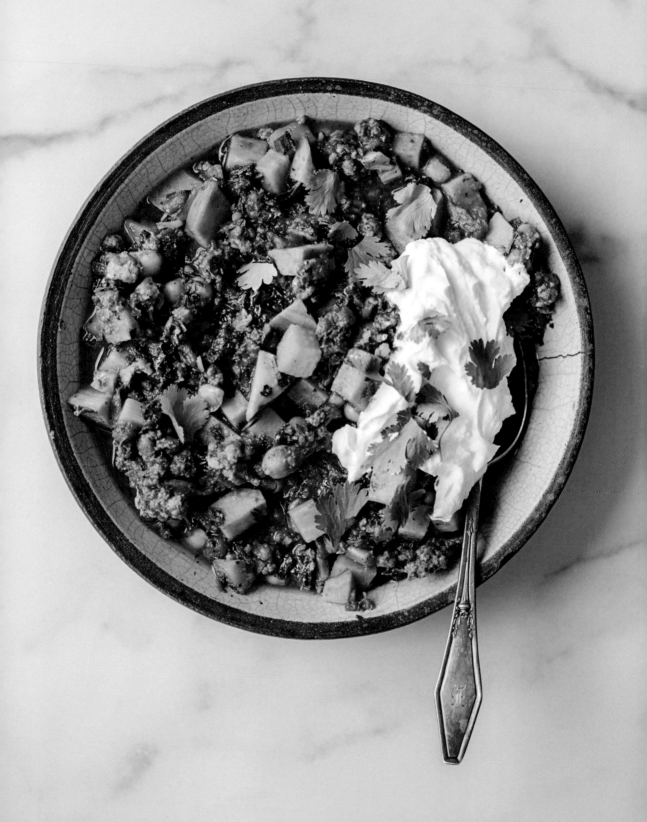

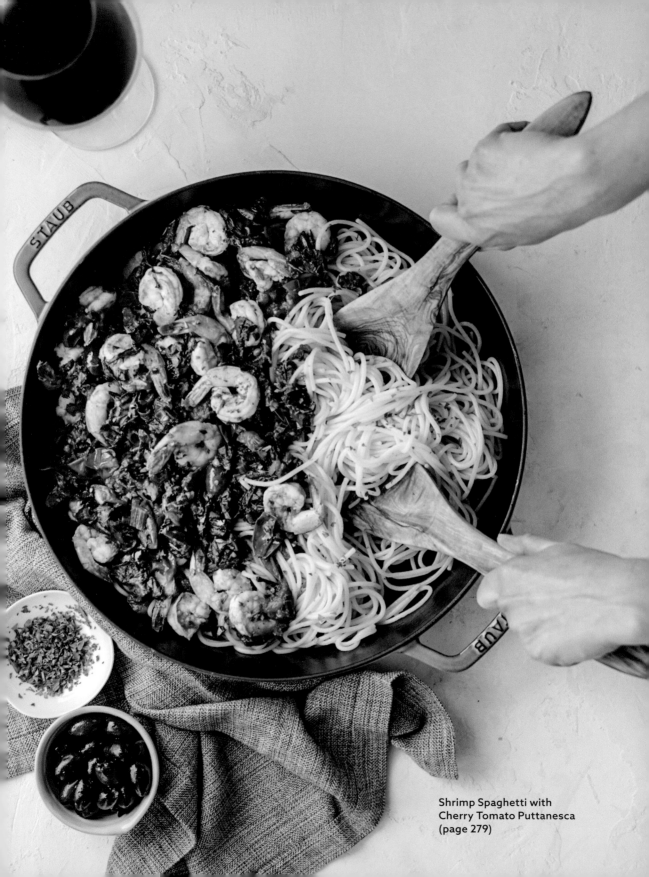

Shrimp Spaghetti with
Cherry Tomato Puttanesca
(page 279)

THE MAIN EVENT

Poodtry, Meat & Seafood Entrées

Lemon-Rosemary Roast Chicken with
Parsnips and Carrots • 241

Chili-Lime Sheet Pan Chicken with
Delicata Squash and Kale • 243

Thai Green Curry Chicken with
Baby Eggplant • 246

Creamy Chicken and
Broccoli Casserole • 248

Turkey-Zucchini Meatballs with
the Simplest Romesco Sauce • 249

Skillet Chicken Cacciatore • 253

Back-Pocket Chicken Paillard with
Sun-Dried Tomato Vinaigrette • 254

Mild and Creamy Butterless
Butter Chicken • 255

Grilled Skirt Steak with Three-Herb
Chimichurri • 256

Beef Negimaki Stir-Fry with
Green Beans and Watercress • 259

Shepherd's Pie with Kale and
Semi-Sweet Potato Mash • 260

Stuffed Collard Greens with
Lamb and Quinoa • 262

Larb Lettuce Wraps • 265

Teriyaki Pork Tenderloin with
Bok Choy and Broccoli • 266

Cider-Dijon Pork Chops with
Silky Cabbage • 268

Sausage and Sweet Pepper Hash • 269

BLT Frittata • 270

Baked Halibut with Green Olive and
Fennel Tapenade • 273

Turmeric-Dill Catfish • 274

Sesame Sheet Pan Salmon
with Radishes • 276

Seared Scallops with
Squash Succotash • 277

Shrimp Spaghetti with
Cherry Tomato Puttanesca • 279

Blackened Salmon Burrito Bowls with
Dirty Quinoa and Cucumber Salsa • 281

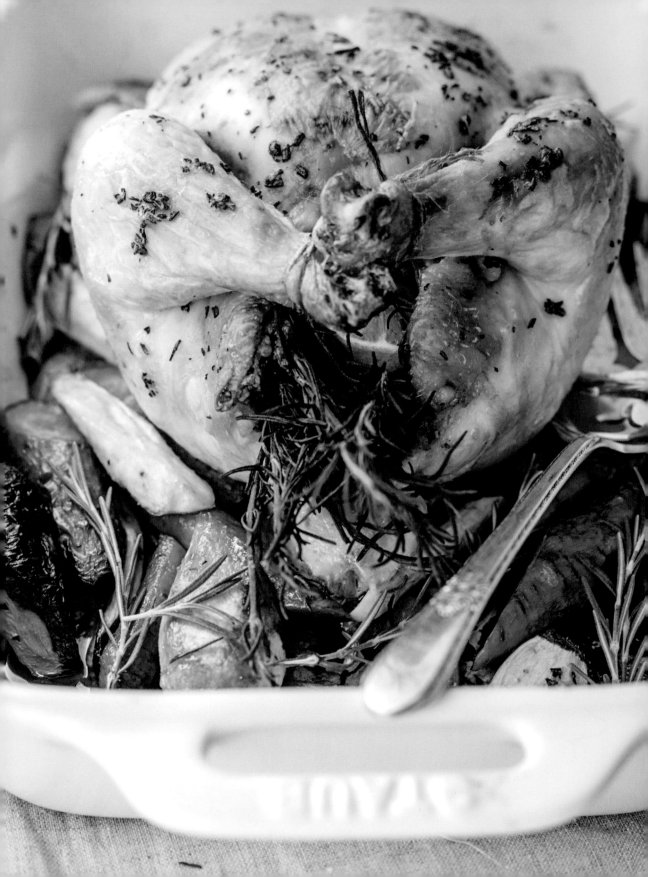

Lemon-Rosemary Roast Chicken with Parsnips and Carrots

Rosemary is one of my favorite all-purpose medicinal herbs with a range of anti-inflammatory compounds that improve digestion. It's also been studied as a natural treatment for *H. pylori* infections. But all of this comes second to the fact that it tastes so darn good. Especially in the fall and winter, I try to pile rosemary onto all my roasted meats and root vegetables. This roast chicken is a double whammy and perfect for a Sunday night. The key to a really flavorful bird is making a compound herb butter and using your fingers to smash it into every crevice beneath the chicken's skin. In this case, I use a combination of ghee and coconut oil, which have a similar texture at room temperature and melt away into the most luscious pan sauce for the vegetables beneath.

MAKES 4 SERVINGS

1 pound carrots (about 8 medium), cut diagonally into 2-inch pieces

1 pound parsnips (about 5 medium), peeled and cut diagonally into 2-inch pieces

1 tablespoon extra-virgin olive oil

Sea salt

1 bunch fresh rosemary (about 8 sprigs)

1 tablespoon coconut oil

1 tablespoon grass-fed ghee

1 (4- to 5-pound) whole chicken

1 lemon, halved

❶ Preheat the oven to 425°F.

❷ Place the carrots and parsnips in a large roasting pan. Toss with the olive oil and ½ teaspoon of salt. Arrange in an even layer.

❸ Remove the leaves from two rosemary sprigs and roughly chop. You should have 2 tablespoons. Transfer the herbs to a small bowl along with the coconut oil, ghee, and ½ teaspoon of salt. Mix thoroughly to combine.

❹ Remove the giblets from the chicken, and trim the wing tips. Rinse the chicken inside and out, and pat the skin dry. Generously salt the inside and outside of the chicken. Stuff the cavity with the remaining rosemary and the lemon halves.

❺ Carefully separate the skin from the chicken breasts, using your fingers, and slather the chicken flesh with the rosemary mixture (about a tablespoon per breast). You'll want to do your best to get it all the way in—but be careful not to pierce the skin! Rub the outside of the skin with the remaining mixture.

❻ Tie the chicken legs together with kitchen string, and tuck the wing tips under the body of the chicken. Place the chicken, breast side up, on top of the veggies in the pan.

recipe continues →

Poultry, Meat & Seafood Entrées

7 Roast in the oven for 1 to 1½ hours, tossing the vegetables once halfway through, until the chicken juices run clear when you cut between the leg and thigh or the internal temperature reads 165°F. Remove from the oven and transfer the chicken to a work surface and allow to rest for at least 15 minutes before carving it. Transfer the chicken pieces to a platter alongside the vegetables. Squeeze the lemon halves from the cavity over the bird and serve immediately topped with the pan drippings.

Onward Add 2 large russet **potatoes**, cut into chunks, to the carrots and parsnips (Step 2).

	LF	SCD	SSFG	BPD1	BPD2	P	SF	YC	HS	Omit parsnips and double carrots ↓	Omit lemon, unless tolerated ↓
										BPD1R	HI

Chili-Lime Sheet Pan Chicken with Delicata Squash and Kale

Sheet pan meals are the gateway drug that will help you fall in love with cooking forever. The key to conceptualizing one is making sure you choose a protein with a cooking time that matches the rest of the ingredients. For instance, bone-in chicken parts usually take forty-five minutes to an hour to get fully tender and crispy, which is why I pair them with sturdy winter squash. Delicata squash is one of my go-to varieties because it doesn't require peeling. If you can't find any at the market, feel free to swap in a pound of red potatoes, parsnips, kabocha squash, or fresh pumpkin cut into small wedges. I prefer dark meat for this sheet pan meal due to the long cooking time, so if opting for breasts, make sure they are bone-in, skin-on.

MAKES 4 SERVINGS

2 small delicata squash (about 1½ pounds), halved lengthwise and seeds scraped out, cut into thin half-moons

Olive oil

Sea salt

2 teaspoons ground cumin

2 tablespoons low-FODMAP hot sauce (I like Cholula), or ¼ teaspoon cayenne pepper

¼ cup freshly squeezed lime juice (from 2 limes)

¼ cup finely chopped fresh cilantro leaves

3 pounds bone-in chicken thighs and drumsticks

1 bunch kale, thick stems removed, roughly chopped (4 cups, packed)

❶ Preheat the oven to 425°F. Line a large, rimmed baking sheet with parchment.

❷ On the prepared baking sheet, toss the squash with 2 tablespoons of olive oil and ½ teaspoon of salt. Arrange in an even layer on the sheet pan.

❸ In a small bowl or 1-cup measure, whisk together the cumin, hot sauce, lime juice, 2 tablespoons of the chopped cilantro, 2 tablespoons of olive oil, and ½ teaspoon of salt until combined.

recipe continues →

4 Arrange the chicken pieces in an even layer on top of the squash. Drizzle the chicken with half of the cumin mixture, and using your hands (or a brush if squeamish), rub the marinade all over the meat. Transfer the sheet pan to the oven and roast for 40 minutes, or until the skin is beginning to brown and the chicken has released some juicy goodness.

5 While the chicken roasts, prep the kale. In a large bowl, combine the chopped leaves with the remaining cumin mixture. Toss until fully coated.

6 Remove the pan from the oven and nestle the marinated kale between the chicken pieces (if it covers the chicken, no worries, but you want the skin to remain crispy if possible). Return the pan to the oven and cook for another 10 minutes, or until the kale is wilted and the top leaves are beginning to crisp.

7 Serve the chicken straight from the pan for a rustic presentation, garnished with the remaining cilantro.

Onward Substitute 1 pound of **cauliflower** florets for the squash (Step 2).

								Omit kale and cilantro ↓	Omit hot sauce or cayenne ↓	
LF	SCD	SSFG	BPD1R	BPD1	BPD2	P	SF	HS	YC	HI

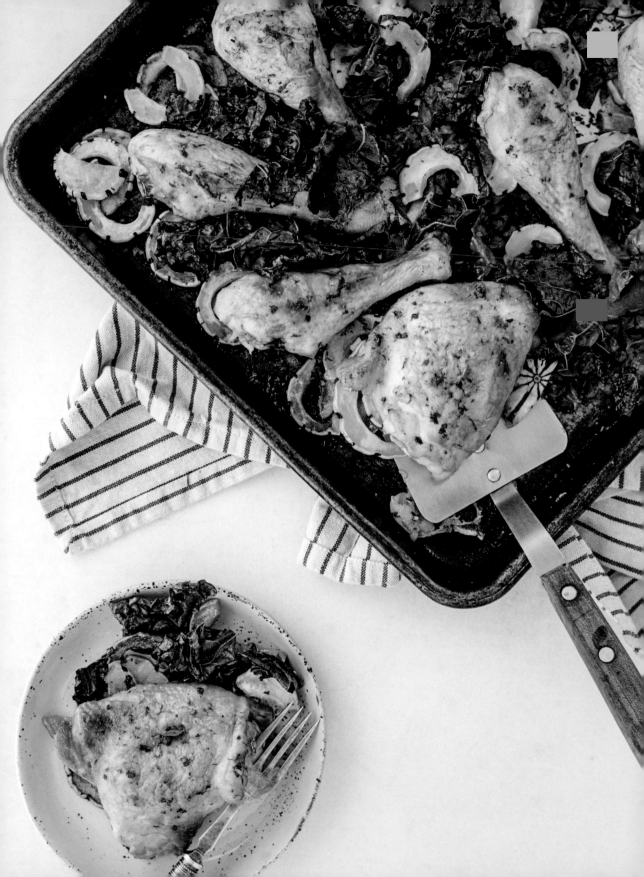

Thai Green Curry Chicken with Baby Eggplant

A homemade Thai green curry paste allows this recipe to be low-FODMAP, sugar-free, and healthy. And yet it comes together quicker than your takeout order would arrive on your doorstep. Since chicken breasts don't have much fat, and therefore dry out more easily, I prefer to cube my chicken on the larger side so that it doesn't overcook. If you want to make your curry look like what you'd get in a Thai restaurant, thinly slice the breasts and poach them in the coconut milk mixture until cooked through, rather than searing first. To speed up your prep time, you can toss the ginger and jalapeño in a small food processor to make the paste. Serve the curry over rice (if tolerated) with extra limes on the side. Or make the Spaghetti Squash Pad Thai (page 204) for a complete takeout fake-out feast.

MAKES 4 SERVINGS

- ¼ cup coconut oil
- 2 pounds chicken breasts (about 4 medium), cut into 2-inch cubes
- Sea salt
- 1 small Japanese or Italian eggplant, halved lengthwise and thinly sliced into half-moons
- 1 (1-inch) piece fresh ginger, minced
- 1 jalapeño pepper, seeds and ribs removed, finely chopped
- 1 teaspoon ground cumin
- ½ teaspoon ground coriander
- ½ teaspoon ground turmeric
- 1 cup full-fat coconut milk
- 1 cup Low-FODMAP Basic Chicken Bone Broth (page 140)
- ¼ cup freshly squeezed lime juice (from 2 limes)
- 1 medium-size red bell pepper, thinly sliced
- 1 cup halved green beans
- ⅓ cup loosely packed torn fresh basil leaves

❶ In a large, nonstick skillet, melt 2 tablespoons of the coconut oil over medium heat. Add the chicken in an even layer. Season generously with salt and cook until golden brown on the first side, about 3 minutes. Flip the chicken and cook for another minute (it doesn't have to be completely cooked through). Transfer from the pan to a large bowl and set aside.

❷ Add the remaining 2 tablespoons of oil to the skillet. When hot, add the eggplant and stir-fry until lightly browned and soft, about 5 minutes. Remove from the pan and set aside in the chicken bowl.

❸ To the pan, add the ginger, jalapeño, ½ teaspoon of salt, and the cumin, coriander, and turmeric and cook until fragrant, 2 minutes (add more oil, if necessary). Pour in the coconut milk, broth, and lime juice, scraping up any brown bits from the bottom of the pan. Bring to a simmer and cook until the liquid has reduced slightly and the broth is a vibrant greenish yellow, 5 minutes.

❹ Carefully add the chicken and eggplant back to the pan, and stir in the bell pepper and green beans; cook for about 5 minutes more, until the vegetables are tender. Remove from the heat and garnish with the basil.

LF	SCD	P	SF	SSFG	BPD1R	BPD1	BPD2	YC	HS	HI
								Use Low-Histamine Stock (page 142) ↓	Omit coriander and green beans; use Low-Histamine Stock (page 142) ↓	Omit jalapeño and eggplant; double bell peppers ↓

Creamy Chicken and Broccoli Casserole

As long as you avoid the 1950s approach to chicken and rice casseroles, they hold a perfectly acceptable place in a low-FODMAP diet. In this version, coconut milk stands in for the usual gloppy can of cream of whatever soup. As discussed on page 128, the ¼ cup low-FODMAP serving of coconut milk is one of the more annoying quantities since a regular can is around 2 cups. Arborio rice, since it's on the starchy side, is ideal for casseroles. But you can also use sushi rice for a similar result: crispy on the outside and sticky in the middle.

MAKES 4 TO 6 SERVINGS

- 1 cup arborio rice
- 2 cups finely chopped broccoli florets (from 1 small crown)
- 4 scallions, green parts only, thinly sliced
- 1 cup full-fat coconut milk
- 2 cups Low-FODMAP Basic Chicken Bone Broth (page 140)
- 2 tablespoons freshly squeezed lemon juice (from ½ lemon)
- 2 tablespoons extra-virgin olive oil
- ½ teaspoon dried thyme
- ¼ teaspoon red pepper flakes
- Sea salt and freshly ground black pepper
- 6 bone-in skin-on chicken thighs (about 2 pounds)

1 Preheat the oven to 400°F.

2 In a large bowl, combine the rice, broccoli, scallions, coconut milk, broth, lemon juice, olive oil, thyme, red pepper flakes, and 1 teaspoon of salt. Fold the ingredients together until well mixed. Transfer to a 12-inch ovenproof skillet or a 9 x 13-inch casserole dish and arrange in an even layer. Nestle the chicken thighs, skin side up, in the rice mixture and season generously with salt and pepper.

3 Bake, uncovered, for 45 minutes, or until the rice is tender and most of the liquid is absorbed. Remove from the oven and allow to rest for 5 minutes. Serve warm with a green salad on the side.

Onward Use the full 14.5-ounce can of **coconut milk** and omit 1 cup of the broth.

		Limit serving of rice to ½ cup ↓		Omit lemon juice, unless tolerated; use Low-Histamine Stock (page 142) ↓
LF	SF	BPD1	BPD2	HI

Turkey-Zucchini Meatballs with the Simplest Romesco Sauce

I learned the secret for these paleo meatballs from my friend Serena Wolf, who is a whiz at making classic comfort food better for you. Chia seeds plump up and develop a gelatinous texture when exposed to liquid. They replace both the usual egg and bread crumbs in this recipe and allow you to sneak in some vegetables (zucchini) without your meatballs becoming soggy. Both the balls and the sauce are fantastic for make-ahead meal prep. Just cook some gluten-free pasta the night of, or omit entirely if you're watching your grains and serve the balls "naked" or over more zucchini in noodle form. The leftover romesco sauce tastes great on scrambled eggs. If your gut is very sensitive, it might be harder to process chia seeds, so use the BPD modification below.

MAKES 4 SERVINGS

▷ Meatballs

1 medium-size zucchini, grated on the largest hole of a box grater (about 1½ cups)

1 pound ground turkey

1 tablespoon chia seeds

2 tablespoons finely chopped fresh mint leaves

½ teaspoon smoked paprika

¼ teaspoon ground cumin

1 teaspoon sea salt

▷ Romesco sauce

1 (16-ounce) jar roasted red peppers, drained

2 tablespoons blanched almonds

¼ cup extra-virgin olive oil

1 tablespoon sherry or red wine vinegar

½ teaspoon sea salt

Pinch of red pepper flakes (optional)

❶ **Make the meatballs:** Preheat the oven to 400°F. Line a baking sheet with parchment paper and set aside.

❷ Gather the grated zucchini in your hands and gently squeeze out some of the water into the sink. Place the zucchini in a medium-size bowl, along with the turkey, chia seeds, mint, smoked paprika, cumin, and salt. With clean hands, mix the turkey until well combined, making sure not to overly break apart the meat. Allow the mixture to rest for at least 10 minutes at room temperature, or longer in the fridge, to give the chia seeds time to activate.

❸ Form the meat into roughly sixteen equal-size balls, about 2 tablespoons of meat in each (I like using an ice-cream scoop to portion). Arrange on the prepared baking sheet and bake in

recipe continues →

Poultry, Meat & Seafood Entrées

the middle of the oven until lightly browned on top and cooked through, about 25 minutes.

4 **Meanwhile, make the sauce:** In a blender or food processor, combine the peppers, almonds, olive oil, vinegar, salt, and red pepper flakes, if using. Puree until smooth, adding a splash of water if necessary to reach your desired consistency.

5 Serve the meatballs warm over your favorite gluten-free pasta, zoodles, or all by themselves "naked" with the romesco drizzled on top.

Onward Add an 8.5-ounce jar of **sun-dried tomatoes** in oil to the romesco (Step 4).

LF	P	SF	Sub ¼ cup of almond flour plus 1 large egg, beaten, for chia seeds ↓					Omit almonds ↓
			SCD	SSFG	BPD1R	BPD1	BPD2	HS

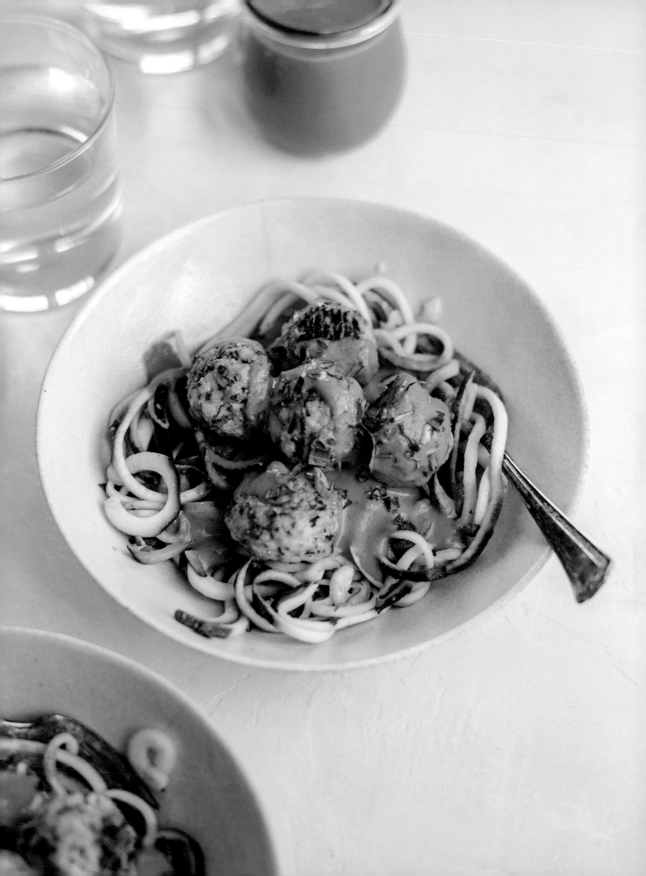

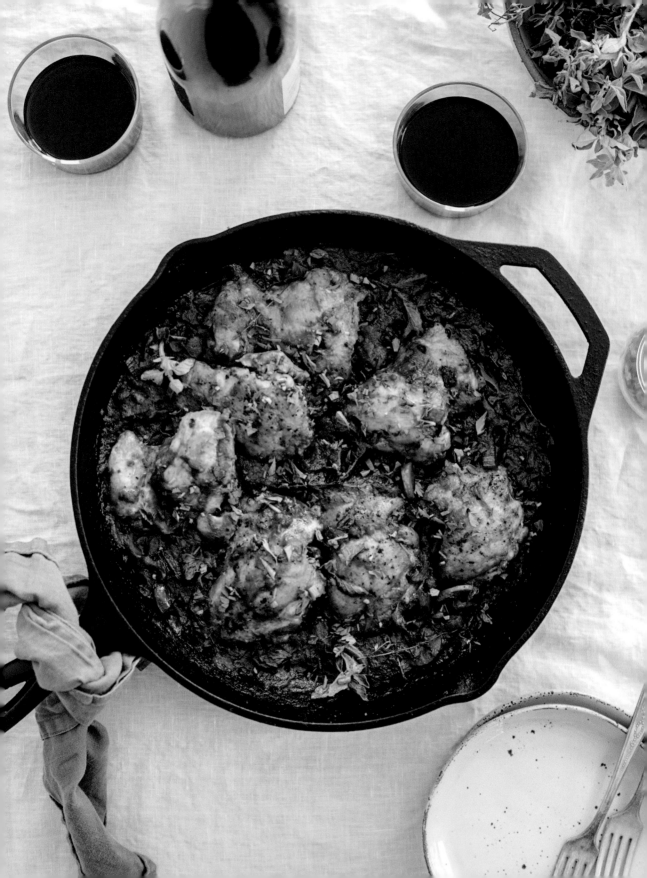

Skillet Chicken Cacciatore

Even without half the usual aromatics, this Italian chicken dish still manages to taste phenomenal, thanks to the power of woody herbs, such as thyme and oregano. I originally developed a version of this recipe for Fody Foods, a brand that makes store-bought versions of many of the recipes in the Foundational Dishes chapter. If you don't feel like making your own Garlic-Infused Oil (page 143), Low-FODMAP Basic Chicken Bone Broth (page 140), or Low-FODMAP Pasta Sauce (page 149), you can easily let Fody do the work for you. Serve the cacciatore alongside gluten-free pasta or the Chicory Salad on page 182.

MAKES 4 SERVINGS

2 tablespoons extra-virgin olive oil

2 pounds boneless, skinless chicken thighs

Sea salt and freshly ground black pepper

2 medium-size carrots, thinly sliced

1 medium-size celery stalk, thinly sliced

1 red bell pepper, diced

¼ teaspoon red pepper flakes

½ cup dry red wine or Low-FODMAP Basic Chicken Bone Broth (page 140)

2 cups Low-FODMAP Pasta Sauce (page 149; see headnote)

4 fresh thyme sprigs, or ¼ teaspoon dried leaves

4 fresh oregano sprigs, or ¼ teaspoon dried leaves

2 tablespoons finely chopped fresh flat-leaf parsley leaves

❶ In a large skillet, heat the oil over medium-high heat. Season the chicken thighs with salt and black pepper and add to the pan in an even layer. Cook the chicken (in batches, if necessary) until a golden brown crust has formed on both sides and the chicken is cooked through, about 10 minutes total. Transfer to a plate and set aside.

❷ Add the carrots, celery, and bell pepper to the pan. Sauté the vegetables, scraping up any brown bits from the bottom of the pan, until soft, about 5 minutes. Season them with 1 teaspoon of salt and the red pepper flakes.

❸ Pour in the red wine or broth and simmer until reduced by at least half, 1 minute. Add the pasta sauce, stirring to combine. Carefully return the chicken to the skillet and nestle it in the sauce, making sure it's fully coated. Tuck the herbs in between the chicken thighs, or sprinkle them over the top if using dried. Simmer over medium-low heat until the sauce has thickened and the chicken is fork-tender, 10 to 15 minutes. Garnish with the parsley and serve directly from the skillet.

Onward Add 8 ounces of cremini **mushrooms**, thinly sliced, with the carrots (Step 2).

					Use Low-Histamine Stock (page 142) instead of wine ↓				
LF	P	SF	SCD	SSFG	BPD1R	BPD1	BPD2	HS	YC

Back-Pocket Chicken Paillard with Sun-Dried Tomato Vinaigrette

When in doubt of what to make for dinner, this grilled chicken breast–salad combo is always a winner, thanks in part to the unexpected dressing. A tricky thing about FODMAPs is that their load differs depending on how a food is prepared. Dried fruit, since the sugars are concentrated, pack a bigger punch than fresh. Take tomatoes, for example. (Yes, tomatoes are a fruit...) The ratio of fructose increases with drying, making more than a three-piece portion high-FODMAP, whereas regular tomatoes are generally in the safe column. One way to enjoy all that sweet, tart goodness that sun-dried tomatoes provide, without overdoing the quantity, is to use them as a condiment.

MAKES 4 SERVINGS

- 4 boneless, skinless chicken breasts
- ¼ cup freshly squeezed lemon juice (from 2 lemons)
- ¾ cup extra-virgin olive oil
- Sea salt
- 8 sun-dried tomatoes packed in oil (see headnote)
- 1 tablespoon sherry or red wine vinegar
- 5 ounces baby arugula (about 5 cups, tightly packed)
- 1 small head radicchio, cored and thinly sliced
- ½ cup walnuts, toasted and chopped

❶ On a clean work surface, working one piece at a time, place the chicken between two pieces of parchment paper and pound with a mallet or bottom of a skillet to an even ½-inch thickness.

❷ Place the chicken breasts in a baking dish or large bowl. Add the lemon juice, ¼ cup of the olive oil, and 1 teaspoon of salt. Flip the chicken breasts around in the marinade until well coated. Set aside for at least 20 minutes or for up to an hour in the fridge.

❸ Meanwhile, in a small food processor or blender, combine the sun-dried tomatoes, vinegar, remaining ½ cup of olive oil, and ½ teaspoon of salt. Puree until the mixture has a smooth, drizzleable consistency, adding more oil as necessary. Set aside.

❹ Heat an indoor grill pan or heavy-bottomed skillet over medium-high. Remove the chicken breasts from the marinade and grill or sear in batches for about 3 minutes per side, until nicely charred and just cooked through. If grilling, rotate the breasts 90 degrees halfway through for a pretty crosshatch!

❺ While the meat rests, combine the arugula, radicchio, and walnuts in a large bowl. Dress with the sun-dried tomato vinaigrette and toss to incorporate.

❻ Divide the chicken paillards among four plates and top with the mixed greens. Serve immediately.

Onward Add 1 cup of rinsed and drained **cannellini beans** or 2 thinly sliced **celery** stalks to the salad (Step 5).

LF	SCD	SSFG	BPD1R	BPD1	BPD2	P	SF

Mild and Creamy Butterless Butter Chicken

If you steer clear of the dishes that have added cream and a little too much butter, Indian cuisine can be incredibly soothing for your gut. The curries and sauces are usually packed to the gills with digestive spices, fresh ginger, and anti-inflammatory turmeric. Butter chicken is one of those generic Americanized dishes that leans heavier on the dairy than the spice blend. I kept my version mild and heat-free, but still relatively creamy thanks to ghee and coconut milk. Add a halved jalapeño to the sauce as it simmers or a few pinches of cayenne to the spice mixture if you want more fire.

MAKES 4 SERVINGS

- ¼ cup grass-fed ghee or coconut oil
- 1 tablespoon ground turmeric
- 2 teaspoons ground cumin
- 1 teaspoon garam masala
- 2 tablespoons minced fresh ginger
- 2 tablespoons tomato paste
- 1 cup full-fat coconut milk
- ½ cup Low-FODMAP Basic Chicken Bone Broth (page 140)
- 2 tablespoons freshly squeezed lemon juice (from ½ lemon)
- 1 teaspoon sea salt
- 2 pounds boneless, skinless chicken thighs, cut into 2-inch pieces
- ¼ cup roughly chopped fresh cilantro leaves

❶ In a large, lidded saucepan, heat the ghee or oil over medium-low heat. Add the turmeric, cumin, garam masala, ginger, and tomato paste. Cook for 2 minutes, or until a fragrant paste forms.

❷ Carefully stir in the coconut milk, broth, lemon juice, and salt. Bring the sauce to a simmer and cook over medium-low heat until slightly reduced and golden in hue, 10 minutes. Fold in the chicken and continue to simmer over medium heat, stirring occasionally, for 10 minutes.

❸ Place the lid on the pan and simmer for another 5 to 10 minutes, or until the chicken is tender enough to break apart with your spatula. Serve immediately with the cilantro as garnish.

Onward Add ½ cup of plain full-fat Greek **yogurt** or 24-Hour Yogurt (page 163) to the finished sauce (end of Step 3) and/or ½ cup of **sweet peas** at the beginning of Step 3.

LF	SCD	SSFG	BPD1R	BPD1	BPD2	P	SF	HI	YC	HS
								Omit tomato paste and lemon juice, unless tolerated; use Low-Histamine Stock (page 142) ↓	Use Low-Histamine Stock (page 142) ↓	Use Low-Histamine Stock (page 142); sub fresh mint for cilantro ↓

Grilled Skirt Steak with Three-Herb Chimichurri

Skirt steak gives you a fantastic bang for your buck at the butcher counter. When cooked properly on a hot cast-iron skillet or charred over an open grill flame, the ribbons of fat keep the meat moist and packed with umami. Flank steak would also work well if you can't find skirt, but might require a few extra minutes of cooking. Not only does the Argentinean-style herb sauce do double duty as a marinade and a topping, it is also a great way to use up whatever leftover herbs you have on hand.

MAKES 4 SERVINGS

- ½ cup finely chopped fresh cilantro leaves
- ¼ cup finely chopped fresh flat-leaf parsley leaves
- 2 tablespoons finely chopped fresh oregano leaves, or 2 teaspoons dried
- ¼ cup red wine vinegar

  Sea salt
- ¼ teaspoon red pepper flakes (optional)

  Olive oil
- 2 pounds grass-fed skirt steak

1 Make the chimichurri: In a medium-size bowl, combine the cilantro, parsley, oregano, vinegar, 1 teaspoon of salt, red pepper flakes (if using), and ½ cup of olive oil.

2 Marinate the steak: Spoon 2 tablespoons of chimichurri into a shallow bowl or baking dish, reserving the rest of the chimichurri for serving. Add the steak and swish around in the marinade until fully covered. Marinate at room temperature for 20 minutes.

3 Grill the steak: Fire up your grill, or heat an indoor cast-iron skillet over a high flame. Remove the meat from the marinade, season with salt on both sides, and add to the grill or skillet, discarding the chimichurri that was used to marinate. Sear the steak on both sides over high heat until nicely browned and slightly firm to the touch, about 3 minutes per side for medium-rare. For a nice crosshatch, rotate the meat 90 degrees on each side halfway through cooking. Remove to a cutting board and allow the meat to rest for at least 10 minutes before thinly slicing against the grain.

4 Serve alongside the reserved chimichurri.

Onward Add 1 minced **garlic** clove to the herbs (Step 1).

| | | | | | | | | Omit red pepper flakes and sub fresh lime juice for vinegar ↓ | |
| LF | SCD | SSFG | BPD1R | BPD1 | BPD2 | P | SF | YC | HI |

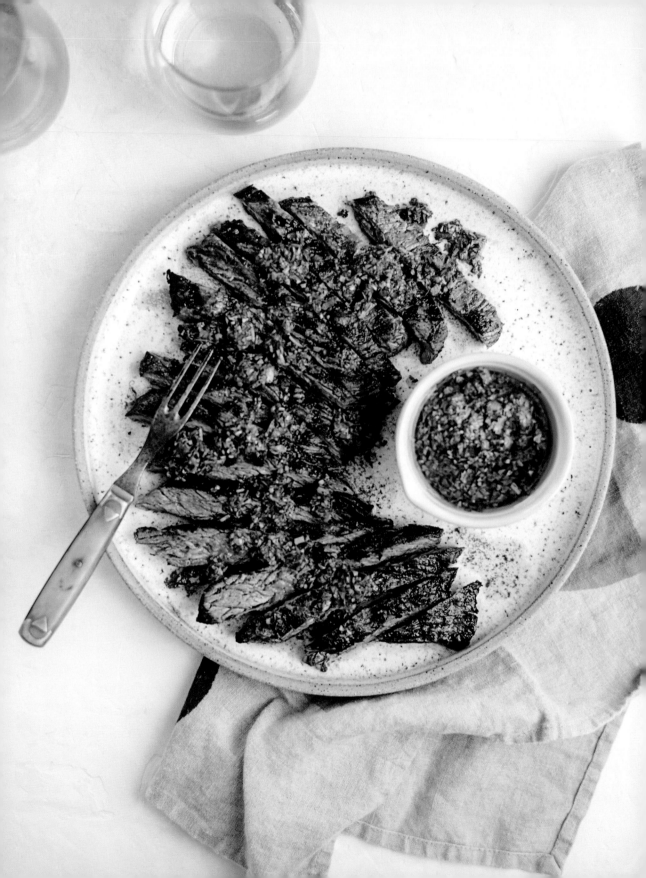

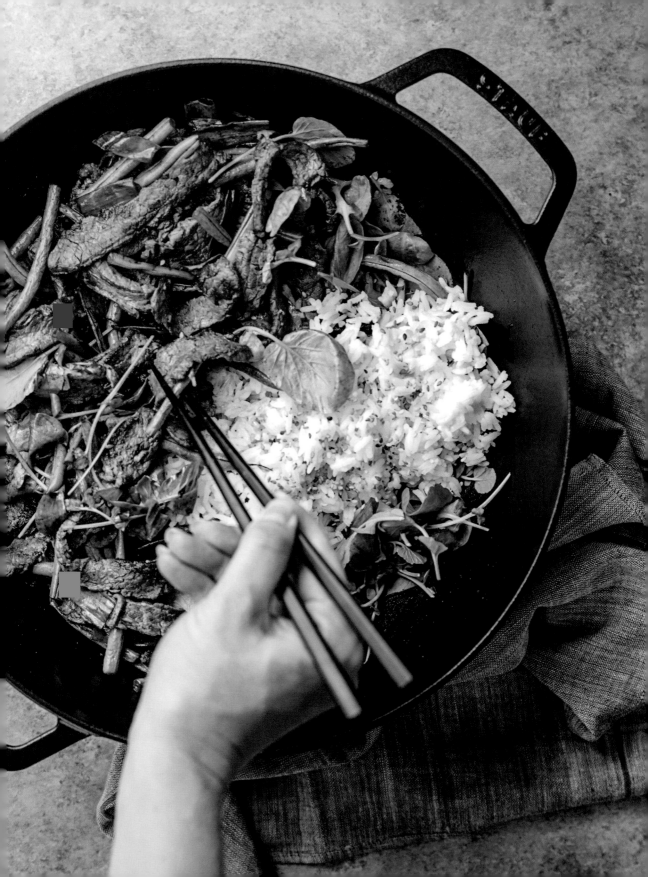

Beef Negimaki Stir-Fry with Green Beans and Watercress

When I was testing dishes for this book, I had my mind set on including a recipe for *negimaki*, the traditional Japanese meat sushi. As I was pounding out the steak and rolling it into tubes, I thought to myself: this is a silly amount of work for dinner, and then proceeded to throw all the ingredients into a skillet and make a delicious stir-fry in under 10 minutes. Instead of the usual whole scallions as the filling, I use just the green parts and bulk it up with French green beans. The stir-fry gets served over a bed of watercress for extra veggies, and since that's what would probably be used as garnish for a plate of negimaki at a Japanese restaurant. White rice, if you can tolerate it, is also perfect for soaking up the sauce.

MAKES 4 SERVINGS

1 pound flank steak

Sea salt

¼ cup sake or dry white wine (optional)

¼ cup gluten-free tamari or coconut aminos

2 tablespoons rice or white wine vinegar

1 tablespoon clover honey or pure maple syrup

Coconut or avocado oil

8 ounces French green beans, cut in half

1 bunch scallions, green parts only, cut into 1-inch pieces

5 ounces watercress (about 4 cups packed)

❶ Slice the steak as thinly as possible against the grain. Season generously with salt. Set aside.

❷ In a small bowl, stir together the sake (if using), tamari, vinegar, and honey until dissolved.

❸ Set a large wok or heavy-bottomed skillet over high heat. Add a thin layer of oil and arrange the steak in an even layer. Brown the meat, flipping once, until there's a dark sear on both sides, about 3 minutes total. Transfer to a bowl.

❹ Add the green beans and sauce to the pan. Simmer vigorously, stirring occasionally, until the sauce has reduced by half and the beans are al dente, about 3 minutes. Return the beef to the pan along with the scallions and toss to coat in the sauce.

❺ To serve, arrange the watercress on a platter and top with the beef stir-fry and sauce. Serve immediately alongside white rice, if you like.

Onward   Add the whole **scallion** and/or 2 cups of chopped **asparagus** or **snow peas** with the green beans (Step 4).

Use pure maple syrup ↓	Use honey, coconut aminos, and white wine vinegar; omit wine ↓					Omit sweetener and alcohol ↓
LF	SCD	SSFG	BPD1	BPD2	P	SF

Shepherd's Pie with Kale and Semi-Sweet Potato Mash

Even though it's traditionally made with milk and flour, shepherd's pie is incredibly simple to adapt to an anti-inflammatory diet. You can adjust the ratio of meat to mash to suit your carb limits, and tweak the latter to include straight spuds or sweet potatoes, depending on your dietary preference. Even prior to experimenting with a low-FODMAP diet, I loved the half-and-half approach of the savory with the sweet. You can make the semi-sweet potato mash on its own as a side—it's a Lapine family Thanksgiving favorite! A note on equipment: using an ovenproof skillet means less cleanup and effort, but if you don't have one, you can assemble the pie in a 9 x 13-inch baking dish. Ground lamb or chicken would also work in place of the beef.

MAKES 6 SERVINGS

- 2 pounds russet potatoes (about 4 medium), peeled and cut into 2-inch chunks
- 1 pound sweet potatoes (about 2 medium), peeled and cut into 2-inch chunks
- Sea salt and freshly ground black pepper
- 2 tablespoons grass-fed ghee

- 4 tablespoons extra-virgin olive oil
- 1½ cups homemade Low-FODMAP Beef or Basic Chicken Bone Broth (pages 142 and 140)
- 1½ pounds grass-fed ground beef (preferably 85% lean)
- 2 medium-size carrots, peeled and finely diced

- ¼ cup tomato paste
- 1 teaspoon paprika
- ½ teaspoon dried thyme, or 1 teaspoon fresh
- 1 small bunch kale, stemmed, thinly sliced into ribbons (3 cups, packed)

❶ Preheat the oven to 400°F.

❷ Place the potatoes and sweet potatoes in a medium-size stockpot and cover with cold water by 2 inches. Season generously with salt and bring to a boil. Simmer until tender, about 15 minutes. Drain and return to the pot. Add the ghee and 2 tablespoons of the olive oil. Mash until the potatoes are smooth and fluffy, adding a splash of broth as necessary to thin them to the desired consistency. Set aside while you prepare the filling.

3 Meanwhile, make the filling: In a large (12-inch or bigger) cast-iron or ovenproof skillet, heat the remaining 2 tablespoons of olive oil over medium-high heat. Add the beef and carrots. Brown the meat, breaking it apart with your spatula into bite-size pieces, until cooked through and charred around the edges, about 7 minutes. Season generously with salt and pepper. Add the tomato paste, paprika, and thyme. Cook for another few minutes, until fragrant and pasty. Carefully fold in the kale and continue to cook the meat mixture until the greens are wilted, 2 minutes more. Pour in the 1¼ cups of broth, scraping up any brown bits from the pan that may have formed. Simmer until the liquid is mostly absorbed but the meat still feels moist and saucy, about 3 minutes.

4 Assemble the pie: Using the back of a wooden spoon or spatula, make sure the meat mixture is spread evenly in the skillet. Scoop the semi-sweet potato mash on top and smooth with your spatula so the meat is mostly covered. You can use a fork to ridge the top and create some texture.

5 Bake the pie: Transfer the skillet to the oven and bake until the meat is bubbling up the sides and the topping has begun to form a light crust, about 20 minutes. For more browning on top, place the pie under the broiler for a few minutes. Serve warm as a one-pan meal, or with a side salad.

Onward Add ½ cup of **sweet peas** to the meat at the end of Step 3.

			Omit sweet potato; limit potato serving to ½ cup ↓	Omit tomato paste; use Low-Histamine Stock (page 142) or water ↓	Sub ground chicken for beef; omit kale; use Low-Histamine Stock (page 142) or water ↓
LF	P	SF	BPD2	HI	HS

Stuffed Collard Greens with Lamb and Quinoa

Cabbage and grape leaves are well loved in Hungarian and Greek cuisine as pockets for rice and meat to steam in. These rolls are no different; I've just swapped out the vehicle for collard greens, which rarely get their due time in the spotlight above the Mason-Dixon Line. Unlike rice, quinoa doesn't swell as much and therefore is less likely to break open the leaves during the cooking process. You could easily use white rice here, or omit the meat and double the grains for a vegetarian version.

MAKES 4 SERVINGS

- 10 collard greens (from 1 to 2 bunches), thick stems removed
- 1 pound ground lamb
- ½ cup quinoa
- ¼ cup finely chopped fresh flat-leaf parsley leaves, plus more for serving
- 2 tablespoons finely chopped fresh mint leaves, or 2 teaspoons dried
- 2 tablespoons extra-virgin olive oil
- 2 teaspoons ground cumin
- ½ teaspoon ground cinnamon
- ¼ teaspoon red pepper flakes
- 1 teaspoon sea salt
- 2 cups Low-FODMAP Pasta Sauce (page 149)

1 Bring a large pot of salted water to a boil while you carefully remove the thicker stems from the collard greens, trying to keep the leaves intact. When the water comes to a boil, add the collard leaves. Blanch for 30 seconds, until soft and pliable, and transfer to a colander. Rinse the greens in cold water to stop the cooking. Shake out excess water and set aside.

2 In a large bowl, combine the lamb, quinoa, parsley, mint, olive oil, cumin, cinnamon, red pepper flakes, salt, and ½ cup of the pasta sauce. Stir until well mixed without overly breaking up the meat—think about it as if you were making meatballs.

3 On a clean work surface, arrange one collard leaf, veiny side up, with the stem end facing you. The leaf may have a big space in the middle where you stemmed it; if it does, pull the two sides of the leaf in toward each other and overlap them slightly. Place 1 to 2 tablespoons of filling (depending on the size of the leaf) on the bottom center of each leaf. Fold the sides over, then roll up, tucking in the sides as you go. The rolls can be slightly loose, leaving room for the quinoa to expand.

4 Pour the remaining pasta sauce into a large, deep, lidded skillet or saucepan and smooth it to cover the whole surface. Place the collard wraps in the pan, seam side down, fitting the stuffed leaves in one snug layer.

5 Add enough water to barely cover the rolls, about 2 cups. Invert an ovenproof plate over the rolls to keep them wrapped and in position, and bring to a simmer over medium heat. Cover the pan, place over low heat, and simmer for 30 minutes, at which point the leaves will be tender and the quinoa cooked. Remove the lid and simmer for another 10 to 15 minutes over low heat, or until the sauce has reduced by half.

6 Remove from the heat and carefully lift the plate off the rolls, using tongs. Serve the rolls warm or at room temperature with the liquid from the pot ladled on top.

Onward Serve with a dollop of **24-Hour Yogurt** (page 163) and/or add 1 **garlic** clove to the filling (Step 2).

					Omit lamb and double quinoa ↓
LF	SF	BPD1	BPD2	YC	V

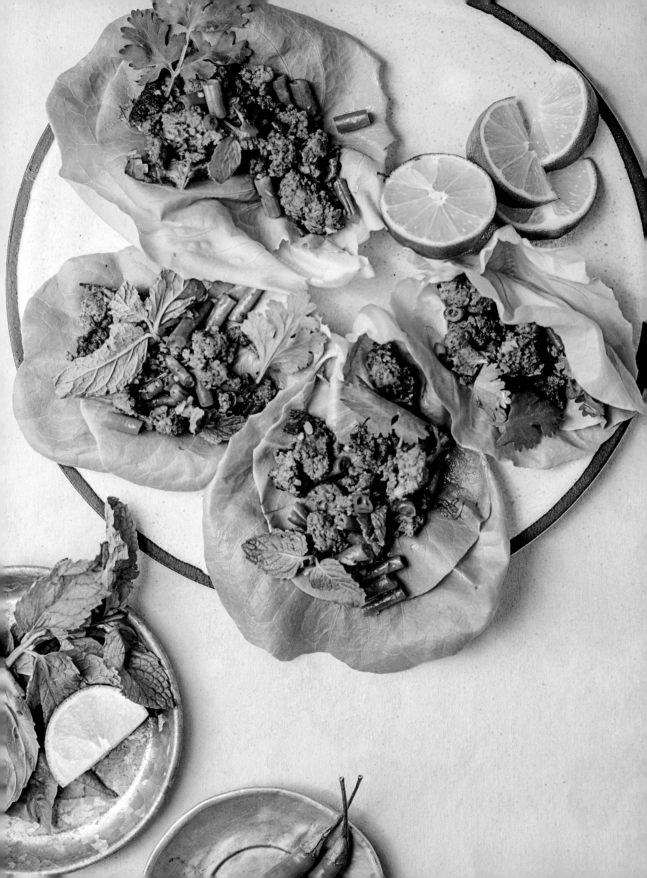

Larb Lettuce Wraps

Authentic Thai food always aims for that perfect balance of sweet, spicy, and tangy. When we're cooking for a SIBO diet, though, we have to be careful of the sweet and the spice, which is why there's no sugar in this minced meat salad. Although a chile pepper is in the ingredient list, listen to your body and know what level of heat you can handle—you're welcome to add even more fire, if you like! For those not watching their grains, serve this alongside white jasmine or sticky rice in addition to the lettuce cups. The most common proteins used for larb are pork and chicken—feel free to use either as substitutes for the beef!

MAKES 4 SERVINGS

1 tablespoon coconut oil

1 pound grass-fed ground beef

Sea salt

1 Thai or serrano chile pepper, ribs and seeds removed, minced

1 tablespoon minced fresh ginger

1 cup finely chopped green beans (about 4 ounces)

½ cup Low-FODMAP Beef or Basic Chicken Bone Broth (pages 142 and 140), or water in a pinch

¼ cup freshly squeezed lime juice (from 2 limes)

2 tablespoons Asian fish sauce (I like Red Boat brand)

½ cup roughly chopped fresh basil, cilantro, or mint leaves (or all three)

1 head Bibb or Boston lettuce, leaves separated, for serving

1 lime, quartered, for serving

1 In a large, nonstick wok or skillet, heat the oil over medium-high heat. Add the beef and brown, breaking it apart with a spatula into bite-size pieces, until no pink remains, about 5 minutes. Season lightly with salt.

2 Add the chile pepper and ginger and cook until fragrant, 1 to 2 minutes more. Add the green beans and pour in the broth or water, lime juice, and fish sauce. Simmer, scraping up any brown bits from the bottom of the pan, until the liquid has reduced slightly but still provides a decent amount of sauce, about 2 minutes. The green beans should still be crunchy.

3 Remove the pan from the heat, add the herbs, and taste for seasoning. Transfer to a serving bowl and serve warm alongside the lettuce leaves and lime wedges.

Onward Add 1 minced **garlic** clove or 1 small thinly sliced **shallot** to the peppers (Step 2).

							Omit hot pepper and fish sauce ↓	
SCD	P	SF	SSFG	BPD1	BPD2	LF	YC	HI

Teriyaki Pork Tenderloin with Bok Choy and Broccoli

Teriyaki sauce is usually chock-full of refined sugar, which isn't great for anyone, especially those of us trying to keep dysbiosis at bay. This homemade version works beautifully as a marinade for any type of meat. Here I use it to give extra flavor and caramelization to a roasted pork tenderloin. The meat cooks up in twenty-five minutes over a bed of broccoli and bok choy, but you can substitute any veggie that roasts in the same amount of time. Similar to leeks, bok choy can be gritty. If you notice any dirt has snuck into the base of the leaves, add the whole lot of sliced bok choy to a bowl of water. Agitate the water so that any dirt falls to the bottom. Then, lift out the greens with your hands (don't drain through a colander!) and pat dry with a clean dish towel. If you can't find full-size heads of bok choy, you can substitute six baby bok choy.

MAKES 4 SERVINGS

- 2 tablespoons pure maple syrup or clover honey
- ¼ cup gluten-free tamari or coconut aminos
- 2 tablespoons minced fresh ginger
- 2 pounds pork tenderloin (about 2 loins)
- 2 heads bok choy (see headnote), thinly sliced widthwise into ribbons
- 1 small broccoli crown, cut into small florets (about 2 cups)
- 2 tablespoons extra-virgin olive oil
- ½ teaspoon sea salt
- Sesame seeds, for garnish (optional)

❶ In a small bowl or 2-cup measure, whisk together the maple syrup, tamari or coconut aminos, and ginger until smooth. Transfer the marinade to a resealable plastic bag. Add the pork and swish it around until coated. Marinate in the refrigerator for at least an hour, preferably overnight.

❷ Preheat the oven to 450°F. Line a baking sheet with parchment. On the prepared baking sheet, toss the bok choy and broccoli with the olive oil and salt until well coated and arrange in an even layer.

❸ Remove the pork from the marinade and set on top of the bok choy mixture. Drizzle the marinade over the veggies. Roast in the oven for 25 minutes, or until the pork is nicely browned on top and firm to the touch, or the internal temperature reads 145°F. Remove the pan from the oven and allow the pork to rest on a cutting board for at least 10 minutes before slicing diagonally on the bias. Serve alongside the roasted bok choy and broccoli with a sprinkle of sesame seeds (if using).

Onward Substitute 8 ounces of **Brussels sprouts**, thinly sliced, for 1 head of bok choy.

Use pure maple syrup ↓	Use clover honey and coconut aminos ↓					Omit maple syrup or honey ↓
LF	P	SCD	SSFG	BPD1	BPD2	SF

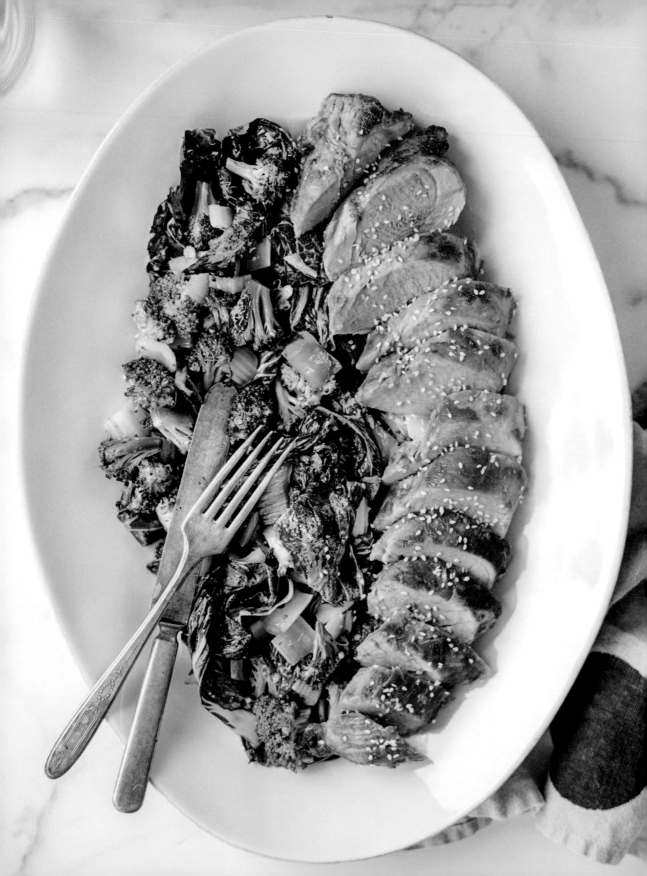

Cider-Dijon Pork Chops with Silky Cabbage

Cabbage is a perfect pairing with pork, which is why I am extra-grateful that you can get away with ¾ cup of it per serving on a low-FODMAP diet. Instead of resorting to store-bought sauerkraut for these pork chops, I use a mustardy pan sauce to create my own briny cooked cabbage and kale mixture. When I served this dish to friends, everyone thought there were onions mixed in. So, needless to say, you won't miss them!

MAKES 4 SERVINGS

- 2 tablespoons Dijon mustard
- 2 tablespoons cider vinegar
- 1 teaspoon clover honey or maple syrup
- 1 teaspoon fresh thyme leaves, or ½ teaspoon dried
- Extra-virgin olive oil
- Sea salt
- 4 boneless pork chops (about 2 pounds), cut 1 inch thick
- 1 tablespoon grass-fed ghee
- 1 small head red or green cabbage (12 ounces), thinly sliced (about 3 cups)
- 1 bunch lacinato kale, thinly sliced (4 cups, packed)
- 1 cup dry red wine or Low-FODMAP Basic Chicken Bone Broth (page 140)

❶ In a medium-size bowl, whisk together the Dijon mustard, vinegar, honey, thyme, 2 tablespoons of olive oil, and 1 teaspoon of salt. Add the pork chops and flip around until well coated in the marinade. Set aside for at least 15 minutes at room temperature, or overnight in the fridge.

❷ In a large, heavy-bottomed skillet (I love cast-iron), heat the ghee over medium heat. Remove the pork chops, shaking off any excess marinade, and reserve the remaining marinade. Brown the meat in batches until golden on both sides and semi-firm, about 4 minutes per side for medium-rare. Transfer to a plate.

❸ Add an additional glug of olive oil to the pan (if needed), along with the cabbage and kale. Sauté over medium heat, stirring occasionally, until soft and wilted, about 7 minutes. Season with ½ teaspoon of salt, pour in the wine, and scrape any remaining marinade into the pan with a rubber spatula. Bring to a simmer and cook over medium heat until most of the liquid is absorbed and the cabbage is very soft, about 10 minutes.

❹ Remove the skillet from the heat. Taste the cabbage for seasoning and add more salt as necessary.

❺ Once the meat has rested for at least 10 minutes, thinly slice the pork chops. Divide the cabbage mixture among four plates and top each with a sliced pork chop along with any drippings. Serve immediately.

Onward Add ½ Granny Smith **apple**, diced, to the cabbage with the wine (Step 3).

Use maple syrup ↓	Use honey ↓		Use honey and omit wine ↓		
LF	SCD	SSFG	BPD1	BPD2	P

Sausage and Sweet Pepper Hash

A perfect weekday breakfast, lunch, or dinner, this hash uses the classic Italian combo of sausage, peppers, and onions—without the onions of course. If you can't handle the heat, use homemade Sweet Italian Sausage (page 155). To make this hash a complete meal, top it with a fried egg and serve alongside a green salad. You can also turn the hash into a frittata by adding eight beaten large eggs to the pan (make sure it's oven-safe) and finishing it under the broiler for two minutes.

MAKES 4 SERVINGS

- 1 pound homemade Hot Italian Sausage (page 155), uncooked
- 2 tablespoons extra-virgin olive oil
- 1 pound russet potatoes (about 2 medium), cut into ½-inch cubes
- 1 teaspoon sea salt
- 2 assorted bell peppers (about 1½ pounds), thinly sliced into strips
- 1 teaspoon smoked paprika
- ⅓ cup roughly chopped fresh basil leaves (optional)

❶ Place a large (12-inch), heavy-bottomed cast-iron or nonstick skillet over medium-high heat. Add the sausage and cook until charred on one side, about 3 minutes. Flip the meat and break it apart with your spatula into bite-size chunks. Cook for another 5 minutes, or until the sausage is browned all over and no longer pink in the center. Transfer the meat to a plate and set aside.

❷ Add the olive oil to the pan along with the potatoes. Cook in an even layer until nicely browned on one side, about 5 minutes. Season with ½ teaspoon of the salt and cook for another 5 minutes, redistributing occasionally. Add the peppers and the remaining ½ teaspoon of salt. Continue to sauté until the peppers are slightly charred and the potatoes are cooked through, about 10 minutes. Return the sausage to the pan and season with the smoked paprika. Sauté for 2 minutes more, or just until the spices are fragrant and the sausage is well integrated. Remove the pan from the heat and fold in the basil (if using).

Onward Brown 1 cup of thinly sliced **Brussels sprouts** along with the potatoes, or substitute half **sweet potatoes** for regular spuds.

LF	P	SF	Limit serving size to 1 cup ↓		Use homemade Sweet Italian Sausage (page 155) made with chicken (not pork) ↓
			YC	BPD2	HI

BLT Frittata

The fact that bacon has a place in your SIBO treatment plan should make everything better. Still, processed meats are labeled by the World Health Organization as known carcinogens, so even more so than any other type of animal product, it's important to buy quality, nitrate-free bacon. Although not too much ends up in the final product, I also look for sugar-free, paleo brands to rule out even more junk. The "lettuce" in our BLT frittata is arugula, which has a wonderful peppery bite to offset the rich bacon.

MAKES 4 SERVINGS

- 4 slices sugar- and nitrate-free bacon
- 8 large eggs
- ½ teaspoon sea salt
- 1 cup cherry tomatoes, halved, or 1 large heirloom tomato, roughly chopped
- 2½ cups baby arugula, tightly packed (about 2.5 ounces)

❶ Preheat the broiler. Line a plate with paper towels.

❷ Place a large (12-inch), ovenproof skillet over medium heat. Add the bacon strips and cook, flipping once or twice, until the fat has been rendered and the meat is nicely browned, about 5 minutes. Transfer with tongs to the paper towel–lined plate.

❸ Meanwhile, in a large bowl, beat the eggs with the salt until the yolk and whites are very well combined.

❹ Pour off all but a thin layer of bacon fat into a jar (you can store for another use). Add the tomatoes to the pan and cook over medium heat, scraping up any brown bits that may have formed, until they have begun to caramelize, about 5 minutes. Fold in the arugula and sauté for 2 minutes more, or until the greens are wilted but not completely shriveled.

❺ Arrange the veggies in an even layer in the pan. Lower the heat to low and pour the eggs over the vegetables, making sure the pan is evenly coated. Cook until the sides are set and there's just a shallow layer of uncooked eggs on the top, about 5 minutes.

❻ Meanwhile, roughly chop the bacon.

❼ Sprinkle the bacon bits over the top of the frittata and transfer the pan to the broiler. Cook for 1 minute, until the top is cooked and beginning to lightly brown. Remove from the oven and allow the frittata to sit in the pan for at least 5 minutes before slicing. Cut into wedges and serve warm.

Onward Omit the arugula and sauté 1 thinly sliced **leek** (as the L, instead of lettuce) with the tomatoes.

LF	SCD	SSFG	BPD1R	BPD1	BPD2	P	SF

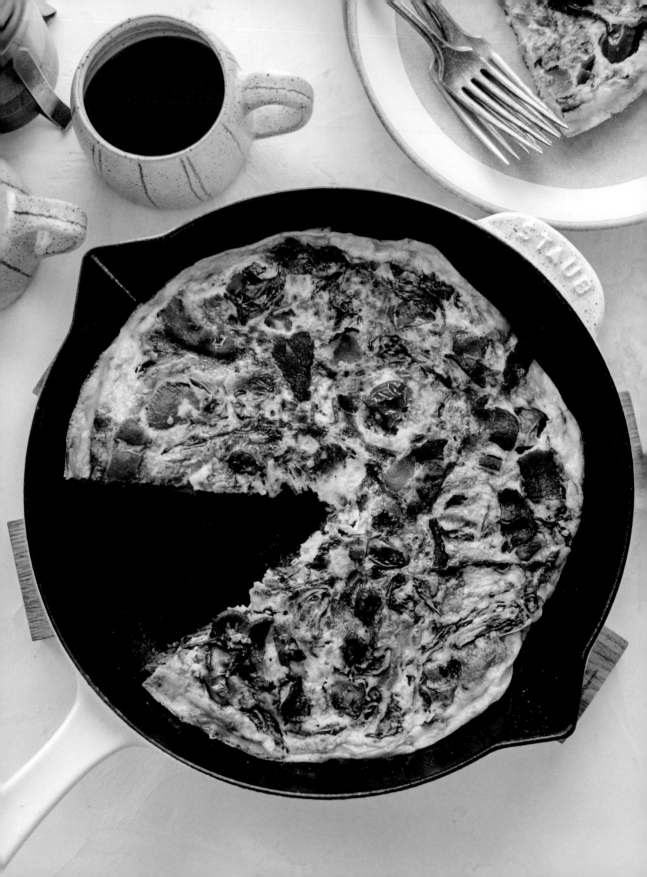

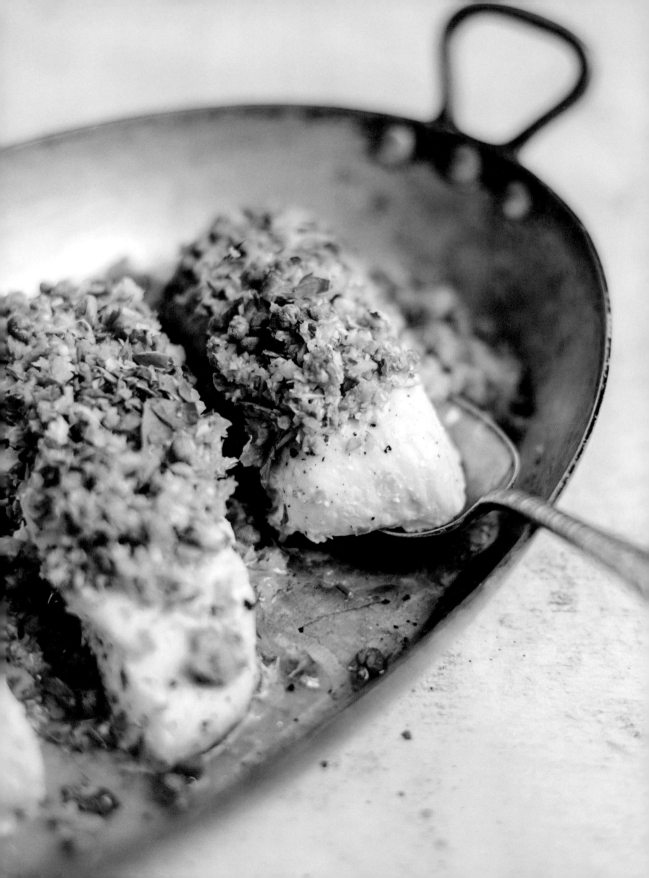

Baked Halibut with Green Olive and Fennel Tapenade

My dad is the king of grilled halibut in the summertime. But when he's too lazy, we just bake it. This dish takes only ten to fifteen minutes in the oven and is perfect for a weeknight meal, while also being fancy enough to serve at a dinner party. Any leftover tapenade can be used as a spread for gluten-free crackers. If you can't find halibut or it's too pricey, any other semi-firm, medium-thickness fish would work. You can also roast the side of fish whole instead of cutting it into individual portions for a more rustic presentation.

MAKES 6 SERVINGS

1 cup pitted green olives

½ medium-size fennel bulb, roughly chopped

¼ cup fresh flat-leaf parsley leaves

2 tablespoons freshly squeezed lemon juice (from ½ lemon)

2 tablespoons capers

¼ cup extra-virgin olive oil, plus more for pan

Sea salt and freshly ground black pepper

6 (6-ounce) halibut, striped bass, or cod fillets

Zest of 1 lemon

❶ Preheat the oven to 400°F.

❷ In a food processor, pulse together the olives, fennel, parsley, lemon juice, capers, and olive oil until finely chopped, but not completely pureed. Season to taste with salt and pepper.

❸ Rinse the fish fillets in cold water and pat dry with a paper towel. Oil a baking sheet or ovenproof skillet with olive oil, and arrange the fish fillets with about an inch of space between them. Season with salt and pepper.

❹ Spoon the tapenade over the fish in a generous pile (2 to 3 heaping tablespoons per fillet), patting it lightly to adhere to the top—but don't worry if any little bits have fallen to the sides.

❺ Bake the halibut for about 15 minutes, or until the fish has fully whitened and is easily flaked with a fork. Sprinkle with the lemon zest and serve immediately.

Onward Add 1 **garlic** clove to the tapenade or ½ cup bread crumbs or panko sprinkled on top.

LF	SCD	SSFG	BPD1R	BPD1	BPD2	P	SF	Sub salmon for halibut ↓
								HS

Turmeric-Dill Catfish

This fish dish from Hanoi (*cha ca la vong*) has popped up on many of the best Vietnamese menus in the States. The base is similar to many dishes from the region: fish sauce, lime juice, and sugar. But turmeric and dill give it a whole new dimension, both bright and pungent at the same time. The deep yellow sauce seeps into everything it sits upon, usually a nest of fresh rice noodles and crunchy greens. When the weather starts to turn springy, I immediately start craving this dish. You simply toss the ingredients together and let it marinate for a few minutes on the counter. Instead of cooking it stovetop, I turn it out on a baking dish and broil it. You can also make it *en papillote* for even less cleanup, and even more Franco-Vietnamese vibes. To bulk it up, serve the catfish as a rice bowl or over gluten-free ramen instead of as lettuce wraps, as recommended.

MAKES 2 TO 4 SERVINGS

¼ cup tightly packed roughly chopped fresh dill

2 tablespoons minced fresh ginger

¼ cup freshly squeezed lime juice (from 2 limes)

2 tablespoons Asian fish sauce (I like Red Boat)

2 tablespoons coconut oil, melted

2 teaspoons pure maple syrup or clover honey

1 teaspoon ground turmeric

¼ teaspoon cayenne pepper (optional)

1 pound catfish, cod, haddock, halibut, or other white semi-firm fish, cut into 2-inch cubes

1 small head bok choy or 3 baby bok choy (1 pound), rinsed well and thinly sliced

1 head Bibb or Boston lettuce, for serving

❶ Preheat the broiler. Line a baking sheet with parchment paper.

❷ In a large bowl, stir together the dill, ginger, lime juice, fish sauce, coconut oil, maple syrup, turmeric, and cayenne, if using. Fold in the fish and set aside to marinate for 10 minutes at room temperature.

❸ Arrange the bok choy in an even layer on the prepared baking sheet. Arrange the fish on top and pour any remaining marinade over the vegetables. Broil until the fillets are cooked through, 5 to 7 minutes.

❹ Serve the fish alongside the lettuce leaves.

Onward Add ½ small **red onion**, thinly sliced, to the marinade.

Use maple syrup ↓		Use honey ↓			Omit cayenne and fish sauce ↓	
LF	SCD	SSFG	BPD1	BPD2	HI	P

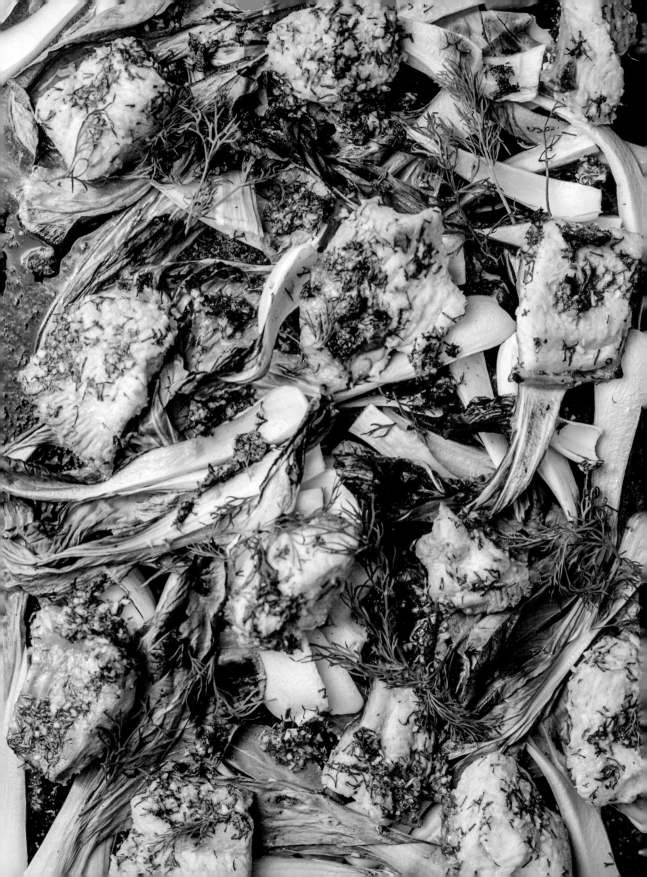

Sesame Sheet Pan Salmon with Radishes

Wild salmon is one of my favorite anti-inflammatory foods. Although some Alaskan salmon is quite pricey, you can usually find great deals on frozen sockeye during the peak of its season, summertime. It's worth it for this pink sheet pan meal, where the salmon is complemented by pink radishes and thinly sliced daikon. Baby turnips or summer squashes are a great swap for the radishes. Serve the fish over white rice, cauliflower rice, or rice noodles, depending on what your diet allows.

MAKES 4 SERVINGS

- 1 pound daikon radishes (about 3 medium), thinly sliced
- 2 bunches pink radishes, quartered
- 4 tablespoons extra-virgin olive oil
- Sea salt
- ¼ cup freshly squeezed lemon juice (from 1 to 2 lemons)
- ¼ cup gluten-free tamari or coconut aminos
- 2 tablespoons toasted sesame oil
- 3 tablespoons finely minced fresh ginger
- 3 tablespoons white or black sesame seeds, or a combination
- 4 (6-ounce) wild salmon fillets, skin-on
- ¼ cup finely chopped fresh cilantro

❶ Preheat the oven to 450°F.

❷ On a baking sheet, toss the daikon and regular radishes with 2 tablespoons of the olive oil and season lightly with salt. Roast in the oven until tender and beginning to shrivel, about 15 minutes.

❸ Meanwhile, in a small bowl, whisk together the remaining 2 tablespoons of olive oil, the lemon juice, tamari or coconut aminos, sesame oil, ginger, and sesame seeds, and ½ teaspoon of salt.

❹ Remove the radishes from the oven, and nestle the salmon fillets, skin side down, into the vegetables, making sure each piece is making contact with the pan. Drizzle half of the marinade over the salmon and radishes. Return the pan to the oven and roast until the salmon is tender, about 10 minutes for medium-rare with just a hint of darker pink in the center.

❺ Stir the cilantro into the remaining marinade and serve alongside the warm salmon.

Onward Add 1 **leek** (white and light green parts), thinly sliced, along with the radishes.

							Use coconut aminos ↓			Omit tamari and coconut aminos; sub lime juice for lemon, unless tolerated ↓	
LF	SF	SCD	SSFG	BPD1	BPD2	P		YC		HI	

Seared Scallops with Squash Succotash

The following instructions, along with a winning combination of ghee and coconut oil, will help you get a perfect brown crust on your scallops every time. But even if you don't manage to do so, piling them high with squash succotash will hide any flaws. I usually make this quick sauté using fresh sweet corn in the summertime, but it also tastes fabulous with yellow squash.

MAKES 4 SERVINGS

- 2 pounds sea scallops
- 2 tablespoons coconut oil
- 2 tablespoons grass-fed ghee
- Sea salt
- 1 medium-size zucchini (about 8 ounces), finely diced
- 2 large summer squash (about 1 pound), finely diced
- ½ teaspoon ground turmeric
- ½ teaspoon ground cumin
- ½ teaspoon smoked paprika
- 2 vine tomatoes, roughly chopped
- 2 tablespoons freshly squeezed lemon juice (from ½ lemon)
- 1 teaspoon clover honey or pure maple syrup
- ¼ cup fresh basil leaves, julienned

❶ Rinse the scallops under cold water and set aside on a clean dish towel. If there is a skinny tendon on the sides of the scallops, remove it and discard.

❷ In large, nonstick or cast-iron skillet, heat 1 tablespoon of the coconut oil and 1 tablespoon of the ghee over medium-high heat. Gently pat the scallops with a paper towel to make sure they are nice and dry and season them with salt. When the oil is quite hot, add the scallops, making sure not to crowd the pan (you will likely need to do this in two batches). DO NOT move the scallops until they have properly browned, 2 to 3 minutes depending on the size of your scallops. When they have a dark brown crust on the bottom, flip them and cook for another minute. The scallops should still be slightly translucent in the center. Transfer the finished scallops to a plate, making sure to put the beautiful seared side facing up. Repeat with the remaining scallops, oil, and ghee.

❸ Lower the heat to medium and add the zucchini and summer squash to the pan. Sauté, stirring occasionally, until tender and beginning to caramelize, about 5 minutes. Add the turmeric, cumin, smoked paprika, and 1 teaspoon of salt. Cook for another minute, or until fragrant. Add the tomatoes and cook for about 3 minutes, or until they have just begun to release their juices. Remove from the heat and stir in the lemon juice, honey, and half of the basil.

❹ Transfer the squash succotash to a platter. Top with the seared scallops, and garnish with the remaining basil. Serve immediately or at room temperature.

Onward Add 2 cups of fresh **sweet corn** kernels with the squash. Omit the honey or maple syrup.

Use maple syrup ↓	Use honey ↓					Omit sweetener ↓		
LF	SCD	SSFG	BPD1	BPD2	P	BPD1R	YC	SF

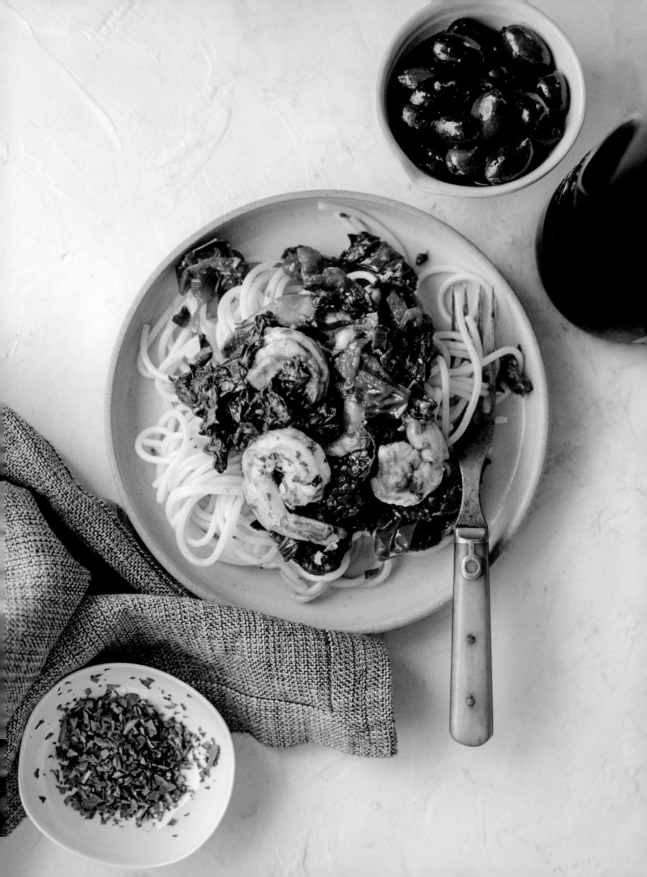

Shrimp Spaghetti with Cherry Tomato Puttanesca

Utilizing the antipasti bar is one of my big strategies for getting around the garlic and onion omission while still packing tons of authentic Italian flavor into my dishes. It also just so happens to be my central strategy for reducing the jars in my fridge and pantry, since capers, olives, and anchovies tend to take up a lot of real estate there. This dish makes for a chunkier version of traditional puttanesca using cherry tomatoes. If fresh tomatoes aren't in season, you can substitute 15 ounces of canned or boxed diced tomatoes. I prefer the latter as tomatoes are quite acidic and have an especially high risk of acquiring leached BPA from the linings of cans. A bunch of chard makes this pasta a complete meal on its own. If you're following a low-carb approach, you can easily serve the shrimp puttanesca over spaghetti squash, zucchini noodles, or cauliflower rice.

MAKES 4 SERVINGS

1 bunch red chard	2 garlic cloves, crushed	1 tablespoon capers
¼ cup extra-virgin olive oil	2 cups cherry tomatoes, halved	12 ounces quinoa spaghetti
1 pound extra-large shrimp (20 count per pound), peeled and deveined	½ cup pitted kalamata olives, roughly chopped	2 tablespoons finely chopped fresh flat-leaf parsley leaves
Sea salt and freshly ground black pepper	2 tablespoons tomato paste	
	2 anchovy fillets, minced	

❶ Bring a large pot of salted water to a boil.

❷ On a work surface, cut the chard leaves from their stems. Thinly slice the stems and roughly chop the leaves. Set both aside separately.

❸ In a large skillet, heat 2 tablespoons of the oil over medium-high heat. Pat the shrimp dry and add to the hot oil in an even layer. Season generously with salt. Cook until the shrimp are light pink and the ends curl in toward each other, 1 to 2 minutes on each side. Remove to a bowl and set aside.

recipe continues →

4 Add the remaining 2 tablespoons of oil to the pan along with the garlic. Lower the heat to low and cook the garlic until golden brown on all sides, 5 minutes. Remove the garlic and discard. Alternatively, you can skip this step and substitute Garlic-Infused Oil (page 143).

5 Add the cherry tomatoes, chard stems, and olives to the pan. Sauté over medium heat until the tomatoes are shriveled and have released their juices, 5 minutes. You can use your spoon or spatula to gently crush the tomatoes and urge them along. Stir in the chard leaves, tomato paste, anchovies, capers, and ½ teaspoon of salt. Gently simmer, stirring occasionally, until the greens are very wilted, about 5 minutes.

6 Meanwhile, cook the pasta according to the package directions. Remove ¼ cup of cooking liquid before draining. Add the drained pasta, reserved cooking liquid, cooked shrimp, and parsley to the pan of puttanesca sauce. Toss until the pasta is well coated. Taste for seasoning and add more salt and pepper as necessary (the anchovies and capers will bring their own salinity). Serve immediately.

Onward Add ½ cup of quartered **artichoke** hearts in oil to the sauce.

		Omit pasta and serve over spaghetti squash ↓					
LF	SF	SCD	SSFG	BPD1R	BPD1	BPD2	P

Blackened Salmon Burrito Bowls with Dirty Quinoa and Cucumber Salsa

This bowl has all the elements of a perfect fish taco: spice, creaminess, crunch, and a pickled punch. It may look like a lot of ingredients and steps, but they are all relatively streamlined and straightforward. Plus, most of the elements can be made in advance. If you're avoiding grains, just omit the quinoa and double up on the lettuces as a bed for your salmon.

MAKES 4 SERVINGS

▷ Quinoa

- 1 tablespoon extra-virgin olive oil
- 1 small red bell pepper, finely diced
- ½ teaspoon ground cumin
- ½ teaspoon smoked paprika
- ½ teaspoon sea salt
- 1 tablespoon tomato paste
- 1 cup quinoa

▷ Salsa

- 2 seedless cucumbers (1¼ pounds), finely diced
- 2 green scallions, thinly sliced
- 1 jalapeño, ribs and seeds removed, minced
- 3 tablespoons finely chopped fresh cilantro leaves
- ¼ cup freshly squeezed lime juice (from 2 limes)

- 2 teaspoons clover honey or pure maple syrup
- ¾ teaspoon sea salt

▷ Salmon

- 1 teaspoon ground cumin
- 1 teaspoon smoked paprika
- 1 teaspoon chili powder
- ¼ teaspoon cayenne pepper (optional)
- 1½ pounds wild salmon fillets

  Extra-virgin olive oil

  Sea salt

▷ To assemble bowls

- 2 heads Little Gem, butter, or Boston lettuce, leaves separated
- 3 cups shredded green cabbage
- 1 cup Creamy Cilantro-Jalapeño Ranch (page 145)
- 1 cup loosely packed fresh cilantro leaves, for serving
- 1 lime, cut into wedges, for serving

❶ Make the quinoa: In a medium-size Dutch oven, heat the olive oil. Sauté the bell pepper until soft, about 5 minutes. Stir in the cumin, paprika, salt, and tomato paste. Cook for another minute, or until fragrant. Add the quinoa and stir until coated in the vegetable mixture. Toast the quinoa, stirring occasionally, for 2 minutes. Add 1¾ cups of water and bring to a boil, cover, and cook until the water has absorbed, about 20 minutes. Stir once and allow the quinoa to sit uncovered until some of the steam has evaporated, about 5 minutes. The quinoa can be made up to 3 days in advance.

recipe continues →

2 **Make the salsa:** In a medium-size bowl, combine the cucumber, scallions, jalapeño, cilantro, lime juice, honey, and salt. Toss to coat and set aside.

3 **Make the salmon:** Preheat the broiler and line a baking sheet with parchment. In a small bowl, stir together the cumin, paprika, chili powder, and cayenne. Arrange the salmon, skin side down, on the prepared baking sheet. Drizzle the fillets with olive oil and season generously with salt, using your fingers to coat the skin thoroughly. Sprinkle the spice mixture evenly over the fillets. Transfer the pan to the oven and broil for 5 minutes, or until the top of the salmon is blackened and the meat is cooked to medium. Set aside to cool.

4 **Assemble the bowls:** Using two forks, flake apart the salmon into bite-size pieces. Discard the skin. Divide the lettuce, cabbage, quinoa, and salmon among four bowls. Top with the cucumber salsa and drizzle with the cilantro ranch. Garnish with cilantro leaves and serve alongside the extra lime wedges.

Onward Divide 1 diced **avocado** or 1 cup of diced **mango** among the bowls.

Use maple syrup ↓	Omit quinoa and double lettuce; use honey ↓				Limit quinoa to ½ cup; use honey ↓		Omit tomato paste, jalapeño, and cayenne; use alternative dressing ↓	Omit quinoa, cilantro, and cabbage ↓	Omit sweetener; use alternative dressing ↓	
LF	P	SCD	SSFG	BPD1R	BPD1	BPD2	HI	HS	YC	SF

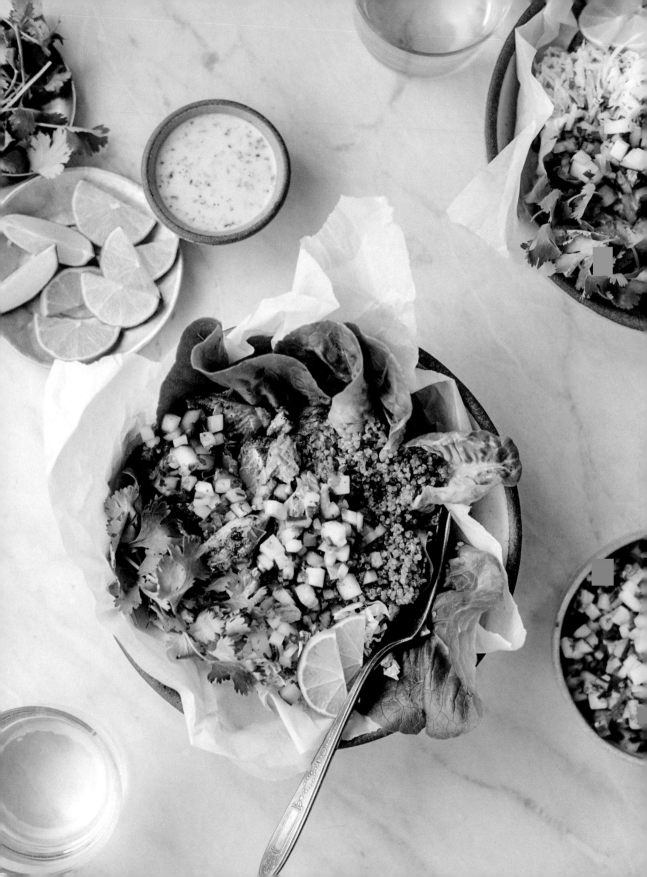

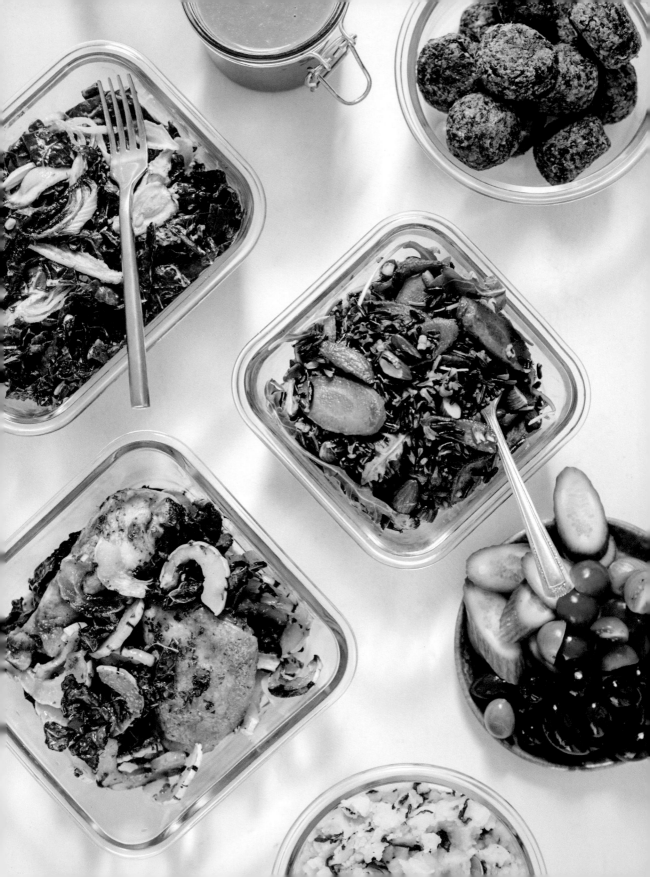

BATCH-COOKING MEAL PLANS & MENUS

THE FOLLOWING BUNDLES OF RECIPES are perfect for your meal prep sessions—making several dishes in one cooking time slot—or if you're in need of guidance for what dishes taste best together. For special diets, make sure you follow the variations specified in the dietary restriction notes for each recipe. The gut-heal bootcamp is made up of the simplest, easiest-to-digest recipes in the book if you're in need of a reset.

GUT-HEAL BOOTCAMP MENU

Week 1	Week 2
Orange Remedy Soup	Kitchen Sink Crucifer Soup
•	•
Green Detox Soup	Greek Chicken Zoodle Soup with Dill
•	•
Pre–Breath Test Chicken Congee	Better-Than-the-Box Yellow Rice Pilaf
•	•
Lemon-Rosemary Roast Chicken with Parsnips and Carrots	Warming Root Vegetable Chicken Tagine with Chard
•	•
Baked Halibut with Green Olive and Fennel Tapenade	Grilled Skirt Steak with Three-Herb Chimichurri

Week 1

Lemon-Rosemary Roast Chicken with
Parsnips and Carrots

•

Spinach-Ghee Mashed Potatoes

•

French Bean and Carrot Salad with
Green Harissa Sauce

•

Green Detox Soup

Week 2

Mild and Creamy Butterless Butter Chicken

•

Turmeric-Ginger Stewed Eggplant

•

Better-Than-the-Box Yellow Rice Pilaf

•

Heat-Free Cucumber Kimchi

•

Nutty Steamed Greens

Week 3

Warming Root Vegetable Chicken Tagine
with Chard

•

Brown Rice Kitchari

•

Marinated Kale with Roasted Fennel,
Parsnips, and Sunflower Seeds

•

Orange Remedy Soup

Week 4

Sesame Sheet Pan Salmon with Radishes

•

Beef Negimaki Stir-Fry with Green Beans
and Watercress

•

Nutty Steamed Greens

•

Kitchen Sink Crucifer Soup

Week 5

Teriyaki Pork Tenderloin with
Bok Choy and Broccoli

•

Thai Green Curry Chicken with Baby Eggplant

•

Spaghetti Squash Pad Thai

•

Zesty Kale Summer Rolls with
Almond-Tamari Dipping Sauce

Week 6

Skillet Chicken Cacciatore

•

Basque Cod, Pepper & Potato Stew

•

Pumpkin-Chive Risotto

•

Chicory Salad with Jammy Eggs and
Bagna Cauda Dressing

Week 7

Grilled Skirt Steak with Three-Herb Chimichurri

•

Summer Squash Moqueca

•

Roasted Tomato-Jalapeño Bisque

•

Southwestern Wedge Salad with
Sweet & Smoky Pepita Brittle

Week 8

Chili-Lime Sheet Pan Chicken with
Delicata Squash and Kale

•

Lamb & Sweet Potato Chili

•

Green Falafel with Magic Tahini Sauce

•

Moroccan Carrot Salad with Wild Rice,
Arugula, and Almonds

VEGETARIAN LOW-FODMAP

Week 1

West African Yam and Peanut Stew

•

Turmeric-Ginger Stewed Eggplant

•

Brown Rice Kitchari

•

Orange Remedy Soup

Week 2

Spaghetti Squash Pad Thai

•

Vietnamese Roasted Eggplant Salad

•

Heat-Free Cucumber Kimchi

•

Gingery Stir-Fried Collards and Quinoa

Week 3

Summer Squash Moqueca

•

Better-Than-the-Box Yellow Rice Pilaf

•

Marinated Kale with Roasted Fennel,
Parsnips, and Sunflower Seeds

•

Green Detox Soup

Week 4

Sweet Potato–Quinoa Burgers with
Sprouts and Spicy Lime Aioli

•

Caper-Herb Potato Salad

•

Moroccan Carrot Salad with
Wild Rice, Arugula, and Almonds

•

Roasted Tomato-Jalapeño Bisque

Week 5

Pumpkin-Chive Risotto

•

Balsamic Roasted Radicchio and Endive

•

Zucchini Carpaccio with Pine Nuts and
Crispy Prosciutto

•

Kitchen Sink Crucifer Soup

Week 6

Green Falafel with Magic Tahini Sauce

•

Millet Tabbouleh

•

French Bean and Carrot Salad
with Green Harissa Sauce

•

Garden Salad with Carrot-Ginger Dressing

BI-PHASIC DIET

Week 1
(BPD1R / Phase 1—Restricted)

Thai Green Curry Chicken
with Baby Eggplant

•

Turmeric-Ginger Stewed Eggplant

•

Garden Salad with Carrot-Ginger Dressing

•

Kitchen Sink Crucifer Soup

Week 2
(BPD1R / Phase 1—Restricted)

Chili-Lime Sheet Pan Chicken with
Delicata Squash and Kale

•

Baked Halibut with Green Olive
and Fennel Tapenade

•

French Bean and Carrot Salad with
Green Harissa Sauce

•

Green Detox Soup

Week 3
(BPD1 / Phase 1—Semi-restricted)

Cider-Dijon Pork Chops with Silky Cabbage

•

Turkey-Zucchini Meatballs with
the Simplest Romesco Sauce

•

Marinated Kale with Roasted Fennel,
Parsnips, and Sunflower Seeds

•

Orange Remedy Soup

Week 4
(BPD1 / Phase 1—Semi-restricted)

Teriyaki Pork Tenderloin
with Bok Choy and Broccoli

•

Larb Lettuce Wraps

•

Better-Than-the-Box Yellow Rice Pilaf

•

Heat-Free Cucumber Kimchi

Week 5
(BPD2 / Phase 2)

Lemon-Rosemary Roast Chicken with
Parsnips and Carrots

•

Stuffed Collard Greens with
Lamb and Quinoa

•

Spinach-Ghee Mashed Potatoes

•

Chicory Salad with Jammy Eggs and
Bagna Cauda Dressing

Week 6
(BPD2 / Phase 2)

Grilled Skirt Steak with
Three-Herb Chimichurri

•

Back-Pocket Chicken Paillard with
Sun-Dried Tomato Vinaigrette

•

Basque Cod, Pepper & Potato Stew

•

Zucchini Carpaccio with
Pine Nuts and Crispy Prosciutto

SIBO-SPECIFIC FOOD GUIDE, SCD & PALEO

Week 1

Thai Green Curry Chicken
with Baby Eggplant

•

Turmeric-Ginger Stewed Eggplant

•

Garden Salad with Carrot-Ginger Dressing

•

Kitchen Sink Crucifer Soup

Week 2

Chili-Lime Sheet Pan Chicken with
Delicata Squash and Kale

•

Baked Halibut with Green Olive and
Fennel Tapenade

•

French Bean and Carrot Salad
with Green Harissa Sauce

•

Green Detox Soup

Week 3

Cider-Dijon Pork Chops with Silky Cabbage

•

Turkey-Zucchini Meatballs with
the Simplest Romesco Sauce

•

Marinated Kale with Roasted Fennel,
Parsnips, and Sunflower Seeds

•

Orange Remedy Soup

Week 4

Teriyaki Pork Tenderloin with
Bok Choy and Broccoli

•

Larb Lettuce Wraps

•

Vietnamese Roasted Eggplant Salad

•

Heat-Free Cucumber Kimchi

Week 5

Beef Negimaki Stir-Fry with
Green Beans and Watercress

•

Turmeric-Dill Catfish

•

Spaghetti Squash Pad Thai

•

Greek Chicken Zoodle Soup with Dill

Week 6

Back-Pocket Chicken Paillard with
Sun-Dried Tomato Vinaigrette

•

Summer Squash Moqueca

•

Southwestern Wedge Salad with
Sweet & Smoky Pepita Brittle

•

Roasted Tomato-Jalapeño Bisque

LOW-HISTAMINE

Week 1

Chili-Lime Sheet Pan Chicken
with Delicata Squash and Kale

•

Better-Than-the-Box Yellow Rice Pilaf

•

French Bean and Carrot Salad
with Green Harissa Sauce

•

Green Detox Soup

Week 2

Mild and Creamy
Butterless Butter Chicken

•

Brown Rice Kitchari

•

Marinated Kale with Roasted Fennel,
Parsnips, and Sunflower Seeds

•

Orange Remedy Soup

Week 3

Creamy Chicken and
Broccoli Casserole

•

Larb Lettuce Wraps

•

Gingery Stir-Fried Collards
and Quinoa

•

Kitchen Sink Crucifer Soup

Week 4

Grilled Skirt Steak with
Three-Herb Chimichurri

•

Blackened Salmon Burrito Bowls with
Dirty Quinoa and Cucumber Salsa

•

Smoky Fingerling Steak Fries

•

Moroccan Carrot Salad with
Wild Rice, Arugula, and Almonds

LOW-SULFUR

Week 1

Skillet Chicken Cacciatore

•

Warming Root Vegetable Chicken Tagine
with Chard

•

Moroccan Carrot Salad
with Wild Rice, Arugula, and Almonds

•

Orange Remedy Soup

Week 2

Mild and Creamy
Butterless Butter Chicken

•

Turmeric-Ginger Stewed Eggplant

•

Better-Than-the-Box Yellow Rice Pilaf

•

Garden Salad with
Carrot-Ginger Dressing

Week 3

Summer Squash Moqueca

•

Vietnamese Roasted Eggplant Salad

•

Millet Tabbouleh

•

Roasted Tomato-Jalapeño Bisque

Week 4

Lemon-Rosemary Roast Chicken
with Parsnips and Carrots

•

Turkey-Zucchini Meatballs
with the Simplest Romesco Sauce

•

Smoky Fingerling Steak Fries

•

Southwestern Wedge Salad
with Sweet & Smoky Pepita Brittle

YEAST- & CANDIDA-FRIENDLY + SUGAR-FREE

Week 1

Seared Scallops with
Squash Succotash

•

French Bean and Carrot Salad
with Green Harissa Sauce

•

Marinated Kale with Roasted Fennel,
Parsnips, and Sunflower Seeds

•

Green Detox Soup

Week 2

Mild and Creamy
Butterless Butter Chicken

•

Turmeric-Ginger Stewed Eggplant

•

Brown Rice Kitchari

•

Orange Remedy Soup

Week 3

Stuffed Collard Greens
with Lamb and Quinoa

•

Basque Cod, Pepper & Potato Stew

•

Millet Tabbouleh

•

Zucchini Carpaccio
with Pine Nuts and Crispy Prosciutto

Week 4

Thai Green Curry Chicken
with Baby Eggplant

•

Sesame Sheet Pan Salmon
with Radishes

•

Better-Than-the-Box Yellow Rice Pilaf

•

Balsamic Roasted Radicchio and Endive

RECIPE INDEX

CAREFUL CARBS

SOUPS & STEWS

THE MAIN EVENT
Poultry, Meat & Seafood Entrées

POULTRY

MEAT

SEAFOOD

RECIPE DIETARY RESTRICTION KEY

LF	**Low-FODMAP (for a list of foods to avoid, see page 83)**
SCD	**Specific carbohydrate diet**
SSFG	**SIBO-specific food guide**
BPD1R	**Bi-phasic diet, Phase 1—Restricted**
BPD1	**Bi-phasic diet, Phase 1—Semi-restricted**
BPD2	**Bi-phasic diet, Phase 2**
P	**Paleo**
V	**Vegetarian / plant-based**
SF	**No added sugar**
HI	**Low-histamine (for a list of foods to avoid, see page 295)**
YC	**Yeast- & candida-friendly (for a list of foods to avoid, see page 296)**
HS	**Hydrogen sulfide–friendly (for a list of foods to avoid, see page 297)**

DIETARY RESTRICTION FOOD LISTS

FOODS TO AVOID FOR A LOW-HISTAMINE DIET (HI)

HIGH-HISTAMINE FOODS

Fermented alcoholic beverages: wine, champagne, beer, and cider

Fermented foods and condiments: sauerkraut, kefir, yogurt, kombucha, kimchi, sour cream, buttermilk, olives, pickles, vinegar, mustard, soy sauce, and other Asian condiments

Cured meats: bacon, salami, deli meats

Canned seafood: tuna, anchovies, sardines

Aged cheeses

Dried fruit: raisins, cherries, apricots, prunes, dates, figs

High-histamine vegetables: avocados, eggplant, spinach, and tomatoes

HISTAMINE-LIBERATING/ RELEASING FOODS

Alcohol

Bananas

Chocolate

Citrus fruits (lime is tolerated by most)

Cow's milk

Eggs

Nuts

Papaya

Pineapple

Shellfish

Strawberries

Wheat germ

DAO-BLOCKING FOODS

Alcohol

Black tea

Energy drinks

Green tea

Maté tea

FOODS TO AVOID FOR YEAST & CANDIDA (YC)

Many candida diets will eliminate all grains, starchy vegetables, and other refined carbs. I've taken a more liberal approach, focusing on the foods that cross-react with yeast and those that are yeast- or mold-containing themselves. For those following a strict low-carb approach, you can reference the specific carbohydrate diet (SCD) dietary label at the bottom of recipes in addition to that for yeast (YC).

Baking yeasts

Bone broth (except homemade low-histamine recipe on page 142)

Bottled fruit and vegetable juices

Canned seafood: tuna, anchovies, sardines, salmon

Cheese

Coffee

Corn

Cured meats: bacon, salami, deli meats

Dairy

Dried fruit

Eggs

Fermented beverages (cider, wine, beer, kombucha)

Fermented condiments (tamari, fish sauce)

Fermented vegetables

Fruit (berries in moderation is okay)

Gluten

Legumes

Mushrooms

Peanuts

Processed starches (flours, pastas, etc.—whole grains in moderation are okay)

Soy

Starchy vegetables— potato, winter squash, sweet potato, parsnip, pumpkin (limited quantities are okay)

Sugar & all sweeteners (see Added Sugar Ingredient List Cheat Sheet, page 298)

Vinegar

HIGH-SULFUR FOODS TO AVOID FOR HYDROGEN SULFIDE SIBO SUFFERERS (HS)

Anything with sulfite on the ingredient list (check your vinegar)

Almonds

Artichokes

Arugula

Asparagus

Bean sprouts

Bok choy

Bone broth

Broccoli

Brussels sprouts

Buckwheat

Cabbage

Cauliflower

Chard

Cheese

Chives

Cilantro

Collagen

Collard greens

Cow's milk

Dried fruit

Eggs

Garlic

Green beans

Jicama

Kale

Leeks

Legumes

Mustard

Mustard greens

Nuts

Onions

Peas

Pork

Quinoa

Radishes (daikon, horseradish, etc.)

Red meat

Rutabaga

Sauerkraut

Scallions

Seafood (except anchovies, clams, herring, mackerel, oysters, sardines, and salmon)

Seaweed

Shallots

Soy

Spinach

Sunchoke (a.k.a. Jerusalem artichoke)

Turnips

Watercress

Wine, beer, and cider

ADDED SUGAR INGREDIENT LIST CHEAT SHEET

Agave nectar/syrup

Barley malt

Beet sugar

Blackstrap molasses

Brown rice syrup

Brown sugar

Buttercream

Cane juice crystals

Cane sugar

Caramel

Carob syrup

Castor sugar

Coconut sugar

Confectioners' sugar (a.k.a. powdered sugar)

Corn syrup

Corn syrup solids

Crystalline fructose

Date sugar

Demerara sugar

Dextrin

Dextrose

Diastatic malt

Ethyl maltol

Evaporated cane juice

Fructose

Fruit juice

Fruit juice concentrate

Galactose

Glucose

Glucose syrup solids

Golden sugar

Golden syrup

Grape sugar

High-fructose corn syrup (HFCS)

Honey

Icing sugar

Invert sugar

Lactose

Maltodextrin

Maltose

Malt syrup

Maple syrup

Molasses

Muscovado sugar

Panela sugar

Raw sugar

Refiner's syrup

Rice syrup

Sorghum syrup

Sucanat

Sucrose

Sugar (granulated or table)

Treacle

Turbinado sugar

Yellow sugar

ELIMINATION DIET REINTRODUCTION WORKSHEET

Use your Symptom and Activity Tracker Worksheet (page 300) to get a full picture of your reintroduction day and log the results in the Symptoms + Notes column.

FOOD + DOSE	DATE AND TIME REINTRODUCED	SYMPTOMS + NOTES
EX: ¼ avocado	5/1, 9 a.m.	A few gurgles but nothing major!

SYMPTOM AND ACTIVITY TRACKER WORKSHEET

TRACK YOUR SYMPTOMS. Write down a time stamp for all that apply:	M	T	W	TH	F	SA	SU
Skin issues: breakouts, rashes, eczema, etc.							
Gas: belching or flatulence							
Heartburn or acid reflux							
Abdominal bloating or distension (upper)							
Abdominal bloating or distension (lower)							
Headaches							
Fatigue							
Back, neck, or joint pain							
Nausea or feeling overly full after eating							
Brain fog or dizziness							
Anxiety or depression							
Sinus congestion, stuffy nose, or itchy eyes							
Other:							
TRACK YOUR POOP. Check all that apply:	M	T	W	TH	F	SA	SU
Diarrhea							
Loose stool							
Dry lumpy rocks							
Constipation							
Poop perfection							
TRACK YOUR SUPPLEMENTS. List all medications, herbs, and vitamins:	M	T	W	TH	F	SA	SU

TRACK YOUR TRIGGER FOODS. Check all that were in your meal today:	M	T	W	TH	F	SA	SU
Corn							
Soy							
Dairy							
Gluten							
Added sugar							
Legumes							
High-FODMAP vegetables							
Other:							
Other:							
Other:							
TRACK YOUR COOKING:	M	T	W	TH	F	SA	SU
I ate _____ meals out.							
TRACK YOUR HYDRATION. Enter your cups/glasses:	M	T	W	TH	F	SA	SU
Coffee and tea							
Alcohol							
Water							
TRACK YOUR SLEEP:	M	T	W	TH	F	SA	SU
_____ hours							
_____ wake-ups in the night							
Rate how you felt in the morning (1–10)							
TRACK YOUR MOVEMENT AND MINDFULNESS. Enter the number of minutes:	M	T	W	TH	F	SA	SU
_____ minutes of _____							
_____ minutes of _____							
FOR THE LADIES, TRACK YOUR CYCLE:	M	T	W	TH	F	SA	SU
Enter what day it is (the first day of your period is 1):							

AN ABBREVIATED LIST OF SIBO-CONCURRENT DISEASES AND CONDITIONS

- Autism

- *C. difficile* infection

- Celiac disease

- Cholelithiasis (gallstones)

- Chronic fatigue syndrome

- Chronic lymphocytic leukemia (CLL)

- Cystic fibrosis

- Diabetes

- Diverticulitis

- Dyspepsia

- Ehlers-Danlos syndrome

- Endometriosis

- Erosive esophagitis

- Fibromyalgia

- Gastroparesis

- Hepatic steatosis

- HIV

- *H. pylori*

- Hypochlorhydria

- Hypothyroid and Hashimoto's thyroiditis

- IBD (Crohn's and ulcerative colitis)

- IBS (irritable bowel syndrome)

- Interstitial cystitis

- Intestinal permeability (leaky gut syndrome)

- Liver disease

- Lyme disease

- Mast cell activation syndrome (MCAS)

- Muscular dystrophy

- Pancreatitis

- Parkinson's disease

- Postural orthostatic tachycardia syndrome (POTS)

- Prostatitis

- Radiation enteropathy

- Restless leg syndrome

- Rheumatoid arthritis

- Scleroderma

- Systemic sclerosis

- Traumatic brain or spinal cord injury

RESOURCES

WEBSITES

SIBO Made Simple by Phoebe Lapine
| https://sibomadesimple.com

Feed Me Phoebe by Phoebe Lapine
| https://feedmephoebe.com/sibo/

The Wellness Project by Phoebe Lapine
| https://www.thewellnessproject.com/

SIBO Info by Dr. Allison Siebecker
| https://www.siboinfo.com

SIBO SOS by Shivan Sarna | https://sibosos.com

A Gutsy Girl by Sarah Kay Hoffman
| https://agutsygirl.com

SIBO Center by NUNM | https://sibocenter.com

The Healthy Gut by Rebecca Coomes
| https://www.thehealthygut.com/

Vital Food Therapeutics by Kristy Regan
| https://vitalfoodtherapeutics.com/

The Gut Solution by Sarah Otto
| https://gutsolutionseries.com/

PODCASTS

SIBO Made Simple by Phoebe Lapine

The Healthy Gut by Rebecca Coomes

Dr. Ruscio Radio by Dr. Michael Ruscio

The SIBO Doctor by Dr. Nirala Jacobi

SIBO SOS Podcast by Shivan Sarna

APPS

FODMAP by Monash University

mySymptoms Food Diary

SPECIAL DIET FOOD LISTS AND DOWNLOADS

Low-FODMAP diet
| https://www.monashfodmap.com/

Low-FODMAP grocery list | https://www
.katescarlata.com/low-fodmapgrocerylist

Bi-phasic diet (BPD) | https://www
.thesibodoctor.com/original-sibo-bi
-phasic-diet/

Bi-phasic low-histamine diet
| https://www.thesibodoctor.com/sibo
-histamine-bi-phasic-diet-download/

Low-histamine diet | https://mastcell360
.com/low-histamine-foods-list/

Low-sulfur diet | https://drruscio.com
/wp-content/uploads/2018/06
/LowSulfurDiet-1.pdf

SIBO-specific food guide (SSFG)
| https://www.siboinfo.com/diet.html

Specific carbohydrate diet (SCD)
| http://www.breakingtheviciouscycle.info/

Gut and psychology syndrome (GAPS)
| http://www.gapsdiet.com/

FURTHER READING

**Mast cell activation syndrome and
histamine intolerance:**
| https://mastcell360.com/mcas-resources/
| http://www.foodlogic.org/

Environmental toxins and mold:
| https://www.amikapadia.com/mold
-information
| https://www.laraadler.com/

LENS and neurofeedback
| https://www.brainresourcecenter.com
| *The Healing Power of Neurofeedback*, by
Stephen Larsen (Rochester, VT: Healing
Arts Press, 2006)

Hypnosis for IBS
| https://healthblog.uofmhealth.org
/digestive-health/gut-directed
-hypnotherapy-ibs-ibd-gerd
| http://www.ibshypnosis.com
/IBStreatments.html

Structural integration
| https://www.theiasi.net
| https://www.rolf.org

Visceral manipulation
| https://www.barralinstitute.com

FINDING A DOCTOR

Academy of Integrative Health and Medicine
| https://aihm.org/

The American Association of Naturopathic
Physicians | https://naturopathic.org

American Board of Physician Specialties
| https://www.abpsus.org/integrative
-medicine-requirements

The Institute for Functional Medicine
| www.functionalmedicine.org

Parsley Health
| https://www.parsleyhealth.com

SIBO SOS | https://sibosos.com

Feed Me Phoebe | https://feedmephoebe.com
/holistic-doctors-integrative-medicine-nyc/

TESTING

Breath Testing—Aerodiagnostics
| https://www.aerodiagnostics.com/

Breath Testing—QuinTron
| https://www.breathtests.com/

Breath Testing—Genova Diagnostics
| https://www.gdx.net/

IBS Smart Test | https://www.ibssmart.com

DNA Stool Test—Onegevity
| https://www.onegevity.com/

PRODUCTS AND SUPPLEMENTS

Phoebe's Favorites
| https://feedmephoebe.com/shop/

Low-FODMAP Pantry
| https://www.fodyfoods.com
| https://casadesante.com

Elemental Diet | https://store.drruscio.com
/products/elemental-heal

Elemental Diet DIY | https://www.siboinfo
.com/elemental-formula.html

Allicin | https://www.allimax.us/Allimed
-Products

Biofilm-busting formulas | Biofilm Defense by
Kirkman Labs; InterFase Plus by Klaire Labs

Digestive enzymes
| Digestzymes by Designs for Health

Probiotics | BioGaia Probiotics; Saccharomyces
Boulardii by Klaire Labs; MegaSpore-Biotic
by Microbiome Labs

Essential oils
| https://www.rockymountainoils.com

Full-spectrum hemp oil
| https://radicalrootsherbs.com

Collagen | https://greatlakesgelatin.com

Partially hydrolyzed guar gum | Perfect Pass
Prebiotic

Water filters | New Wave Enviro 10 Stage Plus;
Pure Effect

Air filters | https://www.intellipure.com

ACKNOWLEDGMENTS

Perhaps the only process that's lonelier than dealing with a chronic illness is writing a book. So I knew if I was going to write another book about chronic illness, I'd need an all-star supporting cast to lean on. I couldn't have asked for a better one this go-round.

The path to this book was paved with rejections from people who thought SIBO was too niche. A huge thank-you to Renée Sedliar for embracing my mission with open arms and an extremely generous word count. You were an essential voice in the ideation and editing process, and all the SIBO Amigos out there can now benefit from your belief.

To Sally Ekus for always supporting my creative whims, no matter where they (or my own health journey) lead.

To Haley Hunt Davis for being an extremely multitalented food artist and agreeing to copilot a very scrappy, DIY photo shoot. The four days we spent cranking and dancing to Noah Cyrus radio in my apartment were my favorite of the whole book process. An additional thank-you to Amelia Arend for your teamwork and superior knife skills, and to Maeve Sheridan for providing my dream props at an insanely kind rate. I can't wait for the day I can afford to hire you to be there in person!

To the whole Hachette Go team for designing the most gorgeous SIBO book in all the land and shepherding it into the world.

To Spruceton Inn for giving me a week of peace and quiet to eat my photo-shoot leftovers and dig in to the rest of the manuscript.

To Erica Adler for testing all the aiolis (among other things) when I really needed a helping hand. I'm so happy to have had you in my corner for the last few years.

To the readers of my site, *Feed Me Phoebe*, who submitted countless comments, messages, and emails about SIBO. You're the reason I looked beyond my own experience and realized there was a need for more answers. Plus, even more gratitude to the seventy-plus of you who were part of my tester tribe—these recipes are so much better for your input and cheerleading.

To my fierce female food friends, who were always there for random questions and spontaneous vent seshes: Serena Wolf, Liz Moody, Talia Pollock, Katie Horwich, and Katie Dalebout, among many others. And a special thank-you to Jessica Murnane and Heather Crosby for also lending me their incomparable eyes and design skills.

To my parents, Sarah and James, for their encouragement and newfound interest in gut stuff. To my mother-in-law, Jane, for being so kind and for keeping us well stocked in monolaurin. And to Cheryl Houser and Debbie Phillips for their mentorship.

To my husband, Charlie, for being the best possible emotional support animal. The process of writing this book overlapped with a pandemic, a terrible loss, and many other extended periods of existential anxiety. Thank you for feeding me and forgiving me when I couldn't clothe myself in anything that didn't involve an elastic waistband. I love your guts the most. And I'm pretty sure your guts love me back for encouraging you to give up dairy.

Finally, I consider myself an expert curator of information, not a SIBO professional in my own right. Needless to say, this book truly wouldn't have been possible without the following medical practitioners who shared their wisdom with me on my podcast, *SIBO Made Simple*, and offline during my own healing period. Thank you for all your research, lectures, resources, and countless hours supporting SIBO Amigos like me: Lara Adler, Delia Ahouandjinou, Dr. Amy Bader, Dr. Maurice Beer, Dr. Susan Blum, David Bouley, Dr. Jolene Brighten, Dr. Will Bulsiewicz, Rebecca Coomes, Dr. Patrick Fratellone, Dr. Mahmoud Ghannoum, Dr. Ilana Gurevich, Jennifer Hanway, Dr. Jason Hawrelak, Dr. Nirala Jacobi, Dr. Ami Kapadia, Dr. Heidi Lovie, Dr. Andrea McBeth, Beth O'Hara, Dr. William Parker, Dr. Jessica Peatross, Dr. Mark Pimentel, Kristy Regan, Dr. Megan Riehl, Dr. Aviva Romm, Dr. Michael Ruscio, Shivan Sarna, Kate Scarlata, Dr. Amy Shah, Dr. Lisa Shaver, Dr. Maya Shetreat, Dr. Allison Siebecker, Heidi Turner, Chloe Weber, and Dr. Jason Wysocki.

A very special thank-you to Dr. Will Cole for giving me an initial nudge of encouragement in Arizona when this book was just a seed of an idea, and for generously seeing it through to its final stages with your foreword. I'm so honored to have you be a part of this project.

BIBLIOGRAPHY

Baker, Sidney MacDonald. *Detoxification and Healing: The Key to Optimal Health.* New York: McGraw Hill Education, 2003.

Barshak, M. B., and M. L. Durand. "The Role of Infection and Antibiotics in Chronic Rhinosinusitis." *Laryngoscope Investigative Otolaryngology* 2, no. 1 (January 2017): 36–42. https://doi.org/10.1002/lio2.61.

Basseri, R. J., B. Basseri, M. Pimentel, K. Chong, A. Youdim, K. Low, L. Hwang, E. Soffer, C. Chang, and R. Mathur. "Intestinal Methane Production in Obese Individuals Is Associated with a Higher Body Mass Index." *Gastroenterology & Hepatology* 8, no. 1 (January 2012): 22–28. https://www.ncbi.nlm.nih.gov/pubmed/22347829.

Belei, Oana, Laura Olariu, Andreea Dobrescu, Tamara Marcovici, and Otilia Marginean. "Is It Useful to Administer Probiotics Together with Proton Pump Inhibitors in Children with Gastroesophageal Reflux?" *Journal of Neurogastroenterology and Motility* 24, no. 1 (January 2018): 51–57. https://doi.org/10.5056/jnm17059.

Borrelli, F., I. Fasolino, B. Romano, R. Capasso, F. Maiello, D. Coppola, P. Orlando, G. Battista, E. Pagano, V. Di Marzo, et al. "Beneficial Effect of the Non-psychotropic Plant Cannabinoid Cannabigerol on Experimental Inflammatory Bowel Disease." *Biochemical Pharmocology* 85, no. 9 (May 1, 2013): 1306–1316. https://doi.org/10.1016/j.bcp.2013.01.017.

Bozek, A., and K. Pyrkosz. "Immunotherapy of Mold Allergy: A Review." *Human Vaccines & Immunotherapeutics* 13, no. 10 (2017): 2397–2401. https://doi.org/10.1080/21645515.2017.1314404.

Cao, Shu-Guang, Wan-Chun Wu, Zhen Han, and Meng-Ya Wang. "Effects of Psychological Stress on Small Intestinal Motility and Expression of Cholecystokinin and Vasoactive Intestinal Polypeptide in Plasma and Small Intestine in Mice." *World Journal of Gastroenterology* 11, no. 5 (February 2005): 737–740. https://doi.org/10.3748/wjg.v11.i5.737.

Chris Kresser. "Biofilm: What It Is and How to Treat It." Kresser Institute. Chris Kresser LLC, March 6, 2018. https://kresserinstitute.com/biofilm-what-it-is-and-how-to-treat-it/.

Cornish, J. A., E. Tan, C. Simillis, S. K. Clark, J. Teare, and P. P. Tekkis. "The Risk of Oral Contraceptives in the Etiology of Inflammatory Bowel Disease: A Meta-analysis." *American Journal of Gastroenterology* 103, no. 9 (September 2008): 2394–2400. https://doi.org/10.1111/j.1572-0241.2008.02064.x.

da Silva, Marco, Antonio Helio, and Peter T. Dorsher. "Neuroanatomic and Clinical Correspondences: Acupuncture and Vagus Nerve Stimulation." *Journal of Alternative and Complementary Medicine* 20, no. 4 (April 2014): 223–240. https://doi.org/10.1089/acm.2012.1022.

Darkoh, Charles, Lenard M. Lichtenberger, Nadim Ajami, Elizabeth J. Dial, Zhi-Dong Jiang, and Herbert L. DuPont. "Bile Acids Improve the Antimicrobial Effect of Rifaximin." *Antimicrobial Agents and Chemotherapy* 54, no. 9 (September 2010): 3618–3624. https://doi.org/10.1128/AAC.00161-10.

Do, Moon Ho, Eunjung Lee, Mi-Jin Oh, Yoonsook Kim, and Ho Young Park. "High-Glucose or -Fructose Diet Cause Changes of the Gut Microbiota and Metabolic Disorders in Mice Without Body Weight Change." *Nutrients* 10, no. 6 (June 2018): 761. https://doi.org/10.3390/nu10060761.

Dominy, Stephen S., Casey Lynch, Florian Ermini, Malgorzata Benedyk, Agata Marczyk, Andrei Konradi, Mai Nguyen, Ursula Haditsch, Debasish Raha, Christina Griffin, et al. "*Porphyromonas gingivalis* in Alzheimer's Disease Brains: Evidence for Disease Causation and Treatment with Small-Molecule Inhibitors." *Science Advances* 5, no. 1 (January 23, 2019). https://doi.org/10.1126/sciadv.aau3333.

Donn, Jeff, Martha Mendoza, and Justin Pritchard. "Pharmaceuticals Lurking in U.S. Drinking Water." NBC News. Associated Press, 2013.

Dukowicz, Andrew C., Brian E. Lacy, and Gary M. Levine. "Small Intestinal Bacterial Overgrowth." *Gastroenterology & Hepatology* 3, no. 2 (February 2007): 112–122.

Erdogan, A., and S. S. Rao. "Small Intestinal Fungal Overgrowth." *Current Gastroenterology Reports* 17, no. 4 (April 2015): 16. https://doi.org/10.1007/s11894-015-0436-2.

Eutamene, Helene, Vassilia Theodorou, Jean Fioramonti, and Lionel Bueno. "Acute Stress Modulates the Histamine Content of Mast Cells in the Gastrointestinal Tract Through Interleukin-1 and Corticotropin-Releasing Factor Release in Rats." *Journal of Physiology* 553, pt. 3 (December 15, 2003): 959–966. https://doi.org/10.1113/jphysiol.2003.052274.

Fahey, Jed W., Katherine K. Stephenson, and Alison J. Wallace. "Dietary Amelioration of Helicobacter Infection." *Nutrition Research* 35, no. 6 (June 2015): 461–473. https://doi.org/10.1016/j.nutres.2015.03.001.

Faresjö, Åshild, Saga Johansson, Tomas Faresjö, Susanne Roos, and Claes Hallert. "Sex Differences in Dietary Coping with Gastrointestinal Symptoms." *European Journal of Gastroenterology & Hepatology* 22, no. 3 (March 2010): 327–333. https://doi.org/10.1097/MEG.0b013e32832b9c53.

Field, Tiffany, Miguel Diego, and Maria Hernandez-Reif. "Preterm Infant Massage Therapy Research: A Review." *Infant Behavior and Development* 33, no. 2 (April 2010): 115–124. https://doi.org/10.1016/j.infbeh.2009.12.004.

Foster, Jane A., and Karen-Anne McVey Neufeld. "Gut-Brain Axis: How the Microbiome Influences Anxiety and Depression." *Trends in Neurosciences* 36, no. 5 (May 2013): 305–312. https://doi.org/10.1016/j.tins.2013.01.005.

Furnari, M., A. Parodi, L. Gemignani, E. G. Giannini, S. Marenco, E. Savarino, L. Assandri, V. Fazio, D. Bonfanti, S. Inferrera, et al. "Clinical Trial: The Combination of Rifaximin with Partially Hydrolysed Guar Gum Is More Effective Than Rifaximin Alone in Eradicating Small Intestinal Bacterial Overgrowth." *Alimentary Pharmacology & Therapeutics* 32, no. 8 (October 2010): 1000–1006. https://doi.org/10.1111/j.1365-2036.2010.04436.x.

Galland, Leo. "Nutrition and Candidiasis." *Journal of Orthomolecular Psychiatry* 14, no. 1 (1985): 50–60. http://www.orthomolecular.org/library/jom/1985/pdf/1985-v14n01-p050.pdf.

Gigli, Stefano, Luisa Seguella, Marcella Pesce, Eugenia Bruzzese, Alessandro D'Alessandro, Rosario Cuomo, Luca Steardo, Giovanni Sarnelli, and Giuseppe Esposito. "Cannabidiol Restores Intestinal Barrier Dysfunction and Inhibits the Apoptotic Process Induced by *Clostridium difficile* Toxin A in Caco-2 Cells." *United European Gastroenterology Journal* 5, no. 8 (December 2017): 1108–1115. https://doi.org/10.1177/2050640617698622.

Godman, Heidi. "Are Sprouted Grains More Nutritious Than Regular Whole Grains?" Harvard Health Publishing. Harvard University, November 6, 2017. https://www.health.harvard.edu/blog/sprouted-grains-nutritious-regular-whole-grains-2017110612692.

Gonsalkorale, W. M., V. Miller, A. Afzal, and P. J. Whorwell. "Long-Term Benefits of Hypnotherapy for Irritable Bowel Syndrome." *Gut* 52, no. 11 (November 2003): 1623–1629. https://doi.org/10.1136/gut.52.11.1623.

Gonsalkorale, W. M. "Gut-Directed Hypnotherapy: The Manchester Approach for Treatment of Irritable Bowel Syndrome." *International Journal of Clinical and Experimental Hypnosis* 54, no. 1 (January 2006): 27–50. https://doi.org/10.1080/00207140500323030.

Grigoleit, H.-G., and P. Grigoleit. "Peppermint Oil in Irritable Bowel Syndrome." *Phytomedicine* 12, no. 8 (August 2005): 601–606. https://doi.org/10.1016/j.phymed.2004.10.005.

Gurav, Abhijit N. "Periodontitis and Insulin Resistance: Casual or Causal Relationship?" *Diabetes and Metabolism Journal* 36, no. 6 (December 2012): 404–411. https://doi.org/10.4093/dmj.2012.36.6.404.

Habib, Navaz. *Activate Your Vagus Nerve*. Brooklyn, NY: Ulysses Press, 2019.

Halmos, Emma P., Claus T. Christophersen, Anthony R. Bird, Susan J. Shepherd, Peter R. Gibson, and Jane G. Muir. "Diets That Differ in Their FODMAP Content Alter the Colonic Luminal Microenvironment." *Gut* 64, no. 1 (January 2015): 93–100. https://doi.org/10.1136/gutjnl-2014-307264.

Hashida, S., E. Ishikawa, N. Nakamichi, and H. Sekino. "Concentration of Egg White Lysozyme in the Serum of Healthy Subjects After Oral Administration." *Clinical and Experimental Pharmacology & Physiology* 29, no. 1–2 (January–February 2002): 79–83. https://www.ncbi.nlm.nih.gov/pubmed/11906463.

Hesselmar, Bill, Anna Hicke-Roberts, and Göran Wennergren. "Allergy in Children in Hand Versus Machine Dishwashing." *Pediatrics* 135, no. 3 (March 2015): e590–e597. https://doi .org/10.1542/peds.2014-2968.

Hesselmar, Bill, Anna Hicke-Roberts, Anna-Carin Lundell, Ingegerd Adlerberth, Anna Rudin, Robart Saalman, Göran Wennergren, and Agnes E. Wold. "Pet-Keeping in Early Life Reduces the Risk of Allergy in a Dose-Dependent Fashion." *PLoS ONE* 13, no. 12 (2018). https://doi .org/10.1371/journal.pone.0208472.

Hill, Peta, Jane G. Muir, and Peter R. Gibson. "Controversies and Recent Developments of the Low-FODMAP Diet." *Gastroenterology & Hepatology* 31, no. 1 (January 2017): 36–45. https://www.ncbi.nlm.nih.gov/pmc/articles /PMC5390324/.

"IARC Monographs Evaluate Consumption of Red Meat and Processed Meat." International Agency for Research on Cancer press release, October 26, 2015. On the IARC website. https:// www.iarc.fr/wp-content/uploads/2018/07 /pr240_E.pdf.

Kajiura, Takayuki, Tomoko Takeda, Shinji Sakata, Mitsuo Sakamoto, Masaki Hashimoto, Hideki Suzuki, Manabu Suzuki, and Yoshimi Benno. "Change of Intestinal Microbiota with Elemental Diet and Its Impact on Therapeutic Effects in a Murine Model of Chronic Colitis." *Digestive Diseases and Sciences* 54 (2009): 1892–1900. https://link.springer.com/article/10.1007 /s10620-008-0574-6.

Katzenberger, R. J., B. Ganetzky, and D. A. Wassarman. "The Gut Reaction to Traumatic Brain Injury." *Fly* 9, no. 2 (2015): 68–74. https:// doi.org/10.1080/19336934.2015.1085623.

Kelesidis, Theodoros, and Charalabos Pothoulakis. "Efficacy and Safety of the Probiotic *Saccharomyces boulardii* for the Prevention and Therapy of Gastrointestinal Disorders." *Therapeutic Advances in Gastroenterology* 5, no. 2 (March 2012): 111–125. https://doi .org/10.1177/1756283X11428502.

Kennedy, Joshua L., and Larry Borish. "Chronic Rhinosinusitis and Antibiotics: The Good, the Bad, and the Ugly." *American Journal of Rhinology & Allergy* 27, no. 6 (November– December 2013): 467–472. https://doi .org/10.2500/ajra.2013.27.3960.

Khalili, Hamed, Leslie M. Higuchi, Ashwin N. Ananthakrishnan, James M. Richter, Diane Feskanich, Charles S. Fuchs, and Andrew T. Chan. "Oral Contraceptives, Reproductive Factors and Risk of Inflammatory Bowel Disease." *Gut* 62, no. 8 (August 2013): 1153–1159. https://doi.org/10.1136/gutjnl-2012-302362.

Kim, Dae Bum, Chang-Nyol Paik, Yeon Ji Kim, Ji Min Lee, Kyong-Hwa Jun, Woo Chul Chung, Kang-Moon Lee, Jin-Mo Yang, and Myung-Gyu Choi. "Positive Glucose Breath Tests in Patients with Hysterectomy, Gastrectomy, and Cholecystectomy." *Gut Liver* 11, no. 2 (March 2017): 237–242. https://doi.org/10.5009 /gnl16132.

Kim, Y., S. C. Park, B. W. Wolf, and S. R. Hertzler. "Combination of Erythritol and Fructose Increases Gastrointestinal Symptoms in Healthy Adults." *Nutrition Research* 31, no. 11 (November 2011): 836–841. https://doi .org/10.1016/j.nutres.2011.09.025.

Korzenik, J., A. K. Koch, and J. Langhorst. "Complementary and Integrative Gastroenterology." *Medical Clinics of North America* 101, no. 5 (September 2017): 943–954. https://doi.org/10.1016/j.mcna.2017.04.009.

Kumamoto, Carol A. "Inflammation and Gastrointestinal Candida Colonization." *Current Opinion in Microbiology* 14, no. 4 (August 2011): 386–391. https://doi.org/10.1016/j .mib.2011.07.015.

Kuo, Braden, Manoj Bhasin, Jolene Jacquart, Matthe A. Scult, Lauren Slipp, Eric Isaac Kagan Riklin, Veronique Lepoutre, Nicole Comosa, Beth-Anne Norton, Allison Dassatti, et al. "Genomic and Clinical Effects Associated with a Relaxation Response Mind-Body Intervention in Patients with Irritable Bowel Syndrome and Inflammatory Bowel Disease." *PLoS ONE* (April 30, 2015). https://doi.org/10.1371/journal .pone.0123861.

Lapine, Phoebe. "SIBO Made Simple | EP 01 | SIBO 101: Root Causes, Testing & The IBS Connection with Dr. Allison Siebecker." *Feed Me Phoebe.* Podcast audio. January 16, 2019. https:// feedmephoebe.com/smsepisode1/.

Lapine, Phoebe. "SIBO Made Simple | EP 02 | How to Treat SIBO Naturally with Dr. Will Cole." *Feed Me Phoebe.* Podcast audio. January 16, 2019. https://feedmephoebe.com/smsepisode2/.

Lapine, Phoebe. "SIBO Made Simple | EP 03 | The Thyroid Thread & What Women Need to Know About SIBO with Dr. Jolene Brighten." *Feed Me Phoebe*. Podcast audio. January 16, 2019. https://feedmephoebe.com/smsepisode3/.

Lapine, Phoebe. "SIBO Made Simple | EP 04 | FODMAP WTF: A Complete Guide to Life Without Fermentable Carbs with Kate Scarlata." *Feed Me Phoebe*. Podcast audio. January 23, 2019. https://feedmephoebe.com/smsepisode4/.

Lapine, Phoebe. "SIBO Made Simple | EP 05 | Intermittent Fasting & Other Strategies for Making the MMC Move Smoothly with Dr. Amy Shah." *Feed Me Phoebe*. Podcast audio. January 30, 2019. https://feedmephoebe.com/smsepisode5/.

Lapine, Phoebe. "SIBO Made Simple | EP 06 | Prebiotic and Probiotic Protocols: A SIBO Management Misnomer with Dr. Jason Hawrelak." *Feed Me Phoebe*. Podcast audio. February 6, 2019. https://feedmephoebe.com/smsepisode6/.

Lapine, Phoebe. "SIBO Made Simple | EP 07 | How Bodywork Can Give Your Intestines a Boost with Dr. Jason Wysocki." *Feed Me Phoebe*. Podcast audio. February 13, 2019. https://feedmephoebe.com/smsepisode7/.

Lapine, Phoebe. "SIBO Made Simple | EP 08 | The Autoimmune-SIBO Connection and How to Heal Leaky Gut with Dr. Susan Blum." *Feed Me Phoebe*. Podcast audio. February 20, 2019. https://feedmephoebe.com/smsepisode8/.

Lapine, Phoebe. "SIBO Made Simple | EP 09 | Feast or Famine: How Your SIBO Diet & Treatment Plans Work in Tandem with Dr. Nirala Jacobi." *Feed Me Phoebe*. Podcast audio. February 27, 2019. https://feedmephoebe.com/smsepisode9/.

Lapine, Phoebe. "SIBO Made Simple | EP 10 | A Patient's Guide to Ridding Your Life of SIBO Without SIBO Taking Over Your Life with Rebecca Coomes." *Feed Me Phoebe*. Podcast audio. March 6, 2019. https://feedmephoebe.com/smsepisode10/.

Lapine, Phoebe. "SIBO Made Simple | EP 12 | Ask a Doctor: All Your Season 1 SIBO Questions Answered." *Feed Me Phoebe*. Podcast audio. March 20, 2019. https://feedmephoebe.com/smsepisode12/.

Lapine, Phoebe. "SIBO Made Simple | EP 13 | Digesting for Two: Infertility, SIBO & What Pregnant Mothers Need to Know About Gut Health with Dr. Aviva Romm." *Feed Me Phoebe*. Podcast audio. May 8, 2019. https://feedmephoebe.com/smsepisode13/.

Lapine, Phoebe. "SIBO Made Simple | EP 14 | The Sleep-Gut Cycle: How Improving Your Sleep Can Heal Your Digestive System with Jennifer Hanway." *Feed Me Phoebe*. Podcast audio. May 15, 2019. https://feedmephoebe.com/smsepisode14/.

Lapine, Phoebe. "SIBO Made Simple | EP 15 | Histamine, SIBO, and Food Sensitivities: What Seasonal Allergies Have to Do with Gut Health with Heidi Turner." *Feed Me Phoebe*. Podcast audio. May 22, 2019. https://feedmephoebe.com/smsepisode15/.

Lapine, Phoebe. "SIBO Made Simple | FP 16 | IBS & Anxiety: Free Your Mind with Hypnotherapy, Your Gut Will Follow with Dr. Megan Riehl." *Feed Me Phoebe*. Podcast audio. May 20, 2019. https://feedmephoebe.com/smsepisode16/.

Lapine, Phoebe. "SIBO Made Simple | EP 17 | The Great SIBO Breath Test Debate: How to Prep, Interpret Your Results, and Look at the Bigger Picture with Dr. Patrick Fratellone." *Feed Me Phoebe*. Podcast audio. June 5, 2019. https://feedmephoebe.com/smsepisode17/.

Lapine, Phoebe. "SIBO Made Simple | EP 18 | Getting Dirty: The Rules of Greater Gut Health to Teach Our Children and Heal Ourselves with Dr. Maya Shetreat." *Feed Me Phoebe*. Podcast audio. June 12, 2019. https://feedmephoebe.com/smsepisode18/.

Lapine, Phoebe. "SIBO Made Simple | EP 23 | Last Resort: The Elemental Diet and Other Strategies for When Your SIBO Won't Quit with Dr. Michael Ruscio." *Feed Me Phoebe*. Podcast audio. July 24, 2019. https://feedmephoebe.com/smsepisode23/.

Lapine, Phoebe. "SIBO Made Simple | EP 26 | Yeast and Other Beasts: The SIBO-Candida Connection, Diet & Treatment of Fungal Overgrowth with Dr. Ami Kapadia." *Feed Me Phoebe*. Podcast audio. November 20, 2019. https://feedmephoebe.com/smsepisode26/.

Lapine, Phoebe. "SIBO Made Simple | EP 30 | Gluten Freedom: Celiac Disease, SIBO & What This Protein Really Does to Our Gut with Dr.

Lisa Shaver." *Feed Me Phoebe.* Podcast audio. January 1, 2020. https://feedmephoebe.com /smsepisode30/.

Lapine, Phoebe. "SIBO Made Simple | EP 36 | Ask a Doctor: The Latest IBS, Methane, and Hydrogen Sulfide Research + All Your Other SIBO Questions Answered with Dr. Mark Pimentel." *Feed Me Phoebe.* Podcast audio. February 19, 2020. https://feedmephoebe.com /smsepisode26/.

Lauritano, E. C., M. Gabrielli, E. Scarpellini, V. Ojetti, D. Roccarina, A. Villita, E. Fiore, R. Flore, A. Santoliquido, P. Tondi, et al. "Antibiotic Therapy in Small Intestinal Bacterial Overgrowth: Rifaximin Versus Metronidazole." *European Review for Medical and Pharmological Sciences* 13, no. 2 (March–April 2009): 111–116. https:// www.ncbi.nlm.nih.gov/pubmed/19499846.

Lee, Han Hee, Yoon Young Choi, and Myung-Gyu Choi. "The Efficacy of Hypnotherapy in the Treatment of Irritable Bowel Syndrome: A Systematic Review and Meta-analysis." *Journal of Neurogastroenterology and Motility* 20, no. 2 (April 2014): 152–162. https://doi.org/10.5056 /jnm.2014.20.2.152.

Lee, H. R., and M. Pimentel. "Bacteria and Irritable Bowel Syndrome: The Evidence for Small Intestinal Bacterial Overgrowth." *Current Gastroenterology Reports* 8, no. 2 (August 2006): 305–311. https://doi.org/10.1007/s11894 -006-0051-3.

Lin, H. C., and M. Pimentel. "Bacterial Concepts in Irritable Bowel Syndrome." *Reviews in Gastroenterological Disorders* 5, suppl. 3 (2005): S3–S9. https://www.ncbi.nlm.nih.gov /pubmed/17713456.

Low, K., L. Hwang, J. Hua, A. Zhu, W. Morales, and M. Pimentel. "A Combination of Rifaximin and Neomycin Is Most Effective in Treating Irritable Bowel Syndrome Patients with Methane on Lactulose Breath Test." *Journal of Clinical Gastroenterology* 44, no. 8 (September 2010): 547–550. https://doi.org/10.1097 /MCG.0b013e3181c64c90.

Lyszkowska, M., K. Popinska, M. Idzik, and P. Ksiazyk. "Probiotics in Children with Gut Failure." *Journal of Pediatric Gastroenterology and Nutrition* 46 (2008): 543.

Mahmood A., A. J. FitzGerald, T. Marchbank, E. Ntatsaki, D. Murray, S. Ghosh, and R. J. Playford. "Zinc Carnosine, A Health Food Supplement That Stabilises Small Bowel Integrity and Stimulates Gut Repair Processes." *Gut* 56, no. 2 (February 2007): 168–175. https://doi .org/10.1136/gut.2006.099929.

Marsh, A., E. M. Eslick, and G. D. Eslick. "Does a Diet Low in FODMAPs Reduce Symptoms Associated with Functional Gastrointestinal Disorders? A Comprehensive Systematic Review and Meta-analysis." *European Journal of Nutrition* 55, no. 3 (April 2016): 897–906. https:// doi.org/10.1007/s00394-015-0922-1.

Mazzawi, Tarek, and Magdy El-Salhy. "Effect of Diet and Individual Dietary Guidance on Gastrointestinal Endocrine Cells in Patients with Irritable Bowel Syndrome (Review)." *International Journal of Molecular Medicine* 40, no. 4 (October 2017): 943–952. https://doi .org/10.3892/ijmm.2017.3096.

McIntosh, Keith, David E Reed, Theresa Schneider, Frances Dang, Ammar H. Keshteli, Giada De Palma, Karen Madsen, Premysl Bercik, and Stephen Vanner. "FODMAPs Alter Symptoms and the Metabolome of Patients with IBS: A Randomised Controlled Trial." *Gut* 66 (2017): 1241–1251. https://gut.bmj.com /content/66/7/1241.

Mena-Sanchez, Guillermo, Nancy Babio, and Jordi Salas-Salvado. "Consuming Fermented Dairy Products Is Associated with a Healthier Life-Style and Greater Adherence to the Mediterranean Diet." Gut Microbiota for Heath. European Society for Neurogastroenterology & Motility, November 12, 2018. https://www .gutmicrobiotaforhealth.com/en/consuming -fermented-dairy-products-is-associated-with -a-healthier-life-style-and-greater-adherence -to-the-mediterranean-diet/.

Menees, Stacy, and William Chey. "The Gut Microbiome and Irritable Bowel Syndrome." *F1000Research* 7 (2018). https://doi .org/10.12688/f1000research.14592.1.

Mesnage, R., E. Clair, S. Gress, C. Then, A. Székács, and G.-E. Séralini. "Cytotoxicity on Human Cells of Cry1Ab and Cry1Ac Bt Insecticidal Toxins Alone or with a Glyphosate-Based Herbicide." *Journal of Applied Toxicology* 33, no. 7 (July 2013): 695–699. https://doi.org/10.1002 /jat.2712.

"Mindfulness Meditation Reduces Severity of IBS in Women, Study Finds." National Center for Complementary and Integrative Health. US Department of Health & Human Services,

National Institutes of Health, September 1, 2011. https://nccih.nih.gov/research/results/spotlight/031912.

Nickmilder, M., S. Carbonnelle, and A. Bernard. "House Cleaning with Chlorine Bleach and the Risks of Allergic and Respiratory Diseases in Children." *Pediatric Allergy and Immunology* 18, no. 1 (February 2007): 27–35. https://doi.org/10.1111/j.1399-3038.2006.00487.x.

Niv, E., A. Halak, E. Tiommny, H. Yanai, H. Strul, T. Naftali, and N. Vaisman. "Randomized Clinical Study: Partially Hydrolyzed Guar Gum (PHGG) Versus Placebo in the Treatment of Patients with Irritable Bowel Syndrome." *Nutrition & Metabolism* 13 (February 6, 2016): 10. https://doi.org/10.1186/s12986-016-0070-5.

Olsen, A. B., R. A. Hetz, H. Xue, K. R. Aroom, D. Bhattarai, E. Johnson, S. Bedi, C. S. Cox Jr., and K. Uray. "Effects of Traumatic Brain Injury on Intestinal Contractility." *Neurogastroenterology & Motility* 25, no. 7 (2013): 593-e463. https://doi.org/10.1111/nmo.12121.

Olsen, Ingar, and Kazuhisa Yamazaki. "Can Oral Bacteria Affect the Microbiome of the Gut?" *Journal of Oral Microbiology* 11, no. 1 (2019). https://doi.org/10.1080/20002297.2019.1586422.

Orme-Johnson, D. W., and R. E. Herron. "Reduced Medical Care Utilization and Expenditures Through an Innovative Approach." *Abstracts of the Association for Health Services Research 14th Annual Meeting* (June 15–17, 1997): 19.

Paddock, Catherine. "New IBD Treatments May Combine Antifungals and Probiotics." Medical News Today. Healthline Media UK Ltd., October 4, 2017. https://www.medicalnewstoday.com/articles/319633.php#1.

Palsson, O. S. "Standardized Hypnosis Treatment for Irritable Bowel Syndrome: The North Carolina Protocol." *International Journal of Clinical and Experimental Hypnosis* 54, no. 1 (January 2006): 51–64. https://doi.org/10.1080/00207140500322933.

Patwardhan, R. V., P. V. Desmond, R. F. Johnson, and S. Schenker. "Impaired Elimination of Caffeine by Oral Contraceptive Steroids." *Journal of Laboratory and Clinical Medicine* 95, no. 4 (April 1980): 603–608. https://www.ncbi.nlm.nih.gov/pubmed/7359014.

Pimentel, M., and S. Lezcano. "Irritable Bowel Syndrome: Bacterial Overgrowth—What's Known and What to Do." *Current Treatment Options in Gastroenterology* 10, no. 4 (August 2007): 328–337. https://doi.org/10.1007/s11938-007-0076-1.

Pimentel, M., E. G. Chow, and H. C. Lin. "Eradication of Small Intestinal Bacterial Overgrowth Reduces Symptoms of Irritable Bowel Syndrome." *American Journal of Gastroenterology* 95, no. 12 (December 2000): 3503–3506. https://doi.org/10.1111/j.1572-0241.2000.03368.x.

Pimentel, M., E. G. Chow, and H. C. Lin. "Normalization of Lactulose Breath Testing Correlates with Symptom Improvement in Irritable Bowel Syndrome. A Double-Blind, Randomized, Placebo-Controlled Study." *American Journal of Gastroenterology* 98, no. 2 (February 2003): 412–419. https://doi.org/10.1111/j.1572-0241.2003.07234.x.

Pimentel, Mark, Edy E. Soffer, Evelyn J. Chow, Yuthana Kong, and Henry C. Lin. "Lower Frequency of MMC Is Found in IBS Subjects with Abnormal Lactulose Breath Test, Suggesting Bacterial Overgrowth." *Digestive Diseases and Sciences* 47, no. 12 (December 2002): 2639–2943. https://doi.org/10.1023/a:1021039032413.

Pimentel, Mark, R. J. Saad, M. D. Long, and S. S. C. Rao. "ACG Clinical Guideline: Small Intestinal Bacterial Overgrowth." *American Journal of Gastroenterology* 114, no. 2 (February 2020): 165–178. https://doi.org/10.14309/ajg.0000000000000501; https://journals.lww.com/ajg/Fulltext/2020/02000/ACG_Clinical_Guideline__Small_Intestinal_Bacterial.9.aspx.

Pimentel, Mark, Soumya Chatterjee, Christopher Chang, Kimberly Low, Yuli Song, Chengxu Liu, Walter Morales, Lemeesa Ali, Sheila Lezcano, Jeffery Conklin, and Sydney Finegold. "A New Rat Model Links Two Contemporary Theories in Irritable Bowel Syndrome." *Digestive Diseases and Sciences* 43, no. 4 (April 2008): 982–989. https://doi.org/10.1007/s10620-007-9977-z.

Pimentel, Mark, Tess Constantino, Yuthana Kong, Meera Bajwa, Abolghasem Rezaei, and Sandy Park. "A 14-Day Elemental Diet Is Highly Effective in Normalizing the Lactulose Breath Test." *Digestive Diseases and Sciences* 49, no. 1 (January 2004): 73–77. https://doi.org/10.1023/b:ddas.0000011605.43979.e1.

Pimentel, Mark, Walter Morales, Ali Rezaie, Emily Marsh, Anthony Lembo, James Mirocha, Daniel A. Leffler, Zachary Marsh, Stacy Weitsman, Kathleen S. Chua, et al. "Development and Validation of a Biomarker for Diarrhea-

Predominant Irritable Bowel Syndrome in Human Subjects." *PLoS ONE* 10, no. 5 (2015). https://doi.org/10.1371/journal.pone.0126438.

Pimentel, Mark, Walter Morales, Venkata Pokkunuri, Constantinos Brikos, Sun Moon Kim, Seong Eun Kim, Konstantinos Triantafyllou, Stacy Weitsman, Zachary Marsh, Emily Marsh, et al. "Autoimmunity Links Vinculin to the Pathophysiology of Chronic Functional Bowel Changes Following *Campylobacter jejuni* Infection in a Rat Model." *Digestive Diseases and Sciences* 60, no. 5 (May 2015): 1195–1205. https://doi.org/10.1007/s10620-014-3435-5.

Ponziani, F. R., F. Scaldaferri, V. Petito, F. Paroni Sterbini, S. Pecere, L. R. Lopetuso, A. Palladini, V. Gerardi, L. Masucci, M Pompili, et al. "The Role of Antibiotics in Gut Microbiota Modulation: The Eubiotic Effects of Rifaximin." *Digestive Diseases* 34, no. 3 (2016): 269–278. https://doi.org/10.1159/000443361.

Ponziani, Francesca Romana, Maria Assunta Zocco, Francesca D'Aversa, Maurizio Pompili, and Antonio Gasbarrini. "Eubiotic Properties of Rifaximin: Disruption of the Traditional Concepts in Gut Microbiota Modulation." *World Journal of Gastroenterology* 23, no. 25 (July 2017): 4491–4499. https://doi.org/10.3748/wjg.v23.i25.4491.

"Post Infectious IBS." About IBS. International Foundation for Gastrointestinal Disorders, Inc., June 15, 2016. https://www.aboutibs.org/what-is-ibs-sidenav/post-infectious-ibs.html.

Prins, Mayumi, Tiffany Greco, Daya Alexander, and Christopher C. Giza. "The Pathophysiology of Traumatic Brain Injury at a Glance." *Disease Models & Mechanisms* 6, no. 6 (2013): 1307–1315. https://doi.org/10.1242/dmm.011585.

Rao, Radha Krishna, and Geetha Samak. "Role of Glutamine in Protection of Intestinal Epithelial Tight Junctions." *Journal of Epithelial Biology & Pharmacology* 5, suppl. 1-M7 (January 2012): 47–54. https://doi.org/10.2174/1875044301205010047.

Rao, Satish, and Ashley James. "248: SIBO and SIFO." Learn True Health. https://www.learntruehealth.com/sibo-and-sifo/.

Rao, Satish S. C., and Jigar Bhagatwala. "Small Intestinal Bacterial Overgrowth: Clinical Features and Therapeutic Management." *Clinical and Translational Gastroenterology* 10, no. 10 (October 3, 2019): e00078. https://doi.org/ 10.14309/ctg.0000000000000078;

https://journals.lww.com/ctg/fulltext/2019/10000/small_intestinal_bacterial_overgrowth__clinical.2.aspx.

Rezaie, Ali, M. Buresi, A. Lembo, H. Lin, R. McCallum, S. Rao, M. Schmulson, M. Valdovinos, S. Zakko, and M. Pimentel. "Hydrogen and Methane-Based Breath Testing in Gastrointestinal Disorders: The North American Consensus." *American Journal of Gastroenterology* 112 (May 2017): 775–784. https://www.ncbi.nlm.nih.gov/pubmed/28323273/.

Romling, U., and C. Balsalobre. "Biofilm Infections, Their Resilience to Therapy and Innovative Treatment Strategies." *Journal of Internal Medicine* 272, no. 6 (December 2012): 541–561. https://doi.org/10.1111/joim.12004.

Santana, Ivone Lima, Letícia Machado Gonçalves, Andréa Araújo de Vasconcellos, Wander José da Silva, Jaime Aparecido Cury, and Altair Antoninha Del Bel Cury. "Dietary Carbohydrates Modulate *Candida albicans* Biofilm Development on the Denture Surface." *PLoS ONE* 8, no. 5 (2013). https://doi.org/10.1371/journal.pone.0064645.

Saraswati, Swami Satyananda. *Asana Pranayama Mudra Bandha*. Munger, India: Yoga Publications Trust, 2008.

Shah, Ayesha, N. J. Talley, M. Jones, B. J. Kendall, M. M. Walker, M. Morrison, and G. J. Holtmann. "Small Intestinal Bacterial Overgrowth in Irritable Bowel Syndrome: A Systematic Review and Meta-analysis of Case-Control Studies." *American Journal of Gastroenterology* 115, no. 2 (February 2020): 190–201. https://doi.org/10.14309/ajg.0000000000000504.

Shah, Eric D., Robert J. Basseri, Kelly Chong, and Mark Pimentel. "Abnormal Breath Testing in IBS: A Meta-analysis." *Digestive Diseases and Sciences* 55, no. 9 (September 2010): 2441–2449. https://doi.org/10.1007/s10620-010-1276-4.

Shahet, Ayesha al. "Small Intestinal Bacterial Overgrowth in Irritable Bowel Syndrome: A Systematic Review and Meta-Analysis of Case-Control Studies." *American Journal of Gastroenterology* 115, no. 2 (February 2020): 190–201. https://doi.org/10.14309/ajg.0000000000000504; https://journals.lww.com/ajg/Abstract/2020/02000/Small_Intestinal_Bacterial_Overgrowth_in_Irritable.11.aspx.

Shiga, Hisashi, Takayuki Kajiura, Junko Shinozaki, Sho Takagi, Yoshitaka Kinouchi, Seiichi Takahashi, Kenichi Negoro, Katsuya Endo, Yoichi Kakuta, Manabu Suzuki, et al. "Changes of Faecal Microbiota in Patients with Crohn's Disease Treated with an Elemental Diet and Total Parenteral Nutrition." *Digestive and Liver Disease* 44, no. 9 (September 2012): 736–742. https://doi.org/10.1016/j.dld.2012.04.014.

Sicard, Jean-Felix, Philippe Vogeleer, Guillaume Le Bihan, Yaindrys Rodriguez Olivera, Francis Beaudry, Mario Jacques, and Josée Harel. "N-Acetyl-glucosamine Influences the Biofilm Formation of *Escherichia coli*." *Gut Pathogens* 10 (2018): 26. https://doi.org/10.1186/s13099-018-0252-y.

Siebecker, Allison, and Steven Sandburg-Lewis. "SIBO: The Finer Points of Diagnosis, Test Interpretation, and Treatment." *Naturopathic Doctor News & Review* (January 2014). https://ndnr.com/gastrointestinal/sibo/.

Staudacher, H. M., and K. Whelan. "The Low FODMAP Diet: Recent Advances in Understanding Its Mechanisms and Efficacy in IBS." *Gut* 66, no. 8 (August 2017): 1517–1527. https://doi.org/10.1136/gutjnl-2017-313750.

Staudacher, H. M., M. C. Lomer, J. L. Anderson, J. S. Barrett, J. G. Muir, P. M. Irving, and K. Whelan. "Fermentable Carbohydrate Restriction Reduces Luminal Bifidobacteria and Gastrointestinal Symptoms in Patients with Irritable Bowel Syndrome." *Journal of Nutrition* 142, no. 8 (August 2012): 1510–1518. https://doi.org/10.3945/jn.112.159285.

Su, Tingting, Sanchuan Lai, Allen Lee, Xingkang He, and Shujie Chen. "Meta-analysis: Proton Pump Inhibitors Moderately Increase the Risk of Small Intestinal Bacterial Overgrowth." *Journal of Gastroenterology* 53, no. 1 (January 2018): 27–36. https://doi.org/10.1007/s00535-017-1371-9.

Suez, Jotham, Niv Zmora, Gili Ziberman-Schapira, Uria Mor, Mally Dori-Bachash, Stavros Bashiardes, Maya Zur, Dana Regev-Lehvi, Rotem Ben-Zeev Brik, Sara Federici, et al. "Post-antibiotic Gut Mucosal Microbiome Reconstitution Is Impaired by Probiotics and Improved by Autologous FMT." *Cell* 174, no. 6 (September 6, 2018): P1406–1423.E16. https://doi.org/10.1016/j.cell.2018.08.047.

Suez, Jotham, Tal Korem, David Zeevi, Gili Zilberman-Schapira, Christoph A. Thaiss, Ori Maza, David Israeli, Niv Zmora, Shlomit Gilad, Adina Weinberger, et al. "Artificial Sweeteners Induce Glucose Intolerance by Altering the Gut Microbiota." *Nature* 514, no. 7521 (October 9, 2014): 181–186. https://doi.org/10.1038/nature13793.

Summers, A. O., J. Wireman, M. J. Vimy, F. L. Lorscheider, B. Marshall, S. B. Levy, S. Bennett, and L. Billard. "Mercury Released from Dental 'Silver' Fillings Provokes an Increase in Mercury- and Antibiotic-Resistant Bacteria in Oral and Intestinal Floras of Primates." *Antimicrobial Agents and Chemotherapy* 37, no. 4 (April 1993): 825–834. https://doi.org/10.1128/aac.37.4.825.

Tabatabaeizadeh, Seyed-Amir, Niayesh Tafazoli, Gordon A. Ferns, Amir Avan, and Majid Ghayour-Mobarhan. "Vitamin D, the Gut Microbiome and Inflammatory Bowel Disease." *Journal of Research in Medical Sciences* 23 (2018): 75. https://doi.org/10.4103/jrms.JRMS_606_17.

Tabibian, N., E. Swehll, A. Boyd, A. Umbreen, and J. H. Tabibian. "Abdominal Adhesions: A Practical Review of an Often Overlooked Entity." *Annals of Medicine and Surgery* 15 (March 2017): 9–13. https://doi.org/10.1016/j.amsu.2017.01.021.

Terciolo, Chloe, Michael Dapoigny, and Frederic Andre. "Beneficial Effects of *Saccharomyces boulardii* CNCM I-745 on Clinical Disorders Associated with Intestinal Barrier Disruption." *Clinical and Experimental Gastroenterology* 12 (2019): 67–82. https://doi.org/10.2147/CEG.S181590.

Valori, R. M., D. Kumar, and D. L. Wingate. "Effects of Different Types of Stress and of 'Protokinetic' Drugs on the Control of the Fasting Motor Complex in Humans." *Gastroenterology* 90, no. 6 (June 1986): 1890–1900. https://doi.org/10.1016/0016-5085(86)90258-1.

Vickhoff, Björn, Helge Malmgren, Rickard Åström, Gunnar Nyberg, Seth-Reino Ekström, Mathias Engwall, Johan Snygg, Michael Nilsson, and Rebecka Jörnsten. "Music Structure Determines Heart Rate Variability of Singers." *Frontiers in Psychology* 4 (2013): 334. https://doi.org/10.3389/fpsyg.2013.00334.

Vlasova, Anastasia N., Sukumar Kandasamy, Kuldeep S. Chattha, Gireesh Rajashekara, and Linda J. Saif. "Comparison of Probiotic Lactobacilli and Bifidobacteria Effects, Immune Responses and Rotavirus Vaccines and Infection in Different Host Species." *Veterinary Immunology and Immunopathology* 172 (April 2016): 72–84. https://doi.org/10.1016/j.vetimm.2016.01.003.

Wang, Peng-fei, Dan-hua Yao, Yue-yu Hu, and Yousheng Li. "Vitamin D Improves Intestinal Barrier Function in Cirrhosis Rats by Upregulating Heme Oxygenase-1 Expression." *Biomolecules and Therapeutics* 27, no. 2 (February 2019): 222–230. https://doi.org/10.4062/biomolther.2018.052.

Yoon, Jin Young, Soo Jung Park, and Jae Hee Cheon. "Effect of Colostrum on the Symptoms and Mucosal Permeability in Patients with Irritable Bowel Syndrome: A Randomized Placebo-Controlled Study." *Intestinal Research* 12, no. 1 (January 2014): 80–82. https://doi.org/10.5217/ir.2014.12.1.80.

Zhang, Luoping, Iemaan Rana, Rachel M. Shaffer, Emanuela Taioli, and Lianne Sheppard. "Exposure to Glyphosate-Based Herbicides and Risk for Non-Hodgkin Lymphoma: A Meta-analysis and Supporting Evidence." *Mutation Research/Reviews in Mutation Research* 781 (July–September 2019): 186–206. https://doi.org/10.1016/j.mrrev.2019.02.001.

Zhang, Mei, and Xiao-Jiao Yang. "Effects of a High Fat Diet on Intestinal Microbiota and Gastrointestinal Diseases." *World Journal of Gastroenterology* 22, no. 40 (October 2016): 805–809. https://doi.org/10.3748/wjg.v22.i40.8905.

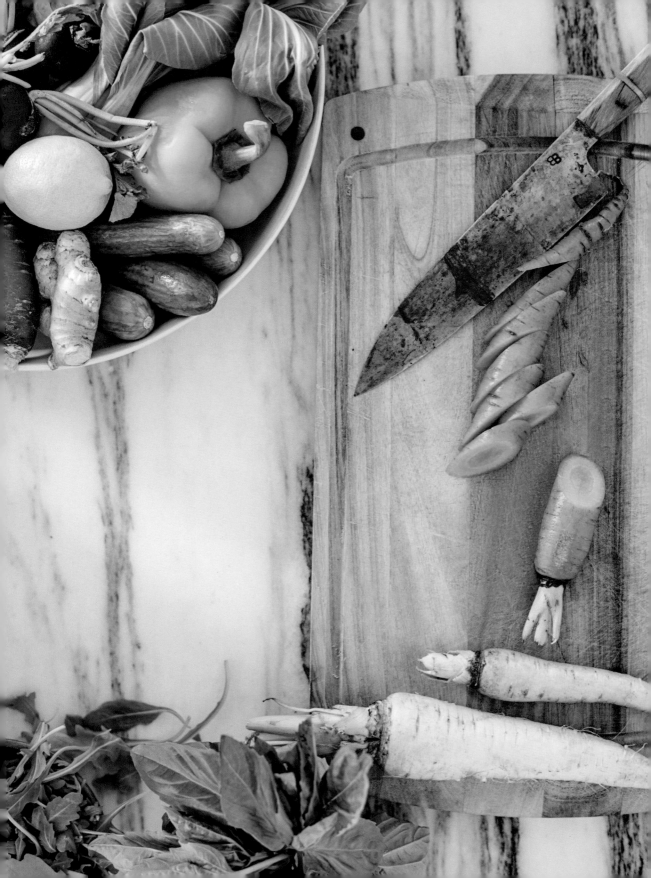

INDEX

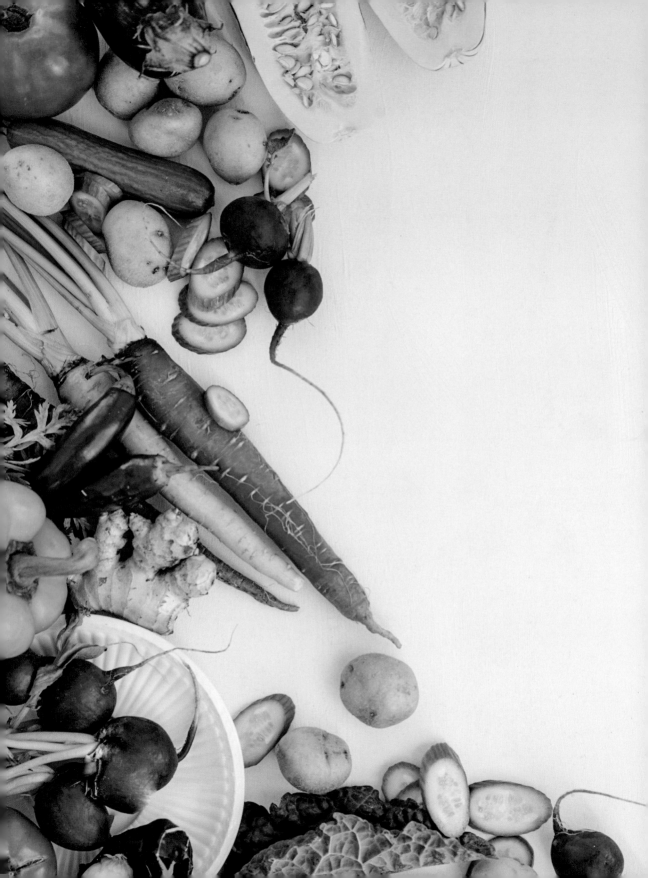